MOLECULAR NUTRITION

MOLECULAR NUTRITION

Mother and Infant

Edited by

MANLIO VINCIGUERRA

Institute for Liver and Digestive Health,
University College London,
London, United Kingdom

&

International Clinical Research Center (FNUSA-ICRC),
St'Anne University Hospital,
Brno, Czech Republic

PAUL CORDERO SANCHEZ

Institute for Liver and Digestive Health,
University College London,
London, United Kingdom

ELSEVIER

ACADEMIC PRESS

An imprint of Elsevier

Academic Press is an imprint of Elsevier
125 London Wall, London EC2Y 5AS, United Kingdom
525 B Street, Suite 1650, San Diego, CA 92101, United States
50 Hampshire Street, 5th Floor, Cambridge, MA 02139, United States
The Boulevard, Langford Lane, Kidlington, Oxford OX5 1GB, United Kingdom

Library of Congress Cataloging-in-Publication Data
A catalog record for this book is available from the Library of Congress

British Library Cataloguing-in-Publication Data
A catalogue record for this book is available from the British Library

ISBN: 978-0-12-813862-5

For information on all Academic Press publications visit our website at https://www.elsevier.com/books-and-journals

Publisher: Charlotte Cockle
Acquisitions Editor: Megan Ball
Editorial Project Manager: Kelsey Connors
Production Project Manager: Sruthi Satheesh
Cover Designer: Christian Bilbow

Typeset by TNQ Technologies

Contents

Contributors

Ishag Adam
Faculty of Medicine, University of Khartoum, Khartoum, Sudan

Antonella Agodi
Department of Medical and Surgical Sciences and Advanced Technologies "GF Ingrassia", University of Catania, Catania, Italy

Martina Barchitta
Department of Medical and Surgical Sciences and Advanced Technologies "GF Ingrassia", University of Catania, Catania, Italy

Zulfiqar A. Bhutta
Centre for Global Child Health, the Hospital for Sick Children, Toronto, ON, Canada; Center of Excellence in Women and Child Health, Aga Khan University, Karachi, Pakistan

Julie Bienertova-Vasku
RECETOX, Faculty of Sciences, Masaryk University, Brno, Czech Republic

Alberto Camacho
Universidad Autonoma de Nuevo Leon, Facultad de Medicina, Departamento de Bioquimica y Medicina Molecular, Monterrey, Nuevo Leon, Mexico; Universidad Autonoma de Nuevo Leon, Unidad de Neurometabolismo, Centro de Investigación y Desarrollo en Ciencias de La Salud, Monterrey, Nuevo Leon, Mexico

Cristina Campoy
Department of Pediatrics, School of Medicine, University of Granada, Granada, Spain; EURISTIKOS Excellence Centre for Pediatric Research, University of Granada, Granada, Spain

Robbi Elizabeth Cárdenas-Pérez
Universidad Autonoma de Nuevo Leon, Facultad de Medicina, Departamento de Bioquimica y Medicina Molecular, Monterrey, Nuevo Leon, Mexico; Universidad Autonoma de Nuevo Leon, Unidad de Neurometabolismo, Centro de Investigación y Desarrollo en Ciencias de La Salud, Monterrey, Nuevo Leon, Mexico

Heriberto Castro
Universidad Autonoma de Nuevo Leon, Facultad de Salud Pública y Nutrición, Centro de Investigación en Nutrición y Salud Pública, Monterrey, Nuevo León, Mexico

Tomás Cerdó
Department of Pediatrics, School of Medicine, University of Granada, Granada, Spain; EURISTIKOS Excellence Centre for Pediatric Research, University of Granada, Granada, Spain

Kimberly D. Charbonneau
Centre for Global Child Health, the Hospital for Sick Children, Toronto, ON, Canada

Mahua Choudhury
Department of Pharmaceutical Sciences, Irma Lerma Rangel College of Pharmacy, Texas A&M Health Science Center, College Station, TX, United States

Fabio Coppedè
Department of Translational Research and of New Surgical and Medical Technologies, Section of Medical Genetics, University of Pisa, Pisa, Italy

Gonzalo Cruz
Centro de Neurobiología y Fisiopatología Integrativa (CENFI), Instituto de Fisiología, Facultad de Ciencias, Universidad de Valparaíso, Valparaíso, Chile

Marloes Dekker Nitert
School of Chemistry and Molecular Biosciences, The University of Queensland, St. Lucia, QLD, Australia

Ana Laura de la Garza
Universidad Autonoma de Nuevo Leon, Facultad de Salud Pública y Nutrición, Centro de Investigación en Nutrición y Salud Pública, Monterrey, Nuevo León, Mexico; Universidad Autonoma de Nuevo Leon, Unidad de Nutrición, Centro de Investigación y Desarrollo en Ciencias de La Salud, Monterrey, Nuevo León, Mexico

Estefanía Diéguez
Department of Pediatrics, School of Medicine, University of Granada, Granada, Spain; EURISTIKOS Excellence Centre for Pediatric Research, University of Granada, Granada, Spain

Mireia Escudero-Marín
Department of Pediatrics, School of Medicine, University of Granada, Granada, Spain; EURISTIKOS Excellence Centre for Pediatric Research, University of Granada, Granada, Spain

Daniela Fernandois
Development and Plasticity of the Neuroendocrine Brain, INSERM, Lille, France

Myriam Gutierrez-Lopez
Universidad Autonoma de Nuevo Leon, Facultad de Salud Pública y Nutrición, Centro de Investigación en Nutrición y Salud Pública, Monterrey, Nuevo León, Mexico

Hamdan Z. Hamdan
Faculty of Medicine, Al-Neelain University, Khartoum, Sudan; Al-Neelain Institute for Medical Research (NIMR), Al-Neelain University, Khartoum, Sudan

Ahmed A. Hassan
Faculty of Medicine, University of Khartoum, Khartoum, Sudan

Olivia Holland
School of Medical Science, Griffith University, Gold Coast Campus, Southport, QLD, Australia

Bruce W. Hollis
Pediatrics Medical University of South Carolina, Charleston, SC, United States

I. Iglesia
Growth, Exercise, Nutrition and Development (GENUD) Research Group, Departamento de Fisiatría y Enfermería, Facultad de Ciencias de la Salud, Universidad de Zaragoza, Zaragoza, España; Instituto Agroalimentario de Aragón (IA2), Universidad de Zaragoza, Zaragoza, España; Fundación del Instituto de Investigación Sanitaria Aragón (IIS Aragón), Zaragoza, España; Red de Salud Materno Infantil y del Desarrollo (SAMID), Red de Salud Materno Infantil y del Desarrollo (SAMID), Instituto de Salud Carlos III, Madrid, España

Gonzalo Jorquera
Centro de Neurobiología y Fisiopatología Integrativa (CENFI), Instituto de Fisiología, Facultad de Ciencias, Universidad de Valparaíso, Valparaíso, Chile

Emily C. Keats
Centre for Global Child Health, the Hospital for Sick Children, Toronto, ON, Canada

SC. Langley-Evans
University of Nottingham, School of Biosciences, Loughborough, United Kingdom

Alicia I. Leikin-Frenkel
The Sackler Faculty of Medicine Ramat Aviv and Bert Strassburger Lipid Center, Sheba, Tel Hashomer Ramat Gan, Israel; The Bert Strassburger Lipid Center, Sheba, Tel Hashomer, Tel Aviv University, Tel Aviv, Israel

Paola Llanos
Instituto de Investigación en Ciencias Odontológicas, Facultad de Odontología, Universidad de Chile, Santiago, Chile

Manuel Maliqueo
Laboratory of Endocrinology and Metabolism, West Division, Faculty of Medicine, Universidad de Chile, Santiago, Chile

Roberta Masella
Italian National Institute of Health, Center for Gender-Specific Medicine, Rome, Italy

Andrea Maugeri
Department of Medical and Surgical Sciences and Advanced Technologies "GF Ingrassia", University of Catania, Catania, Italy

Sunitha Meruvu
Department of Pharmaceutical Sciences, Irma Lerma Rangel College of Pharmacy, Texas A&M Health Science Center, College Station, TX, United States

L.A. Moreno
Growth, Exercise, Nutrition and Development (GENUD) Research Group, Departamento de Fisiatría y Enfermería, Facultad de Ciencias de la Salud, Universidad de Zaragoza, Zaragoza, España; Instituto Agroalimentario de Aragón (IA2), Universidad de Zaragoza, Zaragoza, España; Fundación del Instituto de Investigación Sanitaria Aragón (IIS Aragón), Zaragoza, España; Centro de Investigación Biomédica en Red de Fisiopatología de la Obesidad y Nutrición (CIBERObn), Instituto de Salud Carlos III, Madrid, España

Ximena Palma
Escuela de Nutrición y Dietética, Facultad de Farmacia, Universidad de Valparaíso, Valparaíso, Chile

Mariona Palou
Laboratory of Molecular Biology, Nutrition and Biotechnology (Group of Nutrigenomics and Obesity), University of the Balearic Islands, CIBER de Fisiopatología de La Obesidad y Nutrición (CIBERobn), Instituto de Investigación Sanitaria Illes Balears, Palma de Mallorca, Spain

Andreu Palou
Laboratory of Molecular Biology, Nutrition and Biotechnology (Group of Nutrigenomics and Obesity), University of the Balearic Islands, CIBER de Fisiopatología de La Obesidad y Nutrición (CIBERobn), Instituto de Investigación Sanitaria Illes Balears, Palma de Mallorca, Spain

Catalina Picó
Laboratory of Molecular Biology, Nutrition and Biotechnology (Group of Nutrigenomics and Obesity), University of the Balearic Islands, CIBER de Fisiopatología de La Obesidad y Nutrición (CIBERobn), Instituto de Investigación Sanitaria Illes Balears, Palma de Mallorca, Spain

Catalina Amadora Pomar
Laboratory of Molecular Biology, Nutrition and Biotechnology (Group of Nutrigenomics and Obesity), University of the Balearic Islands, CIBER de Fisiopatología de La Obesidad y Nutrición (CIBERobn), Instituto de Investigación Sanitaria Illes Balears, Palma de Mallorca, Spain

G. Rodríguez-Martínez
Growth, Exercise, Nutrition and Development (GENUD) Research Group, Departamento de Fisiatría y Enfermería, Facultad de Ciencias de la Salud, Universidad de Zaragoza, Zaragoza, España; Instituto Agroalimentario de Aragón (IA2), Universidad de Zaragoza, Zaragoza, España; Fundación del Instituto de Investigación Sanitaria Aragón (IIS Aragón), Zaragoza, España; Red de Salud Materno Infantil y del Desarrollo (SAMID), Red de Salud Materno Infantil y del Desarrollo (SAMID), Instituto de Salud Carlos III, Madrid, España; Departamento de Pediatría, Radiología y Medicina Física, Universidad de Zaragoza, Zaragoza, España; Hospital Clínico Universitario "Lozano Blesa", Zaragoza, España

Rehana A. Salam
Center of Excellence in Women and Child Health, Aga Khan University, Karachi, Pakistan

Carmela Santangelo
Italian National Institute of Health, Center for Gender-Specific Medicine, Rome, Italy

Luis F. Schutz
Department of Pharmaceutical Sciences, Irma Lerma Rangel College of Pharmacy, Texas A&M Health Science Center, College Station, TX, United States

Sue Maye Siow
School of Medical Science, Griffith University, Gold Coast Campus, Southport, QLD, Australia

Carolina Treviño-de Alba
Universidad Autonoma de Nuevo Leon, Facultad de Salud Pública y Nutrición, Centro de Investigación en Nutrición y Salud Pública, Monterrey, Nuevo León, Mexico

Carol L. Wagner
Pediatrics Medical University of South Carolina, Charleston, SC, United States

Series preface

In this series on *Molecular Nutrition*, the editors of each book aim to disseminate important material pertaining to molecular nutrition in its broadest sense. The coverage ranges from molecular aspects to whole organs and the impact of nutrition or malnutrition on individuals and whole communities. It includes concepts, policy, preclinical studies, and clinical investigations relating to molecular nutrition. The subject areas include molecular mechanisms, polymorphisms, single-nucleotide polymorphisms, genome-wide analysis, genotypes, gene expression, genetic modifications, and many other aspects. Information given in the *Molecular Nutrition* series relates to national, international, and global issues.

A major feature of the series that sets it apart from other texts is the initiative to bridge the transintellectual divide so that it is suitable for novices and experts alike. It embraces traditional and nontraditional formats of nutritional sciences in different ways. Each book in the series has both overviews and detailed and focused chapters. *Molecular Nutrition* is designed for nutritionists, dieticians, educationalists, health experts, epidemiologists, and health-related professionals such as chemists. It is also suitable for students, graduates, postgraduates, researchers, lecturers, teachers, and professors. Contributors are national or international experts, many of whom are from world-renowned institutions or universities. It is intended to be an authoritative text covering nutrition at the molecular level.

V.R. Preedy
Series Editor

PART 1

General and introductory aspects

CHAPTER 1

Diet, maternal nutrition, and long-term health consequences: an overview

SC. Langley-Evans
University of Nottingham, School of Biosciences, Loughborough, United Kingdom

Contents

Introduction

Pregnancy is a physiologically and metabolically demanding process for mothers. In addition to the implantation, growth, and development of the fetus, major adaptations must take place in order to accommodate the growth and function of a new organ (the placenta). In humans, increases in maternal body weight and remodeling of body composition (fat accrual) occur from early gestation and are accompanied by an expansion of blood volume, changes in cardiovascular function, and renal and respiratory changes. Metabolically there is a need to drive substrates from maternal to fetal circulation and so an insulin-resistant state must develop [1].

All of these processes are modified by nutrition-related factors and greatly increase demand for nutrients. Some additional demands are readily delivered without any requirement to change intake. For example, additional energy requirements are generally met by reducing physical activity. Other nutrients, however, need to be supplied in greater amounts through increased intake (e.g., additional dietary protein), improved absorption from

Molecular Nutrition
ISBN 978-0-12-813862-5
https://doi.org/10.1016/B978-0-12-813862-5.00001-3

the gut, or release from stores (e.g., calcium release from the skeleton). Although maternal adaptations serve to optimize nutrient bioavailability from the diet, there are many circumstances in which maternal diet is far from optimal for fetal growth and development [1]. For many parts of the world, undernutrition and pregnancy during adolescence, where maternal needs are already high, remain rife. Elsewhere, maternal overweight and obesity have a negative impact.

This chapter will explore the importance of maternal nutritional status during pregnancy, presenting evidence that in addition to determining the outcome of pregnancy, it can set in train changes to fetal development which have a long-lasting impact upon health and well-being [2].

Periconceptual diet and the fetus

Associations between maternal diet and fetal development are most easily demonstrated by considering circumstances in which inadequacy or excess result in congenital defects. Vitamin A from animal sources (retinol), for example, is teratogenic and excessive consumption is associated with craniofacial, central nervous system, and cardiovascular abnormalities. For this reason, pregnant women are advised to avoid rich sources of retinol such as liver, which is particularly enriched with the most potently teratogenic retinol metabolites 13-cis-retinoic acid and 13-cis-4-oxo-retinoic acid [3,4].

The most commonly occurring congenital defects in humans are neural tube defects (spina bifida and ancephaly), which occur in around 4 out of every 1000 pregnancies. The major avoidable risk factors are obesity and low intake of folates. Folates are required for synthesis of nucleotides and cell division, and inadequate supply during the fourth week of human gestation prevents the closure of the neural tube, which goes on to become the spinal cord and brain [5]. Identification of the association between folates and these defects resulted in the recommendation for all women planning to become pregnant to take folic acid supplements for 3 months before conception in the United Kingdom, and the introduction of mandatory folic acid fortification of flour in the United States and many other countries. These measures have been highly effective and within 3 years of introducing folate fortification, the United States saw a 27% reduction in the prevalence of neural tube defects [6,7]. The benefits vary between different ethnic groups, with minimal impact in Black Americans.

This reflects common polymorphisms in genes for key enzymes in folate metabolism, emphasizing that the impact of nutrition is dependent upon other factors.

Neural tube defects are also more common in pregnancies that are complicated by maternal obesity. Women who are obese are more than twice as likely to have a baby with spina bifida and this risk is a consequence of impaired glucose homeostasis and folate metabolism, transport, and storage. Obesity appears to lower the availability of folates to developing embryos, but there is no evidence that public health measures to improve folate status are any less effective in obese compared to lean women [8,9]. Greater risk of neural tube defects is just one aspect of a broad range of negative effects of maternal obesity on pregnancy outcomes, as will be described below.

Associations of specific nutrients with congenital defects are examples of extreme outcomes when maternal nutritional status is poor. The rest of this chapter will focus upon ways in which variation in nutritional quality or quantity can have an impact upon pregnancy outcomes and the long-term disease risk profile of the developing fetus.

Maternal nutrition and pregnancy

The nutritional requirements of pregnancy are considerable. It is estimated that across the whole 9 months of gestation, the additional energy requirement is around 293 MJ (69,982 kcal), which equates to approximately an additional 1.04 MJ/day (249 kcal/day). This is associated with an increase in basal metabolic rate due to the accretion of new tissue and growth of the baby. However, adaptive responses, which include both reduced amounts and reduced intensity of physical activity, mean that in practice no increase in energy intake is required until the third trimester (a modest 0.84 MJ/day—200 kcal/day) [10,11].

Protein requirements for pregnancy are greater than those of nonpregnant women, with an additional 6–10 g/day required. In developed countries where protein intakes are generally excessive (60–110 g/day, versus RNI of 45 g/day), this additional requirement is comfortably achieved without any change in dietary intakes [12]. However, in many parts of the world, women from impoverished backgrounds may struggle to consume sufficient high quality protein to meet demand.

From a metabolic perspective, pregnancy represents a profound shift which favors accretion of protein and the movement of substrates from the maternal to the fetal compartment. A slowing of gastrointestinal mobility ensures that uptake of amino acids is enhanced. Endocrine factors (human chorionic gonadotrophin and placental growth hormone) inhibit deamination of amino acids in the liver, ensuring that circulating amino acids remain high for transfer across the placenta, or for incorporation into expanding maternal tissues and the placenta [1].

In addition to endocrine changes that promote availability of amino acids, pregnancy is associated with increased production of insulin and the development of an insulin-resistant state. This appears to be due to disruption of GLUT4-phosphatidylinositol-3 kinase complex formation and serves to suppress disposal of circulating glucose into maternal muscle and liver. High circulating glucose is then available to the fetal tissues [13].

Micronutrient requirements also increase during pregnancy, with some vitamins being required at levels that are sometimes beyond the capacity of the diet to deliver. Vitamin D, for example, is largely derived from the action of ultraviolet light on the skin (conversion of 7-dehydrocholesterol to vitamin D3) and women in northern latitudes are at risk of seasonal insufficiency [14]. There is evidence that maternal insufficiency is associated with poor bone mineralization in children at age 9, highlighting the important role of vitamin D in formation of the fetal skeleton [15]. In many countries, pregnant women are advised to increase their intakes of vitamin D fortified foods or to take a supplement of 10 μg/day.

The iron requirements of pregnancy are very high, with fetal, placental accrual and expansion of blood volume amounting to approximately 1325 mg which is generally against a background of approximately 560 mg from maternal intake and 500 mg saved through cessation of menstruation. The additional requirements for iron may be achieved with little increase in intake as absorption from the gastrointestinal tract increases markedly (7.3% prepregnancy to 37% in the third trimester) [16]. However, iron deficiency anemia is commonplace in pregnancy, impacting on more than 20% of pregnancies in developed countries and over 50% in many developing countries [17,18]. Iron deficiency is associated with greater risk of preterm birth, low birth weight, and neonatal death. Supplementation is often used to enhance maternal intakes and can be highly effective, but care is required as elevated hemoglobin (>14.5 g/L) is also associated with adverse outcomes of pregnancy [19].

The fetus accumulates large quantities of most minerals during late gestation and skeletal development is highly dependent upon the supply of calcium, phosphorus, copper, zinc, and trace metals. The additional demands are generally met through adaptations in which the absorption of minerals across the digestive tract increases. For example, in women following a western diet, absorption of calcium increases from around 20%–40%. Accompanying the gastrointestinal changes, reabsorption of minerals from the urine increases, thereby conserving minerals in circulation [20]. With the exception of iron (above) and iodine (below), skeletal reserves of minerals are generally sufficient to protect fetal demands against poor maternal intakes.

Iodine is an essential nutrient for fetal development, playing a critical role in the development of the central nervous system. Pregnancy increases requirements by 25 μg/day (UK Reference Nutrient Intake 140 μg/day), and in most parts of the world this can only be achieved through the consumption of fortified sources such as iodized salt, cereals, and products manufactured using iodized salt. In westernized countries, there are major concerns about the prevalence of low maternal iodine intake [21], but the long-term consequences for the developing fetus of subclinical deficiency have not been explored in any depth.

There are of course major global disparities in nutrition. The high nutritional demands of pregnancy mean that mothers and their fetuses are particularly impacted by the great variation in food supply and quality between countries. In westernized countries, there are few concerns about supply of macronutrients but pregnancy is frequently complicated by obesity and poor micronutrient status. In the United States, more than half of pregnant women are overweight or obese [22]. In the United Kingdom, 15%–20% are obese and around 6% enter pregnancy with severe (body mass index (BMI) 35–39.9 kg/m^2) or morbid (BMI>40 kg/m^2) obesity [23].

For pregnant women in developing countries, nutritional status is often compromised by poor intakes, low maternal reserves going into pregnancy, and higher levels of physical activity than are seen in women in developed countries. In developing countries, women are often involved in manual labor, particularly subsistence agriculture, all the way through pregnancy, increasing energy expenditure. In addition, maternal age tends to be lower than is seen in developed countries and so the pregnancy is often competing with ongoing maternal growth for nutrients. Access to high quality protein can be a problem as consumption of animal products is low and for many women a lack of dietary diversity means that protein sources are restricted to a narrow range of plants that may be low in specific amino acids [1]. Micronutrient deficiencies including iron, zinc, and selenium occur with high prevalence and will impact upon fetal development [24,25]. Vitamin A deficiency is a major concern in Africa and South-East Asia, leading to night blindness in women and neonatal death [26].

In countries that undergo rapid economic development, there is generally a nutrition transition where the population shifts from traditional, often plant-based diets, to a western diet. During this transition, as seen in Brazil, India, and China, there is a high prevalence of both over- and undernutrition. The population that moves into expanding urban environments will consume cheaper, low quality, high energy foodstuffs and are prone to obesity, while the rural population remains prone to undernutrition.

Weight gain is a normal feature of pregnancy and occurs in part because of the growth of the conceptus (by the end of gestation approximately 3.5 kg baby, 1 kg placenta, and 1 kg amniotic fluid) and partly because of the expansion of maternal blood and interstitial fluid volume, accretion of adipose tissue, and increased size of the breasts and uterus (approximately 8 kg increase in maternal tissues). This gives a typical gain of around 12.5 kg for a singleton pregnancy. Insufficient or excessive weight gains are associated with poor pregnancy outcomes, so some countries have guidelines on optimal weight gain, which are based on BMI prepregnancy. Women of ideal weight (BMI 18.5–24.9 kg/m^2) should gain between 11 and 16 kg and underweight women (BMI<18.5 kg/m^2) 13–18 kg. With overweight (BMI 25–29.9 kg/m^2) optimal weight gain is 7–11 kg, while for obese women (BMI>30 kg/m^2), weight gain should not exceed 5–9 kg [27]. As will become apparent in the discussion which follows, reducing dietary intake to achieve weight loss during pregnancy is not advisable, so in the United Kingdom, overweight women are advised to lose weight before they become pregnant in order to achieve healthier pregnancy outcomes. A healthy weight is also recommended for women who are trying to conceive as both under- and overweight are associated with subfertility [28].

Obesity in pregnancy or excessive weight gain in pregnancy can have adverse consequences for both mother and fetus. Women who are obese are more likely to have a miscarriage in the first trimester, or intrauterine death (stillbirth) later in pregnancy (Fig. 1.1) [29,30]. During pregnancy,

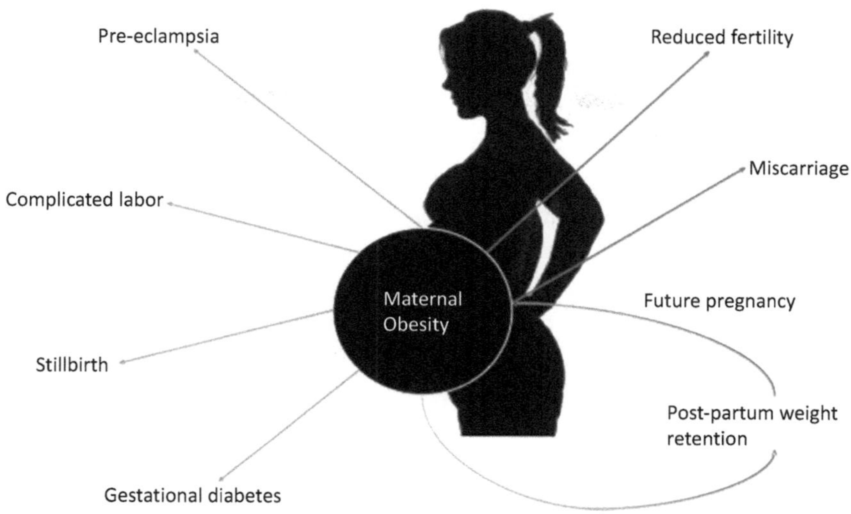

Figure 1.1 ***Impact of maternal obesity.*** Maternal obesity is associated with a number of immediate consequences for the developing fetus. Excessive weight, or weight gain, in pregnancy increases risk of miscarriage and stillbirth and has metabolic and physiological effects that impact upon fetal systems.

obesity is associated with complications such as symphysis pubis dysfunction and hypertensive conditions that threaten maternal and fetal survival; pre-eclampsia and eclampsia [31,32]. Risk of gestational diabetes is increased by more than 2-fold [29,33,34]. Preterm delivery risk is also increased by maternal obesity, either due to spontaneous rupture of membranes or early delivery by cesarian to control preeclampsia [35]. Labor complications are also more likely, with a greater probability of induced labor, cesarian section, and postpartum hemorrhage [36]. Most women retain at least some of the weight gained during pregnancy, so excessive weight gain in pregnancy will promote a higher BMI postpartum. This puts subsequent pregnancies at greater risk (Fig. 1.1) [37].

Developing interventions to minimize the impact of maternal obesity upon pregnancy outcomes and fetal development are currently a high priority in public health. However, large-scale randomized controlled trials that aim to promote more physical activity and improve dietary quality have had variable success, while smaller one-to-one interventions that rely on individuals making small, manageable lifestyle changes have been shown to safely limit pregnancy weight gain and reduce prevalence of hypertensive disorders of pregnancy in severely obese women [29,38].

The early life programming of health and disease

So far, this chapter has provided an overview of the factors which determine nutritional requirements in pregnancy and described some of the immediate consequences of under- and overnutrition for pregnant women and their babies. However, as shown in Fig. 1.2, the consequences of an adverse nutritional environment during fetal development may persist long beyond pregnancy and can impact upon long-term health and well-being. Nutrition is one of a number of factors that can modify the developmental trajectory of the fetus. As fetal life is such a critical phase of development, any compromise in growth or development of organs can be expected to be long-lasting and impact upon physiological and metabolic function in adulthood. One simple manifestation of this effect of nutrition on the fetus is the impact on fetal growth. Growth is genetically determined and yet is readily modified by the prevailing environment. In The Gambia, for example, birth weights of infants vary between the wet season (when agriculture and food storage are problematic and women's weight falls) and the dry season [39]. These differences can be wholly reverse by supplementing maternal diets with protein and energy. Similarly, during the

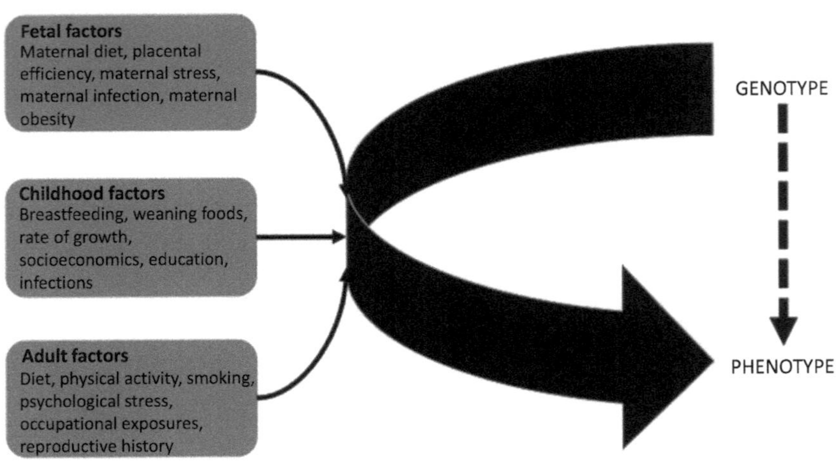

Figure 1.2 ***Factors which impact upon fetal develop influence long-term health.*** The progression from genotype to adult health/disease phenotype is a complex matter. Factors at all stages of life will impact upon expression of the genotype and responses to the environment. These responses will shape future responses as the individual ages. Effectively the phenotype at any stage of life is the result of cumulative environmental exposures across the whole lifespan.

Dutch Famine of 1945, women who were in mid- to late-gestation gave birth to smaller babies than women who gave birth before or after the famine [40]. To some extent, anthropometric measurements at birth provide an indicator of the nutritional environment encountered in utero.

The process through which exposure to an adverse maternal environment has irreversible effects upon fetal development is termed programming [41]. In simple terms, in order to withstand an environment that is less than optimal for development, the fetus must make adaptations which alter the rate of growth and the genetically determined pattern of development. Programming of fetal physiology has a major influence on adult health and well-being and generally we associate exposure to poor maternal diet with increased risk of noncommunicable diseases of adulthood such as coronary heart disease, type-2 diabetes, and chronic kidney disease. Although nutrition is not the only factor that can have a programming effect, it is considered that quantity and quality of nutrition is the most variable factor between pregnancies and is most likely to have a significant impact upon prevalence of disease in human populations.

Epidemiological evidence of early life programming

Some of the earliest indications of a relationship between the intrauterine environment and later health were provided by ecological studies that showed simple correlations between place of birth and the risk of death from coronary heart disease and between the risk of death in infancy and coronary heart disease mortality [42]. For example, in the United Kingdom, there is a well-known North—South divide in cardiovascular disease, with high-risk pockets focused on the industrial cities of the north. The same areas were the places with the highest infant mortality rates in the early 20th century, which can be interpreted as an indicator of a challenging environment for pregnant women and babies. Importantly, individuals who were born in these northern cities who subsequently moved to the south of England retained the high risk associated with their place of birth [42].

Evidence for association between early life environment and later disease risk was strengthened by data from retrospective cohort studies based upon a population from Hertfordshire, UK. Records of weight at birth and infant growth and feeding were available for 16,000 men and women born in Hertfordshire between 1911 and 1930. Although mortality rates for all causes were unrelated to size at birth or in infancy, lower birth weight was associated with increased coronary mortality, blood pressure, type-2 diabetes, and the insulin resistance syndrome [43–46]. Subsequently many similar studies have demonstrated the association between lower weight at birth (but still within the normal range of birth weight and excluding premature birth) and later disease. The US Nurses Health Study reported that among 70,297 women, after adjustment for adult BMI, the risks of coronary heart disease and stroke were both related to weight at birth (relative risk estimate 0.85 per kg increase in birth weight) [47]. A lower weight at birth was also associated with higher blood pressure in adult life. Similarly, the follow-up of 1258 men aged 45–59 in a prospective health study in Caerphilly, Wales, found that lower birth weight was associated with greater coronary heart disease risk, with higher adult BMI exacerbating the effect of prenatal growth [48].

Studies of twins also support the hypothesis factors which constrain fetal growth can program disease in later life. Bo et al. reported that among pairs of both monozygotic and dizygotic twins discordant for impaired glucose tolerance or insulin resistance, the risk of metabolic disturbance was significantly greater in the twin with the lower birth weight in the pair [49]. Metaanalyses of cohort studies that have considered the relationships between birth weight and adult disease show highly robust associations between low birth weight, chronic kidney disease, coronary heart disease, hypertension, and type-2 diabetes [50–52].

Other aspects of anthropometry at birth are predictive of future health and disease. Thinness at birth (measured as ponderal index; weight/length^3) has been found to be inversely related to risk of type-2 diabetes and glucose intolerance. Thinness at birth was also related to risk of coronary heart disease death, type-2 diabetes, and metabolic syndrome if BMI was high in later childhood in a population of Finnish adults [53] and similarly thinness at birth was associated with insulin resistance in 50-year-old British men [54], and glucose homeostasis in children at the age of 7 [55]. Large head circumference in proportion to body length is also a potential disease marker. A large head circumference at birth was associated with greater risk of asthmatic wheeze in 7-year-old children [56]. This may reflect mechanisms which spare the growth of the brain during fetal development, at the expense of the truncal organs.

In the early studies of the Hertfordshire cohort, it was noted that disease in later life was related to weight at 1 year in addition to weight at birth [44]. Individuals who were born small and remained small at 1 year of age were at greater risk of heart disease [57]. This suggested that the postnatal period may also be a window in which adult physiological functions can be programmed. Follow-up of men and woman born in Helsinki in the 1930s showed that women who had developed coronary heart disease had been born smaller and had remained smaller up until the age of 5—6 but had then gained weight very rapidly, such that by age 10—11 they were significantly heavier than girls who had not gone on to develop disease [58]. Similarly, Adair and Cole reported that adolescent boys who were thin at birth had higher blood pressure if they gained weight rapidly between the ages of 8 and 11, but not from birth to 2 year [59]. These studies have led to the idea that fetal growth restraint followed by rapid catch-up growth is a significant determinant of heart disease and diabetes, although few other studies in humans have provided evidence for this.

Collectively these epidemiological observations have paved the way for the developmental origins of disease hypothesis, which postulates that early life factors, particularly nutrition, can predispose individuals to major diseases in adulthood. The programming of disease involves interactions between early life factors and genotype, as shown in Fig. 1.2. Peroxisome proliferator activated receptor-gamma 2 (PPARg2) is a ligand-dependent transcription factor involved in the regulation of lipid metabolism and insulin signaling. The pro12ala polymorphism of PPARg2 is associated with risk of type-2 diabetes, with individuals with the Pro12 variant at greater risk. Studies of the Helsinki birth cohort showed that the effects of low birth weight on future diabetes risk present only in individuals with the Pro12 genotype [60]. Similarly, the relationship between birth weight and degenerative bone disease in elderly individuals is seen only in those carrying a particular variant of the Bsm1 polymorphism of the vitamin D receptor gene [61]. It has been argued that the association between low birth weight and later disease is explained only by genotypes which determine both birth weight and disease risk [62]. There are a number of polymorphisms that are linked to increased risk of type-2 diabetes which also associate with lower birth weight, but the associations tend to be very weak. For example, the high-risk allele for type-2 diabetes at the HHEX-IDE locus is associated with an 81 g lower birth weight [63]. In contrast, it is estimated that risk of diabetes is 23% lower for every 1 kg increase in weight at birth [50].

A genetic explanation of the relationship between birth weight and disease is just one counter to the developmental origins of health hypothesis. It is also argued that maternal undernutrition is not a major driver of birth weight or other features of anthropometry at birth. While a number of studies show that extreme undernutrition can reduce birth weight, the effects are usually small and are only seen in deprived populations. Maternal intakes within the normal range for well-nourished western populations account for only around 6% of variation in birth weight [1]. However, it is important to consider that the nutrition experienced by the fetus is more than just maternal food intake, with influences of maternal stores going into pregnancy, competition between mother and fetus for nutrients (during adolescence, for example), maternal activity, and the quality of placental perfusion.

There are an increasing number of studies in humans which show direct associations between poor maternal nutrition and later disease. A follow-up study of middle-aged men born in Scotland found that blood pressure was related to their mothers' intakes of animal protein and carbohydrate during pregnancy [64]. Offspring of women exposed to the Dutch Famine of 1944–45 were found to have type-2 diabetes (undernutrition in late gestation), impaired renal function (midgestation), and coronary heart disease (early gestation) [40]. More recently, a prospective cohort study reported that blood pressure in infancy was lower in children whose mothers took calcium supplements in pregnancy [65] and that obesity was less prevalent in children whose mothers had higher intakes of n-3 fatty acids [66]. Links between maternal obesity and later disease are demonstrated by a number of studies, including the Amsterdam Born Children and their Development (ABCD) cohort. This showed that BMI and blood pressure in 5- to 6-year-old children were related to maternal prepregnancy BMI [67].

The evidence favoring the developmental origins of health and disease hypothesis from human studies has a number of weaknesses. First and foremost, most of the epidemiology points to associations between anthropometry at birth and later disease and assume that low birth weight, for example, is a proxy for poor maternal nutrition. However, birth weight has complex determinants and the journey to being a low birth weight baby can follow many routes. There is a major lack of studies that are able to directly relate high quality records of maternal nutritional status in pregnancy to health in adult offspring. Observations from historical cohorts such as the Hertfordshire and Helsinki cohorts relate birth weights from the 1920 and 1930s to health measures 60–80 years later. Confounding factors may well influence the observed outcomes, with maternal and childhood infections, social class, quality of the infant diet postnatally, and adult lifestyle factors all being difficult to allow for statistically. It is also inevitable that the long time lag between early life exposure and the emergence of significant disease means that we are only able to relate maternal environments from pre-1950s to adult disease. The factors that may have promoted low birth weight and the patterns of maternal nutrition that were prevalent historically may have no relation to contemporary populations of pregnant women.

Experimental evidence of early life programming

Given the problematic issues with epidemiological observations and the impracticality of running clinical trials to investigate the early life programming of disease states that develop in middle age, animal models have provided an attractive alternative for study [68]. Animal experiments allow all variables to be controlled and to precisely model the impact of under- or overnutrition during pregnancy. Working with short-lived species, these studies can be invasive, performed over a short time span and consider the impact of maternal nutrition across the whole lifespan [69], or across several generations [70].

As shown in Fig. 1.3, animal experiments to model nutritional programming have used a variety of species (rats, mice, guinea pigs, pigs, and sheep) and a great diversity of nutritional challenges. Interestingly, despite the diversity of the challenges applied in pregnancy, the outcomes are

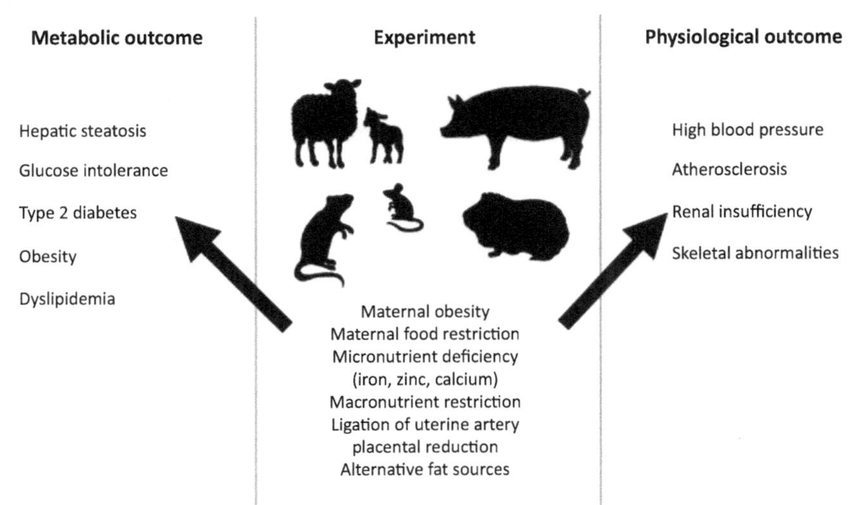

Figure 1.3 ***Experimental models of early life programming.*** Diverse experimental designs using a multitude of nutritional manipulations during pregnancy in animals have shown that consequences for offspring are relatively well conserved.

relatively conserved [71]. Most models, whether inducing obesity through high fat feeding or undernutrition through food restriction, demonstrate that offspring subjected to maternal nutritional insult during pregnancy develop high blood pressure and glucose intolerance [75,76]. With aging, most such animals will display a phenotype of increased adiposity, insulin resistance, and dyslipidemia [72–74]. Renal insufficiency, characterized by reduced nephron numbers and functional deficits, is also a common feature of rodent and sheep models where maternal obesity or nutrient restriction has been applied [75,77,78].

One of the most commonly studied models of nutritional programming utilizes restriction of the protein content of the pregnancy diet in rats [79]. This results in a retardation of fetal growth in late gestation and offspring that develop elevated blood pressure from as early as weaning [80–82]. Initially these offspring have increased insulin sensitivity and show resistance to fat deposition due to suppression of the lipogenic pathway [83]. As they age, these animals become insulin resistant, develop hepatosteatosis, accrue more fat than control animals, and suffer renal failure [73,84]. Their blood pressure remains elevated and this appears to be a product of greater peripheral resistance, strongly driven by altered expression of the key receptors of the renin–angiotensin system [85,86]. Skeletal development is also compromised by the maternal diet and offspring have lower bone mineral content and abnormal formation of the epiphyseal growth plate [87]. Rats exposed to maternal protein restriction in utero have a shorter lifespan than control animals [69,88]. In the atherosclerosis-prone *ApoE*^{3}Leiden* mouse, maternal protein restriction exacerbates atherosclerotic lesion formation [89]. Observations that the effects of maternal protein restriction can be reversed by adding folic acid to the diet, by supplementing with glycine or by blockading maternal glucocorticoid synthesis, have greatly improved mechanistic understanding of early life programming [85,90,91].

Studies which seek to induce obesity in rodents during pregnancy are highly varied in their approach. High fat diets are commonplace, and increasingly researchers are employing the cafeteria diet, in which rats are induced to overfeed through the presentation of a continually changing array of highly palatable, high energy density human foods [92]. Interpretation of such studies can be a challenge as it is difficult to distinguish between the effects of maternal adiposity and the effects of the diets, which often are low in protein and micronutrients, or enriched with particular fatty acids. Typically, however, offspring of mothers fed according to these protocols exhibit high blood pressure and develop an insulin-resistant, obese phenotype. For example, Samuellson et al. found that offspring of mice fed a high fat, high sugar diet were hypertensive, hyperphagic, had dyslipidaemia, and were fatter than offspring of mothers fed a control diet [72]. Similarly, cafeteria feeding in rat pregnancy results in greater adiposity and, with a further high fat challenge in adulthood, insulin resistance in offspring [92]. Clear differences in programmed phenotype resulting from exposure to maternal diet during fetal development and suckling have been identified. Metabolic disturbances are associated with either period, but programming of offspring behavior is strongly linked to the suckling period [92,93].

As rodent species have short lifespans (less than 3 years) and are able to breed within a few weeks of birth, it has been possible to test whether effects of one short period of maternal undernutrition can impact upon physiological or metabolic functions of subsequent generations. Work with zinc restriction in pregnant mice showed that immune function was impacted in not just the immediate offspring (F1 generation) but also the subsequent two (F2 and F3). Harrison and Langley-Evans showed in rats that protein restriction in pregnancy impacted on blood pressure in F1, F2, and F3 and nephron numbers in F1 and F2 [70]. Importantly, the study showed that the programmed phenotype could be transferred down the male as well as the female line. In females, the eggs of the F2 generation are directly impacted by the initial nutritional insult, but for males the result is suggestive of epigenetic memories of the grandmaternal nutritional environment being carried by sperm to the next generation.

Mechanisms of early life programming

In considering how maternal dietary factors can program long-term physiological function and disease risk, it is easiest to think in terms of early life factors setting the functional capacity of tissues and organs (Fig. 1.4). The adaptations that the embryo or fetus makes in order to survive a challenging intrauterine environment enable the development of a level of functional capacity that is sufficient to maintain normal tissue function during the early stages of life, but which with aging and degeneration of systems will result in early loss of function and associated disease.

The programming of functional capacity is driven by a process termed tissue remodeling (Fig. 1.5). This involves changes to the structure of organs

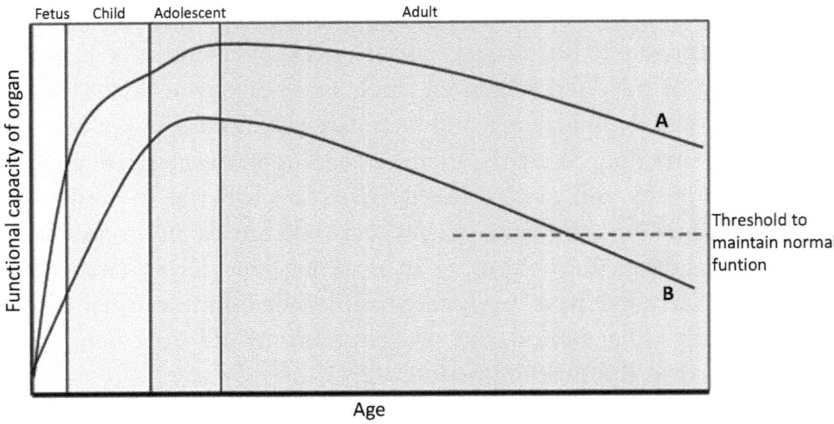

Figure 1.4 ***The concept of functional capacity.*** The functional capacity of an organ or system can be described as its ability to deliver basic requirements. It will vary across the lifespan and decline with age. Factors operating in earlier life stages will determine whether functional capacity remains adequate in older people. Achieving a higher peak functional capacity (A) or slower rate of decline will preserve health for longer than for a lower peak functional capacity (B).

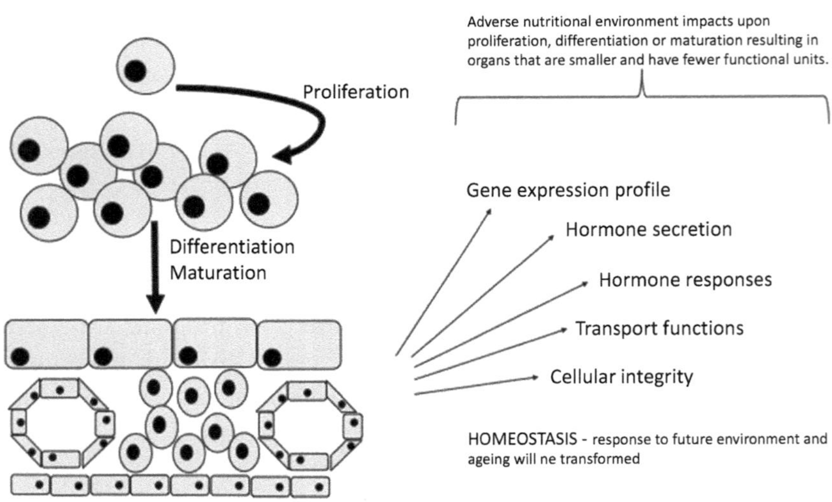

Figure 1.5 ***Tissue remodeling.*** Organs and tissues develop according to a genetically determined pattern during embryonic and fetal life. The formation of mature tissues, which is largely complete before birth in humans, depends upon successive waves of cell proliferation, apoptosis, and differentiation. Disruption of these processes resulting from nutritional insult will result in tissues with fewer functional units.

and tissues due to a lack of substrates, or changes in hormonal or other signaling processes during their phases of cell proliferation, differentiation, and maturation. Disease states that appear to be programmed in utero are exclusively diseases that have their onset in middle age or the later years, which is consistent with an age-related loss of functional reserve. There is a large body of evidence from the animal studies demonstrating tissue remodeling in response to maternal undernutrition. Maternal protein restriction in rat pregnancy remodels hypothalamic structures that regulate food intake [94]. The same maternal insult also remodels the structure of the pancreas [95], with protein-restricted offspring having fewer Islets of Langerhans, which are less vascularized than in controls. In the kidney, nephron number (the key determinant of renal functional capacity) is extremely sensitive to maternal undernutrition and is reduced by maternal food restriction, protein restriction, or iron deficiency during nephrogenesis [75,77,78]. Autopsy studies also suggest an association between nephron number and birth weight in humans [96].

For maternal nutritional status to impact upon organ development through remodeling only a short period of exposure is necessary. It was clear, for example, from the Dutch Famine studies that exposure to maternal undernutrition had effects that depended on the timing of the exposure. It is argued that these periods of exposure to famine coincided with and compromised development of specific systems. Animal studies show that long-lasting effects on physiology and metabolism can stem from extremely short periods of exposure to undernutrition and suggest that the mechanisms which drive programming may be dependent upon transient fluctuations in the environment which impact upon the processes of proliferation or differentiation in tissues (Fig. 1.5). These fluctuations could involve inadequate or excess supply of specific substrates, or changes in maternal—fetal hormone exchanges across the placenta. These will serve to perturb gene expression at critical points in development and remodel the tissues.

Animal studies show that nutritional manipulations during fetal develop have persistent, long-lasting effects on expression of genes in key pathways and processes that regulate blood pressure, vascular endothelial function, glucose homeostasis, insulin signaling, and lipogenesis [97—99]. Of more interest, mechanistically, are the gene expression changes that occur during the period of nutritional insult, as these are the direct responses to nutritional challenges and are most likely to be primary drivers of the programmed response. In the day 13 rat embryo exposed to either protein restriction or maternal iron deficiency, there is evidence that a relatively conserved set of genes that regulate the cell cycle and cytoskeletal remodeling play a key role in the programming response [78]. Similarly, regulation of the cell cycle and maintenance of DNA is perturbed in livers of rat neonates exposed to maternal low protein diets in utero [100]. Effects on the key process of cell division and the integrity of DNA replication would clearly provide a direct link between the maternal diet and tissue remodeling.

The drivers of differential gene expression during development are likely to be variable. It is known, for example, that effects of the maternal diet upon expression of transporters in the placenta will vary transport of substrates from mother to fetus [101,102]. This is likely to impact directly upon nutrient-sensitive transcription factors and suppress or induce pathways and processes. For example, in the rat, exposure to maternal protein restriction is associated with upregulation of genes associated with cholesterol transport across the placenta [101]. This may indicate that maternal undernutrition may in fact increase cholesterol in fetal tissues, which may then impact on cardiovascular development. The same gene loci are also observed to be sensitive to maternal iron deficiency and high fat feeding in rats, and to maternal obesity in humans.

There is also strong evidence that maternal diet regulates metabolism of glucocorticoids in the placenta [85,103,104]. These steroid hormones are powerful regulators of gene expression and promote early maturation of tissues. There is a strong gradient of glucocorticoid concentration across the placenta, with the amount in maternal circulation being orders of magnitude higher than in fetal. This gradient is maintained by 11-beta-hydroxysteroid dehydrogenase 2, which metabolizes active glucocorticoids to inactive forms [104]. With maternal undernutrition, the expression of this enzyme is suppressed, allowing more glucocorticoid to reach the fetal tissues, bringing about altered patterns of gene expression [104]. In the absence of maternal glucocorticoids, the well-established early programming effects of undernutrition are abolished [85].

A growing body of evidence from both human and animal studies supports the hypothesis that maternal nutritional status can impact upon the epigenome (the chemical modifications to bases in DNA and to histone proteins, which modify the transcription of genes). There are numerous reports from animal studies that maternal undernutrition resets DNA methylation and marks of histones in offspring tissue [105,106], and this is matched by data from the Dutch Famine which showed that methylation of genomic DNA from whole blood, at the *Igf2*, locus was reduced in those exposed to famine in utero [107]. There is evidence that some of this is mediated through glucocorticoid-dependent processes [103]. Resetting of epigenetic marks may provide a longer-term cellular memory of the fetal environment and explain some programming of tissue function, a concept that is strongly supported by the observations that effects of maternal undernutrition can be inherited across three generations [70] and that paternal undernutrition can also have a programming effect on offspring [108]. Exploring the relationship between changes to epigenetic marks is problematic as the functional consequences of differential DNA methylation or histone acetylation across a lifespan is difficult to map. It is clear that while fetal and neonatal tissues display differential methylation of DNA, these differentially methylated loci do not always correspond with the genes that are differentially expressed at the same time [106]. Rather than contributing to tissue remodeling, epigenetic responses to maternal nutritional status may also amplify changes in function by altering the capacity of tissues to respond to nutritional challenges later in life.

Conclusions

Nutrition during pregnancy is a complex issue. While pregnancy is highly demanding in terms of additional energy and nutrients to support the physiological and metabolic adaptations of the mother, and the growth and development of the fetus, those nutrient requirements do not depend wholly on food intake. Maternal stores and adaptations to improve efficiency of utilization and uptake play a key role and are difficult to quantify. It should be clear from the above discussion that the nutritional environment is critical for the embryo and fetus, with both under- and overnutrition being associated with risk of fetal death, premature delivery, and low birth weight. Successful fetal adaptations to a suboptimal maternal environment are in themselves hazardous, as in the longer term they increase risk of disease.

The evidence that shows maternal nutrition can program health and disease has changed perspectives of disease etiology. With the recognition that risk of disease is determined not just by interactions of adult lifestyle with the genotype but also by early life experience comes an opportunity to introduce new approaches to the prevention of disease and the promotion of public health.

References

[1] Langley-Evans SC. Pregnancy. In: Nutrition, health and disease. A lifespan approach. Chichester, Sussex, UK: Wiley Blackwell; 2015. p. 61–93.
[2] Langley-Evans SC. Fetal programming of adult disease: an overview. In: Langley-Evans SC, editor. Fetal nutrition and adult disease. Wallingford, Oxfordshire, UK: CABI Publishing; 2004.
[3] Martinez-Frias ML, Salvador J. Megadose vitamin A and teratogenicity. Lancet 1988;1:236.
[4] Martinez-Frias ML, Salvador J. Epidemiological aspects of prenatal exposure to high doses of vitamin A in Spain. Eur J Epidemiol 1990;6:118–23.
[5] Langley-Evans SC, Langley-Evans AJ. Use of folic acid supplements in the first trimester of pregnancy. J R Soc Promo Health 2002;122:181–6.
[6] Honein MA, Paulozzi LJ, Mathews TJ, et al. Impact of folic acid fortification of the US food supply on the occurrence of neural tube defects. J Am Med Assoc 2001;285:2981–6.
[7] Tinker SC, Devine O, Mai C, et al. Estimate of the potential impact of folic acid fortification of corn masa flour on the prevention of neural tube defects. Birth Defects Res A Clin Mol Teratol 2013;97:649–57.
[8] Gao LJ, Wang ZP, Lu QB, et al. Maternal overweight and obesity and the risk of neural tube defects: a case-control study in China. Birth Defects Res A Clin Mol Teratol 2013;97:161–5.
[9] Ray JG, Thompson MD, Vermeulen MJ, et al. Metabolic syndrome features and risk of neural tube defects. BMC Pregnancy Childbirth 2007;7:21.
[10] Durnin JV. Energy requirements of pregnancy. Diabetes 1991;40(Suppl. 2):152–6.
[11] Prentice AM, Goldberg GR. Energy adaptations in human pregnancy: limits and long-term consequences. Am J Clin Nutr 2000;71:1226S–32S.
[12] Millward DJ. Optimal intakes of protein in the human diet. Proc Nutr Soc 1999;58:403–13.
[13] Barbour LA. New concepts in insulin resistance of pregnancy and gestational diabetes: long-term implications for mother and offspring. J Obstet Gynaecol 2003;23:545–9.
[14] MacLennan WJ, Hamilton JC, Darmady JM. The effects of season and stage of pregnancy on plasma 25-hydroxy-vitamin D concentrations in pregnant women. Postgrad Med 1980;56:75–9.
[15] Javaid MK, Crozier SR, Harvey NC, et al. Maternal vitamin D status during pregnancy and childhood bone mass at age 9 years: a longitudinal study. Lancet 2006;367:36–43.
[16] Whittaker PG, Lind T, Williams JG. Iron absorption during normal human pregnancy: a study using stable isotopes. Br J Nutr 1991;65:457–63.
[17] Nisar YB, Dibley MJ. Earlier initiation and use of a greater number of iron-folic acid supplements during pregnancy prevents early neonatal deaths in Nepal and Pakistan. PloS One 2014;9. e112446.
[18] Gomes da Costa A, Vargas S, Clode N, et al. Prevalence and risk factors for iron deficiency anemia and iron depletion during pregnancy: aprospective study. Acta Med Port 2016;29:514–8.
[19] Scholl TO, Reilly T. Anemia, iron and pregnancy outcome. J Nutr 2000;130:443S–7S.
[20] Chapman AB, Abraham WT, Zamudio S, et al. Temporal relationships between hormonal and hemodynamic changes in early human pregnancy. Kidney Int 1998;54:2056–63.
[21] Marchioni E, Fumarola A, Calvanese A, et al. Iodine deficiency in pregnant women residing in an area with adequate iodine intake. Nutrition 2008;24:458–61.

[22] Ogden CL, Carroll MD, Fryar CD, et al. Prevalence of obesity among adults and youth: United States, 2011-2014. NCHS Data Brief; 2015. p. 1–8.
[23] Heslehurst N, Rankin J, Wilkinson JR, et al. A nationally representative study of maternal obesity in England, UK: trends in incidence and demographic inequalities in 619 323 births, 1989-2007. Int J Obes 2010;34:420–8.
[24] Mishra V, Thapa S, Retherford RD, Dai X. Effect of iron supplementation during pregnancy on birthweight: evidence from Zimbabwe. Food Nutr Bull 2005;26:338–47.
[25] Melse-Boonstra A, Gowachirapant S, Jaiswal N, et al. Iodine supplementation in pregnancy and its effect on child cognition. J Trace Elem Med Biol 2012;26:134–6.
[26] Christian P, West Jr KP, Khatry SK, et al. Night blindness during pregnancy and subsequent mortality among women in Nepal: effects of vitamin A and beta-carotene supplementation. Am J Epidemiol 2000;152:542–7.
[27] Institute of Medicine. Weight gain during pregnancy: reexamining the guidelines. Washington DC: National Academies Press; 2009.
[28] Dag ZO, Dilbaz B. Impact of obesity on infertility in women. J Turk Ger Gynecol Assoc 2015;16:111–7.
[29] McGiveron A, Foster S, Pearce J, et al. Limiting antenatal weight gain improves maternal health outcomes in severely obese pregnant women: findings of a pragmatic evaluation of a midwife-led intervention. J Hum Nutr Diet 2015;28:29–37.
[30] Chu SY, Kim SY, Lau J, et al. Maternal obesity and risk of stillbirth: a metaanalysis. Am J Obstet Gynecol 2007;197:223–8.
[31] Rasmussen S, Irgens LM, Espinoza J. Maternal obesity and excess of fetal growth in pre-eclampsia. BJOG 2014;121:1351–7.
[32] Madan J, Chen M, Goodman E, et al. Maternal obesity, gestational hypertension, and preterm delivery. J Matern Fetal Neonatal Med 2010;23:82–8.
[33] Bowers K, Laughon SK, Kiely M, et al. Gestational diabetes, pre-pregnancy obesity and pregnancy weight gain in relation to excess fetal growth: variations by race/ethnicity. Diabetologia 2013;56:1263–71.
[34] Ray JG, Vermeulen MJ, Shapiro JL, et al. Maternal and neonatal outcomes in pregestational and gestational diabetes mellitus, and the influence of maternal obesity and weight gain: the DEPOSIT study. Diabetes Endocrine Pregnancy Outcome Study in Toronto. QJM 2001;94:347–56.
[35] Nohr EA, Bech BH, Vaeth M, et al. Obesity, gestational weight gain and preterm birth: a study within the Danish National Birth Cohort. Paediatr Perinat Epidemiol 2007;21:5–14.
[36] Blomberg M. Maternal obesity and risk of postpartum hemorrhage. Obstet Gynecol 2011;118:561–8.
[37] Merlino A, Laffineuse L, Collin M, et al. Impact of weight loss between pregnancies on recurrent preterm birth. Am J Obstet Gynecol 2006;195:818–21.
[38] Dodd JM, Cramp C, Sui Z, et al. The effects of antenatal dietary and lifestyle advice for women who are overweight or obese on maternal diet and physical activity: the LIMIT randomised trial. BMC Med 2014;12:161.
[39] Ceesay SM, Prentice AM, Cole TJ, et al. Effects on birth weight and perinatal mortality of maternal dietary supplements in rural Gambia: 5 year randomised controlled trial. BMJ 1997;315:786–90.
[40] Roseboom T, de Rooij S, Painter R. The Dutch famine and its long-term consequences for adult health. Early Hum Dev 2006;82:485–91.
[41] Langley-Evans SC. Nutrition in early life and the programming of adult disease: a review. J Hum Nutr Diet 2015;28:1–14.
[42] Osmond C, Barker DJP, Slattery JM. Risk of death from cardiovascular-disease and chronic-bronchitis determined by place of birth in England and Wales. J Epidemiol Community Health 1990;44:139–41.

[43] Osmond C, Barker DJP, Winter PD, et al. Early growth and death from cardiovascular-disease in women. Br Med J 1993;307:1519–24.
[44] Hales CN, Barker DJP, Clark PMS, et al. Fetal and infant growth and impaired glucose-tolerance at age 64. Br Med J 1991;303:1019–22.
[45] Phipps K, Barker DJP, Hales CN, et al. Fetal growth and impaired glucose-tolerance in men and women. Diabetologia 1993;36:225–8.
[46] Barker DJP, Hales CN, Fall CHD, et al. Type 2 (Non-Insulin-Dependent) diabetes-mellitus, hypertension and hyperlipemia (Syndrome-X) - relation to reduced fetal growth. Diabetologia 1993;36:62–7.
[47] Curhan GC, Chertow GM, Willett WC, et al. Birth weight and adult hypertension and obesity in women. Circulation 1996;94:1310–5.
[48] Frankel S, Elwood P, Sweetnam P, et al. Birthweight, body-mass index in middle age, and incident coronary heart disease. Lancet 1996;348:1478–80.
[49] Bo S, Cavallo-Perin P, Scaglione L, et al. Low birthweight and metabolic abnormalities in twins with increased susceptibility to Type 2 diabetes mellitus. Diabet Med 2000;17:365–70.
[50] Whincup PH, Kaye SJ, Owen CG, et al. Birth weight and risk of type 2 diabetes A systematic review. Jama-J Am Med Assoc 2008;300:2886–97.
[51] Zhang Y, Li H, Liu SJ, et al. The associations of high birth weight with blood pressure and hypertension in later life: a systematic review and meta-analysis. Hypertens Res 2013;36:725–35.
[52] White SL, Perkovic V, Cass A, et al. Is low birth weight an antecedent of CKD in later life? A systematic review of observational studies. Am J Kidney Dis 2009;54:248–61.
[53] Eriksson JG, Forsen T, Tuomilehto J, et al. Effects of size at birth and childhood growth on the insulin resistance syndrome in elderly individuals. Diabetologia 2002;45:342–8.
[54] Phillips DIW, Barker DJP, Hales CN, et al. Thinness at birth and insulin-resistance in adult life. Diabetologia 1994;37:150–4.
[55] Law CM, Barker DJP, Hales CN, et al. Insulin-resistance in 7 Year-old children who were thin at birth. Pediatr Res 1994;35. 263-263.
[56] Carrington LJ, Langley-Evans SC. Wheezing and eczema in relation to infant anthropometry: evidence of developmental programming of disease in childhood. Matern Child Nutr 2006;2:51–61.
[57] Barker DJP, Fall CHD. Fetal and infant origins of cardiovascular-disease. Arch Dis Child 1993;68:797–9.
[58] Forsen T, Eriksson JG, Tuomilehto J, et al. Growth in utero and during childhood among women who develop coronary heart disease: longitudinal study. Br Med J 1999;319:1403–7.
[59] Adair LS, Cole TJ. Rapid child growth raises blood pressure in adolescent boys who were thin at birth. Hypertension 2003;41:451–6.
[60] Eriksson JG, Lindi V, Uusitupa M, et al. The metabolic effects of the Pro12Ala Polymorphism of the PPAR gamma 2 gene interact with size at birth. Diabetologia 2002;45:A125–6.
[61] Jordan KM, Syddall H, Dennison EM, et al. Birthweight, vitamin D receptor gene polymorphism, and risk of lumbar spine osteoarthritis. J Rheumatol 2005;32:678–83.
[62] Hattersley AT, Tooke JE. The fetal insulin hypothesis: an alternative explanation of the association of low birthweight with diabetes and vascular disease. Lancet 1999;353:1789–92.
[63] Horikoshi M, Yaghootkar H, Mook-Kanamori DO, et al. New loci associated with birth weight identify genetic links between intrauterine growth and adult height and metabolism. Nat Genet 2013;45:76–U115.

[64] Campbell DM, Hall MH, Barker DJP, et al. Diet in pregnancy and the offspring's blood pressure 40 years later. Br J Obstet Gynaecol 1996;103:273–80.
[65] Bakker R, Rifas-Shiman SL, Kleinman KP, et al. Maternal calcium intake during pregnancy and blood pressure in the offspring at age 3 years: a follow-up analysis of the Project Viva cohort. Am J Epidemiol 2008;168:1374–80.
[66] Donahue SM, Rifas-Shiman SL, Olsen SF, et al. Associations of maternal prenatal dietary intake of n-3 and n-6 fatty acids with maternal and umbilical cord blood levels. Prostaglandins Leukot Essent Fatty Acids 2009;80:289–96.
[67] Gademan MG, van Eijsden M, Roseboom TJ, et al. Maternal prepregnancy body mass index and their children's blood pressure and resting cardiac autonomic balance at age 5 to 6 years. Hypertension 2013;62:641–7.
[68] McMullen S, Mostyn A. Animal models for the study of the developmental origins of health and disease. Proc Nutr Soc 2009;68:306–20.
[69] Sayer AA, Dunn R, Langley-Evans S, et al. Prenatal exposure to a maternal low protein diet shortens life span in rats. Gerontology 2001;47:9–14.
[70] Harrison M, Langley-Evans SC. Intergenerational programming of impaired nephrogenesis and hypertension in rats following maternal protein restriction during pregnancy. Br J Nutr 2009;101:1020–30.
[71] McMullen S, Langley-Evans SC, Gambling L, et al. A common cause for a common phenotype: the gatekeeper hypothesis in fetal programming. Med Hypotheses 2012;78:88–94.
[72] Gopalakrishnan GS, Gardner DS, Dandrea J, et al. Influence of maternal pre-pregnancy body composition and diet during early-mid pregnancy on cardiovascular function and nephron number in juvenile sheep. Br J Nutr 2005;94:938–47.
[73] Jackson AA, Dunn RL, Marchand MC, et al. Increased systolic blood pressure in rats nduced by a maternal low-protein diet is reversed by dietary supplementation with glycine. Clin Sci 2002;103:633–9.
[74] Langley SC, Jackson AA. Increased systolic blood-pressure in adult-rats induced by fetal exposure to maternal low-protein diets. Clin Sci 1994;86:217–22.
[75] Samuelsson AM, Matthews PA, Argenton M, et al. Diet-induced obesity in female mice leads to offspring hyperphagia, adiposity, hypertension, and insulin resistance - a novel murine model of developmental programming. Hypertension 2008;51:383–92.
[76] Gambling L, Dunford S, Wallace D, et al. Postnatal effects of prenatal iron deficiency in the rat. Pediatr Res 2003;53:30a–1a.
[77] Bellinger L, Sculley DV, Langley-Evans SC. Exposure to undernutrition in fetal life determines fat distribution, locomotor activity and food intake in ageing rats. Int J Obes 2006;30:729–38.
[78] Fernandez-Twinn DS, Wayman A, Ekizoglou S, et al. Maternal protein restriction leads to hyperinsulinemia and reduced insulin-signaling protein expression in 21-mo-old female rat offspring. Am J Physiol-Reg I 2005;288:R368–73.
[79] Langley-Evans SC, Welham SJM, Jackson AA. Fetal exposure to a maternal low protein diet impairs nephrogenesis and promotes hypertension in the rat. Life Sci 1999;64:965–74.
[80] Swali A, McMullen S, Hayes H, et al. Cell cycle regulation and cytoskeletal remodelling are critical processes in the nutritional programming of embryonic development. PloS One 2011;6.
[81] Langley-Evans SC, Gardner DS, Jackson AA. Association of disproportionate growth of fetal rats in late gestation with raised systolic blood pressure in later life. J Reprod Fertil 1996;106:307–12.
[82] Langley-Evans SC, Phillips GJ, Jackson AA. In utero exposure to maternal low protein diets induces hypertension in weanling rats, independently of maternal blood pressure changes. Clin Nutr 1994;13:319–24.

[83] Langley-Evans SC, Welham SJ, Sherman RC, et al. Weanling rats exposed to maternal low-protein diets during discrete periods of gestation exhibit differing severity of hypertension. Clin Sci (Lond) 1996;91:607−15.
[84] Erhuma A, Salter AM, Sculley DV, et al. Prenatal exposure to a low-protein diet programs disordered regulation of lipid metabolism in the aging rat. Am J Physiol Endocrinol Metab 2007;292:E1702−14.
[85] Joles JA, Sculley DV, Langley-Evans SC. Proteinuria in aging rats due to low-protein diet during mid-gestation. J Dev Orig Hlth Dis 2010;1:75−83.
[86] McMullen S, Langley-Evans SC. Maternal low-protein diet in rat pregnancy programs blood pressure through sex-specific mechanisms. Am J Physiol-Reg I 2005;288:R85−90.
[87] Swali A, McMullen S, Langley-Evans SC. Prenatal protein restriction leads to a disparity between aortic and peripheral blood pressure in Wistar male offspring. J Physiol-London 2010;588:3809−18.
[88] Mehta G, Roach HI, Langley-Evans S, et al. Intrauterine exposure to a maternal low protein diet reduces adult bone mass and alters growth plate morphology in rats. Calcif Tissue Int 2002;71:493−8.
[89] Langley-Evans SC, Sculley DV. The association between birthweight and longevity in the rat is complex and modulated by maternal protein intake during fetal life. FEBS Lett 2006;580:4150−3.
[90] Yates Z, Tarling EJ, Langley-Evans SC, et al. Maternal undernutrition programmes atherosclerosis in the ApoE*3-Leiden mouse. Br J Nutr 2009;101:1185−94.
[91] Engeham SF, Haase A, Langley-Evans SC. Supplementation of a maternal low-protein diet in rat pregnancy with folic acid ameliorates programming effects upon feeding behaviour in the absence of disturbances to the methionine-homocysteine cycle. Br J Nutr 2010;103:996−1007.
[92] Akyol A, McMullen S, Langley-Evans SC. Glucose intolerance associated with early-life exposure to maternal cafeteria feeding is dependent upon post-weaning diet. Br J Nutr 2012;107:964−78.
[93] Wright TM, Voigt JP, Langley-Evans SC. Alterations to feeding behaviour in offspring induced by maternal exposure to a high caloric diet throughout lactation. Eur J Med Res 2010;15. 185-185.
[94] Plagemann A, Waas T, Harder T, et al. Hypothalamic neuropeptide Y levels in weaning offspring of low-protein malnourished mother rats. Neuropeptides 2000;34:1−6.
[95] Snoeck A, Reusensbillen B, Remacle C, et al. Effect of protein-deprivation during pregnancy in the fetal endocrine pancreas in rats. Diabetologia 1989;32. A543-A543.
[96] Hughson M, Farris 3rd AB, Douglas-Denton R, et al. Glomerular number and size in autopsy kidneys: the relationship to birth weight. Kidney Int 2003;63:2113−22.
[97] Erhuma A, McMullen S, Langley-Evans SC, et al. Feeding pregnant rats a low-protein diet alters the hepatic expression of SREBP-1c in their offspring via a glucocorticoid-related mechanism. Endocrine 2009;36:333−8.
[98] McMullen S, Gardner DS, Langley-Evans SC. Prenatal programming of angiotensin II type 2 receptor expression in the rat. Br J Nutr 2004;91:133−40.
[99] Sandovici I, Hammerle CM, Cooper WN, et al. Ageing is associated with molecular signatures of inflammation and type 2 diabetes in rat pancreatic islets. Diabetologia 2016;59:502−11.
[100] Altobelli G, Bogdarina IG, Stupka E, et al. Genome-wide methylation and gene expression changes in newborn rats following maternal protein restriction and reversal by folic acid. PloS One 2013;8.

[101] Daniel Z, Swali A, Emes R, et al. The effect of maternal undernutrition on the rat placental transcriptome: protein restriction up-regulates cholesterol transport. Genes Nutr 2016;11:27.

[102] Nusken E, Gellhaus A, Kuhnel E, et al. Increased rat placental fatty acid, but decreased amino acid and glucose transporters potentially modify intrauterine programming. J Cell Biochem 2016;117:1594–603.

[103] Bogdarina I, Haase A, Langley-Evans S, et al. Glucocorticoid effects on the programming of AT1b angiotensin receptor gene methylation and expression in the rat. PloS One 2010;5.

[104] Langley-Evans SC, Phillips GJ, Benediktsson R, et al. Protein intake in pregnancy, placental glucocorticoid metabolism and the programming of hypertension in the rat. Placenta 1996;17:169–72.

[105] Lillycrop KA, Lapham A, O'Neil D, et al. Maternal protein restriction decreases global histone H3 K27 methylation in the liver of adult offspring through the altered expression of specific microRNAs. J Dev Orig Hlth Dis 2011;2. S19-S19.

[106] Lillycrop KA, Slater-Jefferies JL, Hanson MA, et al. Induction of altered epigenetic regulation of the hepatic glucocorticoid receptor in the offspring of rats fed a protein-restricted diet during pregnancy suggests that reduced DNA methyltransferase-1 expression is involved in impaired DNA methylation and changes in histone modifications. Br J Nutr 2007;97:1064–73.

[107] Heijmans BT, Tobi EW, Stein AD, et al. Persistent epigenetic differences associated with prenatal exposure to famine in humans. Proc Natl Acad Sci U S A 2008;105:17046–9.

[108] Watkins AJ, Sinclair KD. Paternal low protein diet affects adult offspring cardiovascular and metabolic function in mice. Am J Physiol Heart Circ Physiol 2014;306:H1444–52.

CHAPTER 2

Benefits of breastfeeding in infant health: a role for milk signaling peptides

Catalina Picó, Mariona Palou, Catalina Amadora Pomar, Andreu Palou
Laboratory of Molecular Biology, Nutrition and Biotechnology (Group of Nutrigenomics and Obesity), University of the Balearic Islands, CIBER de Fisiopatología de La Obesidad y Nutrición (CIBERobn), Instituto de Investigación Sanitaria Illes Balears, Palma de Mallorca, Spain

Contents

Metabolic programming in the immediate postnatal life

Prenatal and early postnatal periods have been revealed as critical stages of development, where nutritional and other environmental factors may have a profound influence on health [1,2]. Accordingly, exposure to an unfavorable environment during this critical window can lead to lasting or permanent effects on the structure and function of the body, resulting in detrimental effects on metabolic health in the long-term, a concept referred to as "metabolic programming" [3]. Namely, for a given genotype there

Molecular Nutrition
ISBN 978-0-12-813862-5
https://doi.org/10.1016/B978-0-12-813862-5.00002-5

will be a range of possible phenotypes in response to distinct environmental exposures, including nutritional, social, psychological, physical, and lifestyle factors during early life and infancy that can modify or condition the ability to respond to new metabolic challenges in adulthood (Fig. 2.1). Interactions between pre- and postnatal environment may also be determinant of future metabolic health. For instance, accelerated postnatal growth after growth restriction during fetal life (so-called "catch-up" growth) has been associated with adverse outcomes in later life [4].

Mechanisms of metabolic programming remain incompletely understood, but there is growing evidence that epigenetic mechanisms (DNA methylation, histone modification, and noncoding RNAs) may facilitate developmental plasticity by encoding information from an organism's early life to coordinate future gene activity and phenotypes in later-life environments without altering the gene sequence [5–7]. Other potential mechanisms accounting for metabolic programming may involve

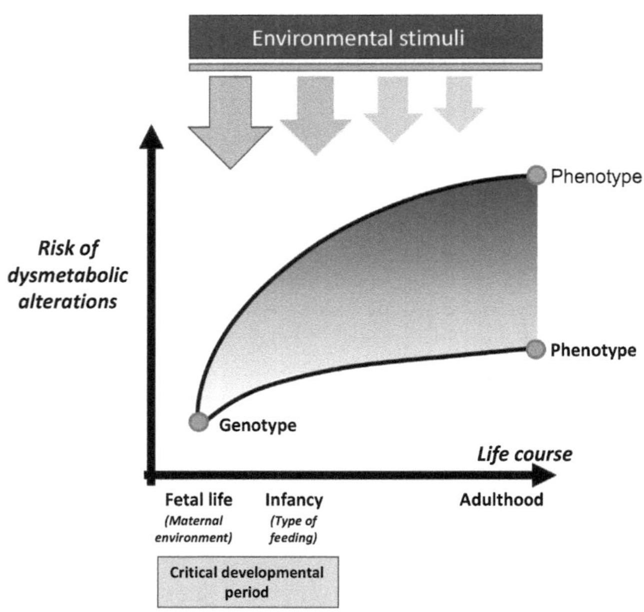

Figure 2.1 ***Effects of environmental stimuli on phenotype and risk of metabolic alterations.*** The phenotype in adulthood is mainly influenced by the genotype and by nutrition and other environmental factors during the whole life, but especially during perinatal life, which is a critical period of developmental plasticity. Therefore, an individual can experience different developmental trajectories in response to specific environmental conditions and acquire a variety of phenotypes with lifelong consequences on their metabolic health.

permanent structural changes in key organs involved in energy metabolism, such as brain and adipose tissue. These changes may cause permanent alterations in number of cells, affect vascularization or innervation of organs, and/or determine changes in the juxtaposition of different cell types within an organ [8].

In humans, the impact of nutritional influence on disease programming during gestation has been evidenced in several epidemiological studies. The most emblematic example is the Dutch famine, where poor maternal nutrition in the first and second trimesters of gestation during World War II resulted in increased incidence of obesity, cardiovascular disease, and diabetes in adult descendants compared with descendants whose mothers did not experience poor nutrition during pregnancy [9]. This has been explained by the "thrifty phenotype hypothesis" proposed by Barker and colleagues, suggesting that poor nutrition during gestation leads to metabolic adaptations in order to maximize survival chances under conditions of food scarcity after birth [10,11]. However, if adequate or abundant nutrition is received later on, such metabolic adaptations in individuals can lead to a greater propensity to adult-onset obesity and related metabolic disorders [10,11]. This hypothesis has provided a plausible explanation of the link between low birth weight and later risk of developing features related with the metabolic syndrome [12].

In mammals, organ development is not completed at birth and continues in the immediate postnatal period. Nutrition during this stage, particularly during lactation, is also important in triggering metabolic programming effects; therefore, infant feeding practices are highly relevant. However, compared to studies addressing environmental effects during fetal life, studies on metabolic programming during early postnatal life are scarce. In general, animal studies have shown that severe under- or overnourishment in the immediate postnatal life, e.g., by adjustment of litter size in rodents, results in adverse effects, such as growth retardation (large litter) or increased body weight gain, hyperinsulinemia, and hyperleptinemia (small litter) [2,13]. Notwithstanding, mild calorie restriction in rat dams during lactation has been reported to protect offspring against obesity and insulin resistance in later life [14]. Other studies in rats have also shown that an increased proportion of carbohydrates taken during the immediate postnatal period induce adaptations predisposing to adult-onset obesity [15]. Therefore, alterations in the amount or composition of food intake in early life may have adverse effects on offspring metabolic health during adulthood.

In humans, what is clearly established is that breastfeeding represents optimal nutrition during immediate postnatal life. A number of epidemiological studies have clearly documented that breastfeeding, compared with formula feeding, represents a protective factor against obesity and related metabolic disorders [16]. Breast milk is considered the ideal combination of nutrients and other bioactive compounds, such as growth factors and hormones, which may affect infant growth and development (Fig. 2.2). Notably, breast milk composition is not uniform, and may be affected by maternal environment. Thus, the beneficial effects of breastfeeding might be influenced by the mother's metabolic state. In fact, despite the well-known beneficial effects of breastfeeding, some animal studies have shown that lactation by a diabetic, obese, or malnourished mother might alter the quality of breast milk and have an impact on the metabolic state of the offspring [17].

These aspects, particularly the beneficial effects of breastfeeding as compared with formula feeding, the potential mechanisms responsible for beneficial health outcomes, and the role of some bioactive peptides present in breast milk that could be considered as a link between maternal nutrition and/or status and metabolic programming in offspring will be discussed below.

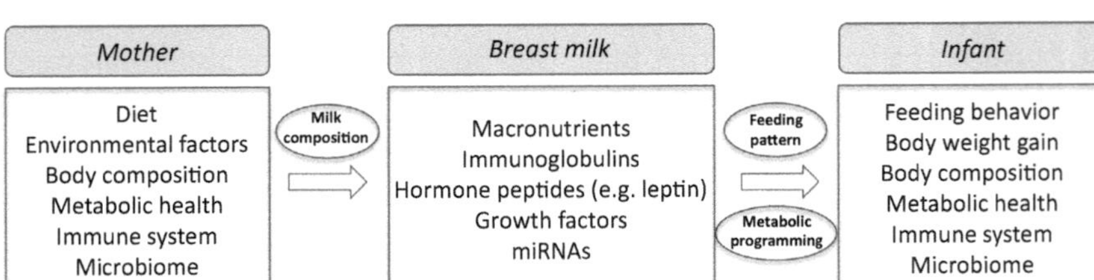

Figure 2.2 ***Mother-infant interaction through breast milk during the immediate postnatal period and consequences in infants.*** Breast milk represents a way of maternal signaling to infants during immediate postnatal life. It contains all nutrients necessary for adequate postnatal growth, but also has a number of bioactive compounds that provide regulation of infant growth trajectory, acquisition of adequate metabolic function, immune protection, and a favorable gut microbiome, all of them in a programmed manner according to the changing circumstances of the infant's development. Maternal environmental conditions can affect breast milk production and composition, which in turn can have life-long effects on infant health, e.g., through effects on feeding patterns, growth trajectory, and/or metabolic programming.

Benefits of breastfeeding on infant metabolic health

Breast milk, the first natural food for mammals, is largely and universally accepted as the best choice for nutrition during an infant's first year of life. The World Health Organization (WHO) recommends exclusive breastfeeding up to 6 months of age, with continued breastfeeding along with appropriate complementary foods up to 2 years or beyond [18].

Maternal milk has the nutritive function of promoting adequate postnatal growth and meeting the complete nutritional needs of infants [19,20]. Even more, breast milk can experience different modifications in its composition to better adapt to infants' requirements depending on individual conditions [21], acting as a truly functional food [22]. Lipids represent the major source of energy in breast milk, contributing to 44% of total energy supplied [23]. They are also an important source of key nutrients for infants: essential fatty acids, phospholipids, liposoluble vitamins, and precursors for the synthesis of eicosanoid hormones [24]. Lactose is the most abundant carbohydrate in breast milk, although small amounts of galactose, fructose, and oligosaccharides are also found [25]. Regarding protein content, mature human milk contains 8%–9% of proteins with balanced amino acids to meet the nutritional needs of infants [25].

However, breast milk provides much more than traditionally considered nutrients. It is a source of maternal immunoglobulins (e.g., secretory IgA), which prime the neonatal and infant immune system and compensate for deficiencies in the neonate [26]. In addition, it also contains bioactive factors that are able to inhibit inflammation and enhance antibody production – such as antioxidants, interleukins, etc. [27] – as well as growth factors and hormones involved in energy metabolism, such as epidermal growth factor (EGF), leptin, adiponectin, etc., which may also be important in the development of the neonate [28,29]. The stomach of infants is able to absorb in its intact form some of these bioactive peptides that are broken in the stomach of adults by digestive mechanisms. The high permeability of the gastrointestinal tract in neonates, together with the immaturity of digestive mechanisms, favors the nondigestive pathway for the absorption of active peptides [30,31]. miRNAs are also emerging as bioactive components of breast milk; they are abundantly present in milk and have been proposed to exert tissue-specific immunoprotective and developmental functions in infants [32].

Therefore, besides ensuring essential nutrients to infants, breastfeeding has been associated with a number of short- and long-term beneficial

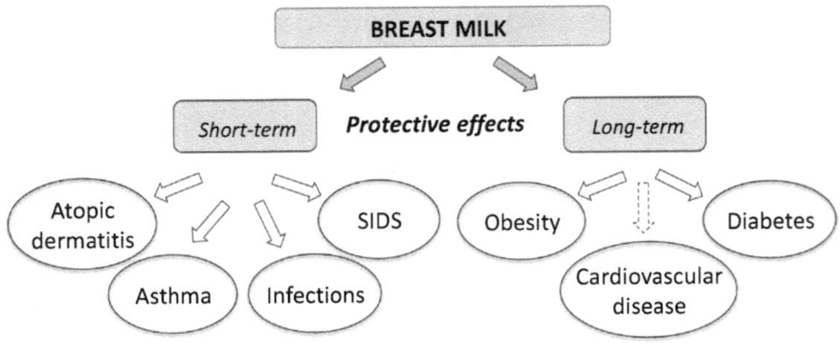

Figure 2.3 ***Breast milk short- and long-term protective effects on infant health.*** Short-term benefits of breast milk include protection against infections, asthma, atopic dermatitis, and sudden infant death syndrome (SIDS). In the long-term, breastfeeding confers certain protection against obesity and type 1 and 2 diabetes, and may have modest effects against cardiovascular disease risk factors.

outcomes for both children and their mothers [33] (Fig. 2.3). For mothers, the benefits associated to the history of lactation include a reduced risk of type 2 diabetes, and of breast and ovarian cancer, while early interruption of breastfeeding or no breastfeeding has been related to a higher risk of maternal postpartum depression [33]. Moreover, faster maternal weight loss postpartum is also one of the benefits for lactating mothers [33].

Focusing on the effects of breastfeeding on infant's health, breastfeeding has been shown to have distinct short-term advantages. Breastfed children, compared with formula-fed infants, show lower risk of different infections, including acute otitis media, nonspecific gastroenteritis, and severe lower respiratory tract infections [33,34]. The likelihood of developing atopic dermatitis and asthma (young children) is also reduced by breastfeeding, in comparison to formula feeding [33,34]. Importantly, the risk of sudden infant death syndrome (SIDS), which is the leading cause of infant mortality between 1 and 12 months of age, is also reduced by breastfeeding in developed countries, such as the United States [33,34].

Breast milk also impacts infant microbiota. There is a close association between mother's microbiota, human milk oligosaccharide composition, and infant gut microbiota [35]. It has been reported that exclusively breastfed infants, compared to nonexclusively breastfed ones, have higher gut bacterial diversity and relative abundance of Bacteroidetes and Firmicutes in the first 6 months of life [36]. These differences in gut microbiota persist after 6 months of age. This seems to be of interest since a healthy gut microbiota profile may contribute to improving host metabolism through dynamic changes in metabolites, nutrients, and vitamins, and to maintaining energy homeostasis [37]. In fact, alterations in microbiota profile have been related to the development of some diseases, and have been postulated as an important factor for obesity development [38,39]. Additionally, longer duration of exclusive breastfeeding can be related to reduced diarrhea-related gut microbiota dysbiosis [36].

Among the long-term health outcomes of breastfeeding, one of the most important benefits is probably the prevention of obesity and related diseases. Breastfeeding, compared with formula feeding, may have a protective role against obesity, as well as other metabolic diseases such as diabetes, hypertension, and cardiovascular disease [40–44]. However, some controversy remains [33,34], and the relevant findings and evidence relating breastfeeding to the incidence of metabolic health diseases in adult life are further discussed.

Breastfeeding, compared to infant formula feeding, improves the later metabolic health of infants, particularly by reducing the risk of developing obesity and diabetes in adulthood.

Obesity

Obesity is one of the major health problems throughout the world [45], whose prevalence nearly tripled between 1975 and 2016 [46]. In 2016, 39% of adults over 18 years were overweight and about 13% of the world's adult population were obese [46]. Current obesity treatment strategies, mainly based on food intake control, seem to be not enough to deal with this multifactorial disorder of pandemic prevalence. The fact that obesity may be strongly influenced by nutrition during fetal and early postnatal life opens an important window of opportunities for intervention in the battle against this global epidemic.

Hence, there is strong confirmation from multiple population studies showing that breastfeeding compared with infant formula feeding confers reliable protection from later overweight/obesity [33]. Concretely, two - decades ago, von Kries and collaborators, in a cross-sectional study carried out in more than 9000 children 5–6 years old, found a lower prevalence of obesity in breastfed children compared with infant formula–fed ones [41]. Later on, another cohort study including more than 9000 boys and 7000 girls, aged 9–14 years, also showed that breastfed infants had a lower risk of being overweight during older childhood and adolescence compared with formula-fed ones [42]. Armstrong and Reilly also found a positive correlation between breastfeeding and the reduction of the risk of obesity in 32,000 Scottish children 3–4 years old [43]. Two meta-analyses analyzing the effects of breastfeeding against the risk of obesity concluded that breastfeeding is indeed a significant protective factor against childhood obesity [47,48]. Horta and collaborators [47] also showed that breastfeeding was associated with a 13% reduction in overweight/obesity, in subjects aged 1–9, 10–19, and more than 20 years (from 105 studies). Moreover, these authors also found decreased odds of developing type 2 diabetes associated to breastfeeding, by the analysis of 11 studies in subjects aged 10–19 and more than 20 years [47].

Notably, not only the fact of receiving breast milk or not, but also the duration of breastfeeding appears to be strongly related to its protective effect against excess body weight. This has been addressed in several studies [41,42]. Moreover, in a meta-analysis where the relationship between the duration of breastfeeding and the prevalence of obesity was analyzed, the authors found a positive, strong, time-dependent association between the longer duration of breastfeeding and the lower risk of obesity [44]. Few studies have found no such clear association [49,50].

Potential mechanisms involved in the beneficial effects of breastfeeding compared with formula feeding against overweight/obesity in adulthood may be attributed to differences in feeding patterns between both types of feeding [51], and to the caloric content and macronutrient composition of breast milk compared to commercial infant formula [52]. However, strong evidence is recently emerging supporting the role of specific bioactive components, which are functionally present in breast milk but not in infant formula [29]. These aspects, and particularly the potential role of leptin and main milk-derived hormones on later metabolic health of infants, are further discussed in the next section of the present chapter.

Type 1 and type 2 diabetes

Diabetes is a major cause of blindness, kidney failure, heart attacks, stroke, and lower limb amputation. Worldwide prevalence of diabetes in adults aged 18 years and over has risen during the last few decades (e.g., from 4.7% in 1980 to 8.5% in 2014) [53]. In 2015, diabetes was the direct cause of 1.6 million deaths, and in 2012 high blood glucose was the cause of another 2.2 million deaths [54]. Interestingly, the risk has been related to lack of breastfeeding not only for type 2 but also for type 1 diabetes.

Type 1 diabetes is an immune-mediated disease caused by the destruction of the β cells in the pancreatic islets, which produce insulin. Exogenous agents, such as dietary factors and viruses, may trigger the immune-mediated process that leads to β cell destruction [55]. Most of the evidence relating breastfeeding to type 1 diabetes has been obtained from retrospective control studies, showing infants who were breastfed for more than 3 months had lower incidence of type I diabetes, compared to those who were breastfed for less than 3 months [33,34]. The protection offered by breast milk against type 1 diabetes has been related to an improvement in the immune response provided by secretory immunoglobulin A antibodies, enhancement of the infant's own immune response, and also increased β-cell proliferation, which has been described in breastfed infants compared with formula-fed infants [56]. A delay in the introduction of foreign antigens from food could be another factor [55].

Regarding type 2 diabetes, both a family history of the disease and being overweight or obese are usually related to the development of type 2 diabetes in both adults and children. Maternal gestational diabetes also results in higher rates of obesity and type 2 diabetes in their children [57]. In addition, early food intake patterns, particularly the type of infant feeding—breast milk versus infant formula —may also influence the risk of type 2 diabetes. In fact, breastfeeding compared with infant formula feeding is associated with a reduced risk of developing type 2 diabetes later in life [33,34]. Notably, longer exposure to breastfeeding is also associated with a greater reduction of the risk of developing type 2 diabetes [47]. The putative mechanisms of the protector effects of breast milk against type 2 diabetes are not yet well understood.

Risk of cardiovascular disease

Cardiovascular disease (CVD) is the first cause of mortality worldwide [58], and dislipidemia, abnormal levels of blood pressure, and obesity in adults are main risk factors for CVD [59,60].

It is well-accepted that high serum cholesterol levels are a risk factor for CVD [59,61]. In this sense, breastfeeding has been reported to be associated with increased levels of total and LDL-cholesterol in infancy but with lower levels in adulthood/adult life, suggesting that breastfeeding could be related to long-term beneficial effects for cardiovascular health in adulthood [62]. Notably, the reduction in cholesterol concentration in breastfed individuals compared with formula-fed ones in adulthood was found to be more pronounced in a subgroup of studies in which comparisons were based on exclusive breastfeeding versus formula feeding [63]. However, this association is not clearly established. Horta and collaborators recently described no association between breastfeeding and total cholesterol levels [47].

Regarding blood pressure, within certain margins, the risk for CVD could be doubled by every 20 mm Hg increase in systolic blood pressure and 10 mm Hg in diastolic blood pressure [64]. In this regard, breastfeeding, compared with infant formula feeding, has been related to a small reduction in systolic and diastolic blood pressure in adulthood [65,66]. Therefore, despite the difficulty of a correct interpretation of results from different studies and the fact that the possibility of publication bias and confounding factors cannot be excluded, this reduction in blood pressure may have limited but important effects on public health [65]. Breastfeeding has been suggested to influence blood pressure via a variety of mechanisms [65], including reducing the intake of sodium in infancy; increasing intake of long-chain polyunsaturated fatty acids (LC-PUFA), which are of relevance as structural components of membranes in tissue systems; and providing protection against insulin resistance, a process which may in turn increase blood pressure through different mechanisms. Levels of docosahexaenoic acid (DHA) and other LC-PUFAs in breast milk are highly influenced by dietary intake of lactating mothers [67].

Notwithstanding the aforementioned studies showing a certain improvement in adult blood lipid profile and modest effects regarding blood pressure by breastfeeding, the beneficial effects on CVD risk in adult life are not completely demonstrated. In this regard, Martin and coworkers [68] analyzed the relationship of breastfeeding with all-cause CVD, and ischemic heart disease mortality in cohorts born between 1904 and 1939, but no clear association was found. This aspect would need further study in current conditions of infant feeding and in well-designed study cohorts. However, it should be taken into account the protection of breastfeeding against obesity development, as obesity itself is a main risk factor for CVD [60]. Therefore, it is a fact that breastfeeding is able to decrease the predisposition to overweight and obesity later in life (see above) and could have an impact on the predisposition to CVD, which should not be ignored. This association, breastfeeding-obesity-CVD, is an issue that needs to be addressed in future studies.

Mechanisms underlying health outcomes of breastfeeding

The underlying mechanisms involved in the long-term benefits of breast milk compared with infant formula, particularly the prevention of obesity, are still a matter of debate. Besides potential sociobiological differences —such as socioeconomic and demographic factors, or health behaviors that may be different between mothers of breast- and formula-fed infants —and the effects of mother-child interaction, several factors have been proposed as potential contributors:

- Differences in feeding patterns. Breastfed infants exhibit greater frequency of intake and decreased meal size compared with formula-fed infants [51]. This means formula-fed infants generally consume a higher volume of milk compared with formula-fed infants.
- Differences in caloric content and macronutrient intake. The composition of human milk varies throughout lactation, according to the infant's age. Mean energy content of breast milk (colostrum, transitional milk, and mature milk) reported from different studies is lower than conventional infant formula [52]. Mean protein concentration of colostrum and transitional milk is higher in breast milk than formula (mainly because of the great content of immunoglobulins and lactoferrin), while the protein content of mature milk is slightly lower [52]. Therefore, also considering the greater volume intake, formula-fed infants generally have higher energy and protein intake than breastfed infants [69]. These differences seem to be of particular relevance during the first weeks of life. Both factors are likely to contribute to the greater weight gain in formula-fed infants compared with breastfed infants during early infancy, a critical period of growth that may lead to programming of long-term obesity [52,70,71]).
- Specific milk bioactives. Health benefits of breastfeeding may also rely on specific milk components, such as endogenously synthesized peptide hormones or cytokines involved in body weight control. Indeed, there is a growing number of hormones, such as leptin, insulin, adiponectin, ghrelin, resistin, insulin-like growth factor-1, copeptin, apelin, and nesfatin, among others, described to be secreted into breast milk (see Refs. [29,72,73]), which differentiate human milk from commercially available infant formula; however, for most of them there is a lack of studies aimed at elucidating the effects they may have on the

newborn. It should be noted that most of the bioactive peptides present in breast milk may not be present, or at least not in the active form, in infant formula, due to the pasteurization process. Moreover, these hormones from cow's milk may have no biological activity in humans. Among these compounds, leptin seems to be the most biologically relevant, since there is direct cause-effect demonstration from animal studies and indirect evidence from human studies of the critical role during the early postnatal period in metabolic programming of the neonate [29,74]. There is also some, more limited, evidence of the potential role of other hormones with a relevant function in energy metabolism, such as insulin, adiponectin, and ghrelin [72], although the concrete role they exert as milk components is to date less known. In general, milk-derived hormones can exert direct effects on intestinal epithelial cells, but may also be absorbed into the circulation. In fact, it is biologically plausible that orally ingested bioactive peptides may be able to enter the infant's circulation and exert potential outcomes on infant health [31]. This may be accomplished due to the low acidity of the stomach and the immaturity of digestive enzymes in neonates [30]. In addition, the colostrum and early milk have high concentrations of the protease inhibitor α1-antitrypsin. Therefore, some peptides may resist proteolytic degradation and remain intact through the gastrointestinal tract. Moreover, the high permeability of the gastrointestinal tract in newborn infants favors the nondigestive pathway for the absorption of peptides by paracellular diffusion [31]. Transfer from maternal milk to infant circulation has been experimentally demonstrated in animals for some of the above mentioned hormones, such as leptin [75,76].

Regarding the health benefits of breastfeeding, it must be considered that breast milk composition is not uniform; rather, it is produced by women with markedly varying genotypes, phenotypes, and environmental factors, such as diet, that may influence milk production and the concentration of bioactive components. Therefore, these changes are expected to impact infant health. Moreover, factors influencing breast milk composition may, in turn, affect infant outcomes independently of their effect on breast milk composition. Taken together, these aspects make it difficult to decipher the specific effects of breast milk components, and unequivocally attribute to changes in such components that lead to different health outcomes in children [31].

The question as to why breast milk is a protective factor against obesity in children or in later life may be explained, but only in part, because of the presence of hormones/cytokines acting as appetite regulating hormones, thus suppressing excess body weight gain or fat mass gain at an early age [73]. However, the role of milk bioactives may go beyond their influence on the regulation of food intake and body weight during lactation, as they might also affect the development and metabolic programming of the newborn, and hence may be important in the context of metabolic plasticity [29]. The potential role of the most promising milk-derived hormones in the development of the neonate and factors potentially affecting their levels in milk are addressed below.

Milk-derived peptide hormones potentially influencing infant development and metabolic programming

Leptin

Leptin is a 16-kDa polypeptide (167 amino acids) hormone mainly produced by the adipose tissue, with an important role in the central regulation of energy balance, by decreasing food intake and increasing energy expenditure [77,78]. This hormone is also produced by other tissues, such as stomach [79–82], placenta [83], and mammary epithelium [75,84,85], and is present in breast milk [75,84]. Leptin present in milk comes from production in the mammary epithelial cells but it is also transferred from maternal blood [84], although the relative contribution of each component is not fully known [86]. Notably, as occurring with other bioactive peptides, leptin is not present in infant formula, or at least not in the active form.

Considerable variability has been described in the literature for the concentration of leptin in milk, ranging from mean values of around 0.2–1.4 ng/mL [75,87] to higher values of around 10 mg/mL [84]. Differences may be attributed to methodological aspects, such as the type of assay and the breast milk fractions used—e.g., whole milk or skim milk samples [88]. In fact, some authors have reported greater leptin concentrations in whole milk compared with skimmed milk [84]. Differences may also depend on variations due to biological rhythms and the period of lactation, as described in animal models [89]. Regardless of methodological aspects, there is clear evidence that the amount of leptin present in breast milk is not uniform. Obese mothers have greater amounts of leptin in milk than normal-weight mothers, and a positive association between maternal BMI and breast milk leptin concentration has been consistently reported in most studies [90]. Leptin concentration in milk is also correlated with plasma leptin levels [87]. Therefore, the amount of leptin supplied to an infant through breast milk depends on the mother's adiposity, although whether the functionality of leptin is maintained in obesity or other metabolic alterations is not known.

Leptin present in breast milk seems to be critical for the development of the neonate [29]. Animal studies have shown that leptin, taken orally at physiological doses in the early postnatal period, rather than playing a main role in energy balance, has an essential neurotrophic action and is an important signal for the development of hypothalamic circuits involved in food intake and body weight control [29,71]. In rodents, this activity is restricted to a critical period during lactation that coincides with a transient increase in plasma leptin levels, the so-called leptin surge [91,92]. A lack of leptin during early life in rodents, or alterations or disruptions in leptin surge due to adverse perinatal conditions, such as maternal undernutrition [93], compromises the neuronal organization of hypothalamic nuclei involved in food intake control and other regulatory centers, affecting sensitivity to this hormone in adulthood and impairing energy balance regulation [91,94].

Animal studies have provided direct evidence of the essential role of leptin during the suckling period. Neonate rats supplemented with physiological doses of leptin (comparable to those in breast milk) during the suckling period are protected from age-related overweight and metabolic alterations associated with the intake of an obesogenic diet in adulthood [74,95,96]. These studies showed that leptin during this period may be important in both regulating neonate food intake and affecting the developmental events involved in the central control of energy balance [74]. In addition, animals treated with leptin showed increased insulin sensitivity [95] and a better capacity to handle excess fuel [96], which may be related to greater peripheral leptin sensitivity. Thus, besides central effects, leptin intake during the suckling period may also exert regulatory effects at the peripheral level, thereby protecting animals against metabolic disorders related to high-fat diet feeding, such as hepatic lipid accumulation [71].

The long-term beneficial effects of leptin intake at physiological levels during early postnatal life may be attributed, at least in part, to an imprinted greater sensitivity to the central and peripheral actions of leptin.

Nevertheless, leptin during the suckling period may determine different outcomes in adulthood depending on dose, route of administration, and timing of exposure [92]. In fact, unlike the above-described beneficial effects of leptin supplementation during the suckling period programming a lean phenotype, injection of leptin at pharmacologic doses in neonate rats has been shown to result in adult obesity [97]. In general, injection of leptin producing far greater concentrations of circulating leptin in the offspring than those achieved through oral leptin administration or its delivery in milk determines negative effects in offspring.

In humans, several independent studies have provided limited indirect evidence of the potential role of breast milk leptin during lactation [29]. Miralles et al. [87] first described the existence of a negative association between breast milk leptin levels and body weight—related parameters in infants in a group of nonobese women. Other studies reported similar results in different cohorts [28,98—102], thereby suggesting that the intake of moderate amounts of milk-borne maternal leptin provides moderate protection to infants from excess weight gain. Interestingly, some studies have reported no differences in leptin concentration in milk ingested by obese and nonobese infants or no clear correlation between milk leptin and anthropometric measures in infants [103—107], which is suggestive that in obesity other factors may affect the outcome. It must be considered that, besides the potential effects of leptin, anthropometric parameters in infants are predicted by maternal body weight and adiposity. Therefore, the fact that leptin concentration is a factor that differentiates the milk of obese women from that of lean women complicates the investigation of the effects of leptin on body weight and infant adiposity [108]. Thus, excess maternal adiposity may mask the effects of the greater intake of leptin during the lactation period regarding body weight of infants. Other explanations, such as (i) possible adverse effects of excess leptin intake during lactation favoring the development of leptin resistance, (ii) interactions with other components whose concentrations in milk are also affected by maternal adiposity and/or maternal diet, (iii) modifications in milk leptin due to an altered hormonal milieu cannot be ruled out. However, such possibilities have not been specifically addressed so far. At any rate, the recommendation of breastfeeding over formula feeding should be emphasized, regardless of leptin concentration in milk and/or maternal adiposity [29].

Direct cause-effect demonstration in rodents and limited indirect evidence from human studies support the essential role of milk leptin in the prevention of excess body weight gain.

Leptin intake during the suckling period may also be of interest to reverse postnatal sequels induced by an adverse gestational environment [29]. Studies in animal models with a greater propensity to obesity-related metabolic disturbances due to calorie restriction during gestation have shown that leptin may reverse most of the programmed adverse health outcomes, such as insulin resistance, hypertriglyceridemia, hepatic steatosis, and adipose tissue inflammation, thereby improving energy homeostasis and metabolic control [109]. The trophic action of leptin may be considered among the potential underlying mechanisms. In fact, leptin supplementation throughout lactation has been shown to restore hypothalamic structure [110] and sympathetic innervation of white adipose tissue (WAT) [111] and the stomach [112], which had been altered in the offspring of rats exposed to moderate calorie restriction during gestation. Therefore, leptin during lactation may play a master role in programming mechanisms and structures involved in body weight control, favoring a better control of energy balance in adulthood.

The potential role of breast milk leptin in programming later metabolic health of infants, as deduced from direct cause-effect demonstration in animal models and limited evidence from human studies, is summarized in Fig. 2.4.

Insulin

Insulin is a pancreas-derived hormone with a well-known role in blood glucose homeostasis and liver metabolism. Besides its peripheral action, insulin acts as an adiposity-signaling stimulus to the brain, playing an important role in the central control of energy homeostasis, as does leptin [113]. Circulating insulin is transported through the blood-brain barrier and acts on its receptor in the hypothalamus to lower food intake and body weight, by regulation of neurotransmitters [113].

Insulin was identified in human milk about three decades ago [114], although its function in the newborn has not yet been clearly defined. Given the established role of insulin in the maturation of intestinal epithelium [115] and in the development of pancreatic amylase [116], several authors have proposed that milk-derived insulin may have a role in the development of intestinal epithelium in neonates [117]. Studies performed in calves and piglets have also demonstrated the presence of epithelial cell insulin receptors in the intestine, and insulin has been suggested to play a role in influencing small intestine growth and development

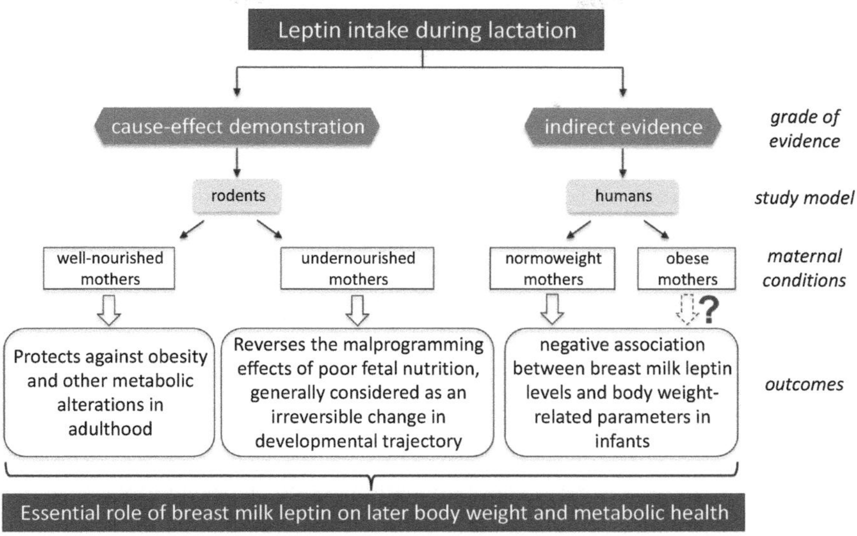

Figure 2.4 ***Essential role of leptin during lactation in programming later metabolic health of infants.*** There is a direct cause-effect demonstration in animal models that leptin intake during the suckling period confers protection against obesity and related metabolic alterations in adulthood in the offspring of well-nourished mothers, and also reverses malprogramming effects of poor fetal nutrition, generally considered as an irreversible change in developmental trajectory. Human studies have also provided indirect evidence of the potential role of leptin during lactation, since breast milk leptin levels have been reported to be negatively correlated with body-weight-related parameters in infants, particularly in those nourished by normal weight mothers. Potential beneficial effects of a greater leptin supply during lactation (e.g., infants nourished by obese mothers) have not been clearly established.

[118,119]. In this regard, a human study suggests that breast milk insulin and leptin may independently influence infant gut microbiome and reduce intestinal inflammation [120].

Insulin is present in breast milk at concentrations similar to serum levels in healthy mothers [100]. This suggests pancreas-derived insulin must be transported into human milk, but the specific transporter involved has not been fully characterized [117]. Notably, the existence of no significant difference between the levels of insulin in the milk of control mothers and mothers with type 1 diabetes suggests the exogenous insulin used for type 1 diabetes treatment is transported into milk with similar affinity to endogenous insulin in mothers without diabetes [117].

Maternal metabolic status before and/or during pregnancy has been reported to affect insulin concentration in breast milk. Concretely, higher pregravid BMI and/or maternal BMI during lactation, gravid hyperglycemia, and insulin resistance (gestational diabetes) have been associated with higher insulin concentration in mature milk [102,121,122]. This association was not found in some studies for early milk samples [121], which may be tentatively explained by the high variation of insulin concentration in milk during the first week of lactation [108]. Other authors have also described a greater concentration of insulin in breast milk of overweight/obese mothers (about 7 times higher) than in normal weight mothers at 6 weeks postpartum [123]. However, results are controversial and no significant correlation between maternal BMI and breast milk insulin has been found in other studies [100,124]. Therefore, the evidence for an association between maternal BMI and insulin concentration in breast milk is still controversial [31]. It has been suggested that some unknown factors may influence the transfer of circulating insulin into breast milk, in some cases attenuating the association between maternal BMI and human milk insulin concentration [108].

There are few studies examining the association between breast milk insulin concentration and infant outcomes. Notably, in a pilot study, a negative association was reported between breast milk insulin concentration and body weight, weight-for-length z-score, BMI-for-age z-score, and total lean mass in infants from both normal weight and obese mothers at the age of 1 month, suggesting that breast milk insulin may play a role in the accrual of fat and lean body mass in infants [100]. Indeed, in this study milk leptin was also negatively associated with infant BMI-for-age z-score, but not with lean body mass, and TNFα was also negatively associated with lean body mass [100]. Considering that insulin was positively associated with milk leptin and with TNFα, it seems to be difficult to decipher what effects may be attributed to each hormone. More recent studies have also examined the relation between milk insulin and infant growth, but no definitive conclusion can be deduced [102,122]. One of the studies reported a U-shaped association between breast milk insulin and infant body composition, with intermediate concentrations predicting the lowest infant weight—for length and BMI z-scores at 4 and 12 months [102]. In another study with women with and without gestational diabetes mellitus, breast milk insulin was inversely associated with head circumference in infants at the age of 3 months, but no significant association was found with weight-for-height [122]. Therefore, the question still remains as to whether there is a relationship between infant growth and breast milk–derived insulin.

Adiponectin

Adiponectin is a 244 amino acid protein and to date the most abundant peptide secreted by the adipose tissue, and one of the most abundant proteins in human circulation. In addition to adipocytes, other cell types, such as endothelial cells and skeletal and cardiac myocytes, also produce this cytokine [125]. Adiponectin plays a significant role in the regulation of glucose and lipid homeostasis via its insulin-sensitizing properties. Serum levels of adiponectin are higher in lean individuals and in those with greater sensitivity to the action of insulin, and lower levels have been associated with the development of type 2 diabetes and metabolic syndrome (see Ref. [126]). In fact, adiponectin exhibits antidiabetic, antiatherogenic, and antiinflammatory effects [127].

Given the importance of adiponectin in the regulation of metabolism, the discovery of its presence in breast milk opened many expectations concerning its possible influence on the growth and adiposity of offspring [128]. Adiponectin is present in human milk at concentrations that vary considerably throughout lactation, and there is also high interindividual variation. The concentration of breast milk adiponectin ranges between 4 and 88 ng/mL, and the average is approx. 19 ng/mL, which is more than 40 times that of other major cytokines in milk such as leptin and ghrelin [19]. In breastfed infants, serum adiponectin is related to the concentration of adiponectin in the milk that is consumed, suggesting it can be transported across the intestinal mucosa [19].

Although adiponectin levels in plasma are inversely related to fat mass and insulin resistance [129], the relationship between BMI and milk adiponectin levels remains inconclusive [90]. Namely, some studies have found a positive association between adiponectin levels in milk and maternal adiposity [122,130], while others have found no clear relationship [102]. Studies in animals are limited, but adiponectin levels in milk have been reported to be effectively higher in rats made obese by cafeteria diet feeding and moved to a normal fat diet 1 month before mating, so-called postcafeteria model, in agreement with the presence of greater adiposity [131].

Milk adiponectin might influence infant growth and development, although the concrete relationship is still a controversial issue. High levels of milk adiponectin have been associated with lower weight gain of infants during the first 6 months of life [132], but with an accelerated weight trajectory during the second year—i.e., increased weight-for-age and weight-for-length z scores—compared with infants exposed to low milk adiponectin [133]. In addition, it has been shown that there is a greater risk of being overweight at 2 years of age with increasing breast milk adiponectin concentrations [103]. In another study, adiponectin was inversely associated with infant weight-for-height during the first 3 months of age [122]. Therefore, milk-borne adiponectin may play both a downregulating role in infant growth during the first months and an accelerating role during the second year. However, other studies have reported no significant association between adiponectin in milk and infant body composition at the age of 1 year [102]. Thus, regarding obesity prevention, it could be deduced from some studies that high levels of adiponectin in maternal milk may be a risk factor for childhood overweight, and that infants might benefit from the intake of milk with a low adiponectin content. It could also be possible that the effects observed to be associated with milk adiponectin could be caused or modulated by other factors, such as other milk hormones whose levels are affected by maternal body weight [19]. Therefore, although results are promising, the exact role of adiponectin during early postnatal life and the consequences of changes in its intake in later adiposity need to be further explored.

So far, no studies have been published in animal models to specifically address the role of adiponectin during the suckling period in later obesity. Nevertheless, in post-cafeteria rats (see description above), the presence of greater adiponectin levels in milk has not been associated with harmful effects in offspring, despite maternal overweight [131]. It has been speculated that the potential adverse effects of greater adiponectin levels are counterbalanced by concomitant exposure to higher leptin levels during this period [131]. This possibility, together with the deciphering of the direct effects of adiponectin during lactation, requires further investigation.

Ghrelin

Ghrelin is a 28 amino acid peptide hormone synthesized primarily in the gut that is an endogenous ligand of the released growth hormone secretagogue receptor (GHSR) [134]. Ghrelin circulates in acylated and unacylated forms. In the acylated form, the third amino acid (usually a serine, but it depends on the species) is esterified by a fatty acid, and this modification is essential for its activity [135]. The acylated form is involved in the short-term regulation of food intake, acting as an appetite-stimulating hormone. It also has other metabolic effects, including the modulation of glucose homeostasis, stimulation of liver gluconeogenesis, improvement of skeletal muscle mitochondrial function, and increase in fat mass; therefore, besides its action as an anorexic hormone, it may be involved in the long-term regulation of energy homeostasis and body weight (reviewed by Ref. [136]). Unacylated ghrelin has no orexigenic effects, although more recent studies have attributed to this form a direct role in the modulation of energy metabolism in skeletal muscle, by reducing skeletal muscle reactive oxygen species generation, and improving tissue inflammation and insulin signaling and action [136].

Although ghrelin was initially described to be produced by the stomach, ghrelin and its mRNA have been detected in numerous tissues, including breast [137], and it is also present in breast milk [137,138]. The sources of breast milk ghrelin seem to be both maternal serum and breast tissue itself [139]. The amount of total ghrelin in breast milk is around 1 ng/mL, of the same order as leptin [73]. Levels of total ghrelin in breast milk appear to be comparable with maternal serum and infant serum, although some authors have reported higher levels in breast milk compared to levels in maternal blood [140]. Some studies have also described greater levels of active ghrelin (the acylated form) in breast milk compared to levels in maternal blood [139–141], suggesting an enrichment in this ghrelin isoform in breast milk. Different results among studies may be related to the commercial kits and experimental conditions [141]. A positive correlation has been described between total and active ghrelin concentrations and the time of lactation [140].

Ghrelin in breast milk may also have a plausible role in infant growth and development during early postnatal life, although the concrete effects are still uncertain. A negative correlation has been described between active ghrelin levels in breast milk and BMI of infants in their first month of life [139]. However, in the same study, active ghrelin levels at 4 months were positively related to weight gain of infants during the study period [139]. In another study, ghrelin levels in the first 2 months of lactation were described to be greater in the milk consumed by infants with highest weight gain [104]. Other studies have reported no significant relation between breast milk ghrelin and infant growth [122]. Therefore, more studies are needed in order to establish a clear relationship between milk ghrelin levels and weight gain trajectory in infants.

In summary, various milk hormones with a demonstrated role in energy homeostasis may also play a key role in infant growth and development, and exert long-term programming effects, potentially accounting for the beneficial effects of breastfeeding compared with formula feeding. However, with the exception of leptin for which there are animal studies providing cause-effect demonstration of its role during this period, corroborated by human studies in the absence of maternal confounding conditions, such as obesity or diabetes, the concrete function of the other hormones is as yet unknown. Therefore, more studies are needed to provide conclusive evidence of the effects of breast milk hormones on infant body composition, as well as the possible determinants of their levels in milk, including maternal diet and obesity.

Acknowledgments

Spanish Government: AGL2015-67019-P (MINECO/FEDER, UE) and PGC2018-097436-B-I00 (MCIU/AEI/FEDER, UE). CIBER de Fisiopatología de la Obesidad y Nutrición is an initiative of the ISCIII. The Laboratory of Molecular Biology, Nutrition and Biotechnology is a member of the European Research Network of Excellence NuGO.

Conflict of interest

A.P. and C.P. are authors of a patent held by the University of the Balearic Islands entitled "Use of leptin for the prevention of excess body weight and composition containing leptin" (WO 2006089987 A1) (Priority data: February 23, 2005).

References

[1] Langley-Evans SC. Developmental programming of health and disease. Proc Nutr Soc 2006;65(1):97–105.
[2] Armitage JA, Taylor PD, Poston L. Experimental models of developmental programming: consequences of exposure to an energy rich diet during development. J Physiol 2005;565(Pt 1):3–8.
[3] McMillen IC, Robinson JS. Developmental origins of the metabolic syndrome: prediction, plasticity, and programming. Physiol Rev 2005;85(2):571–633.
[4] Eriksson JG, et al. Catch-up growth in childhood and death from coronary heart disease: longitudinal study. BMJ 1999;318(7181):427–31.
[5] Jaenisch R, Bird A. Epigenetic regulation of gene expression: how the genome integrates intrinsic and environmental signals. Nat Genet 2003;33(Suppl. l):245–54.
[6] Feinberg AP. Phenotypic plasticity and the epigenetics of human disease. Nature 2007;447(7143):433–40.
[7] Hochberg Z, et al. Child health, developmental plasticity, and epigenetic programming. Endocr Rev 2011;32(2):159–224.
[8] Waterland RA, Garza C. Potential mechanisms of metabolic imprinting that lead to chronic disease. Am J Clin Nutr 1999;69(2):179–97.
[9] Ravelli GP, Stein ZA, Susser MW. Obesity in young men after famine exposure in utero and early infancy. N Engl J Med 1976;295(7):349–53.
[10] Hales CN, Barker DJ. The thrifty phenotype hypothesis. Br Med Bull 2001;60:5–20.
[11] Barker DJ, et al. Fetal origins of adult disease: strength of effects and biological basis. Int J Epidemiol 2002;31(6):1235–9.

[12] Hales CN, et al. Fetal and infant growth and impaired glucose tolerance at age 64. BMJ 1991;303(6809):1019–22.
[13] Remmers F, Fodor M, Delemarre-van de Waal HA. Neonatal food restriction permanently alters rat body dimensions and energy intake. Physiol Behav 2008;95(1–2):208–15.
[14] Palou M, et al. Moderate caloric restriction in lactating rats protects offspring against obesity and insulin resistance in later life. Endocrinology 2010;151(3):1030–41.
[15] Srinivasan M, et al. A high-carbohydrate diet in the immediate postnatal life of rats induces adaptations predisposing to adult-onset obesity. J Endocrinol 2008;197(3):565–74.
[16] Kramer MS. "Breast is best": the evidence. Early Hum Dev 2010;86(11):729–32.
[17] Patel MS, Srinivasan M. Metabolic programming in the immediate postnatal life. Ann Nutr Metab 2011;58(Suppl. 2):18–28.
[18] WHO. The World Health Organization's infant feeding recommendation. 2002 10/11/2018. Available from: https://www.who.int/nutrition/topics/infantfeeding_recommendation/en/.
[19] Newburg DS, Woo JG, Morrow AL. Characteristics and potential functions of human milk adiponectin. J Pediatr 2010;156(2 Suppl. l):S41–6.
[20] Martin CR, Ling PR, Blackburn GL. Review of infant feeding: key features of breast milk and infant formula. Nutrients 2016;8(5).
[21] Bitman J, et al. Comparison of the lipid composition of breast milk from mothers of term and preterm infants. Am J Clin Nutr 1983;38(2):300–12.
[22] Lonnerdal B. Breast milk: a truly functional food. Nutrition 2000;16(7–8):509–11.
[23] Mosca F, Gianni ML. Human milk: composition and health benefits. Pediatr Med e Chir 2017;39(2):155.
[24] Zou L, Pande G, Akoh CC. Infant formula fat analogs and human milk fat: new focus on infant developmental needs. Annu Rev Food Sci Technol 2016;7:139–65.
[25] Jenness R. The composition of human milk. Semin Perinatol 1979;3(3):225–39.
[26] Van de Perre P. Transfer of antibody via mother's milk. Vaccine 2003;21(24):3374–6.
[27] Hanson LA, Korotkova M. The role of breastfeeding in prevention of neonatal infection. Semin Neonatol 2002;7(4):275–81.
[28] Fields DA, et al. Associations between human breast milk hormones and adipocytokines and infant growth and body composition in the first 6 months of life. Pediatr Obes 2017;12(Suppl. 1):78–85.
[29] Palou M, Pico C, Palou A. Leptin as a breast milk component for the prevention of obesity. Nutr Rev 2018.
[30] Henderson TR, et al. Gastric proteolysis in preterm infants fed mother's milk or formula. Adv Exp Med Biol 2001;501:403–8.
[31] Fields DA, Schneider CR, Pavela G. A narrative review of the associations between six bioactive components in breast milk and infant adiposity. Obesity 2016;24(6):1213–21.
[32] Alsaweed M, et al. MicroRNAs in breastmilk and the lactating breast: potential immunoprotectors and developmental regulators for the infant and the mother. Int J Environ Res Publ Health 2015;12(11):13981–4020.
[33] Ip S, et al. A summary of the Agency for Healthcare Research and Quality's evidence report on breastfeeding in developed countries. Breastfeed Med 2009;4(Suppl. 1):S17–30.
[34] Ip S, et al. Breastfeeding and maternal and infant health outcomes in developed countries. Evid Rep Technol Assess 2007;(153):1–186.

[35] Wang M, et al. Fecal microbiota composition of breast-fed infants is correlated with human milk oligosaccharides consumed. J Pediatr Gastroenterol Nutr 2015;60(6):825–33.
[36] Ho NT, et al. Meta-analysis of effects of exclusive breastfeeding on infant gut microbiota across populations. Nat Commun 2018;9(1):4169.
[37] Althani AA, et al. Human microbiome and its association with health and diseases. J Cell Physiol 2016;231(8):1688–94.
[38] Pascale A, et al. Microbiota and metabolic diseases. Endocrine; 2018.
[39] Omer E, Atassi H. The microbiome that shapes us: can it cause obesity? Curr Gastroenterol Rep 2017;19(12):59.
[40] Weyermann M, Rothenbacher D, Brenner H. Duration of breastfeeding and risk of overweight in childhood: a prospective birth cohort study from Germany. Int J Obes 2006;30(8):1281–7.
[41] von Kries R, et al. Breast feeding and obesity: cross sectional study. Br Med J 1999;319(7203):147–50.
[42] Gillman MW, et al. Risk of overweight among adolescents who were breastfed as infants. Jama 2001;285(19):2461–7.
[43] Armstrong J, Reilly JJ. Breastfeeding and lowering the risk of childhood obesity. Lancet 2002;359(9322):2003–4.
[44] Harder T, et al. Duration of breastfeeding and risk of overweight: a meta-analysis. Am J Epidemiol 2005;162(5):397–403.
[45] Bray GA, et al. Obesity: a chronic relapsing progressive disease process. A position statement of the World Obesity Federation. Obes Rev 2017;18(7):715–23.
[46] WHO. Obesity and overweight. 2018 10/11/2018. Available from: http://www.who.int/news-room/fact-sheets/detail/obesity-and-overweight.
[47] Horta BL, Loret de Mola C, Victora CG. Long-term consequences of breastfeeding on cholesterol, obesity, systolic blood pressure and type 2 diabetes: a systematic review and meta-analysis. Acta Paediatr 2015;104(467):30–7.
[48] Yan J, et al. The association between breastfeeding and childhood obesity: a meta-analysis. BMC Publ Health 2014;14:1267.
[49] Michels KB, et al. A longitudinal study of infant feeding and obesity throughout life course. Int J Obes 2007;31(7):1078–85.
[50] Grummer-Strawn LM, et al. Does breastfeeding protect against pediatric overweight? Analysis of longitudinal data from the centers for disease control and prevention pediatric nutrition surveillance system. Pediatrics 2004;113(2):e81–6.
[51] Sievers E, et al. Feeding patterns in breast-fed and formula-fed infants. Ann Nutr Metab 2002;46(6):243–8.
[52] Hester SN, et al. Is the macronutrient intake of formula-fed infants greater than breast-fed infants in early infancy? J Nutr Metab 2012;2012:891201.
[53] Sarwar N, et al. Diabetes mellitus, fasting blood glucose concentration, and risk of vascular disease: a collaborative meta-analysis of 102 prospective studies. Emerging Risk Factors, Collaboration. Lancet 2010;375(9733):2215–22.
[54] Forouhi NG, Wareham NJ. Epidemiology of diabetes. Medicine 2014;42(12):698–702.
[55] Virtanen SM, Knip M. Nutritional risk predictors of beta cell autoimmunity and type 1 diabetes at a young age. Am J Clin Nutr 2003;78(6):1053–67.
[56] Juto P. Human milk stimulates B cell function. Arch Dis Child 1985;60(7):610–3.
[57] Lindsay RS, et al. Secular trends in birth weight, BMI, and diabetes in the offspring of diabetic mothers. Diabetes Care 2000;23(9):1249–54.
[58] WHO. Cardiovascular diseases (CVDs). 2017 10/11/2018. Available from: http://www.who.int/news-room/fact-sheets/detail/cardiovascular-diseases-(cvds).

[59] Lowe LP, et al. Impact of major cardiovascular disease risk factors, particularly in combination, on 22-year mortality in women and men. Arch Intern Med 1998;158(18):2007–14.
[60] Scaglione R, et al. Obesity and cardiovascular risk: the new public health problem of worldwide proportions. Expert Rev Cardiovasc Ther 2004;2(2):203–12.
[61] Stamler J, et al. Relationship of baseline serum cholesterol levels in 3 large cohorts of younger men to long-term coronary, cardiovascular, and all-cause mortality and to longevity. J Am Med Assoc 2000;284(3):311–8.
[62] Owen CG, et al. Infant feeding and blood cholesterol: a study in adolescents and a systematic review. Pediatrics 2002;110(3):597–608.
[63] Owen CG, et al. Does initial breastfeeding lead to lower blood cholesterol in adult life? A quantitative review of the evidence. Am J Clin Nutr 2008;88(2):305–14.
[64] Chobanian AV, et al. The seventh report of the joint national committee on prevention, detection, evaluation, and treatment of high blood pressure: the JNC 7 report. J Am Med Assoc 2003;289(19):2560–72.
[65] Martin RM, Gunnell D, Smith GD. Breastfeeding in infancy and blood pressure in later life: systematic review and meta-analysis. Am J Epidemiol 2005;161(1):15–26.
[66] Owen CG, et al. Effect of breast feeding in infancy on blood pressure in later life: systematic review and meta-analysis. BMJ 2003;327(7425):1189–95.
[67] Sherry CL, Oliver JS, Marriage BJ. Docosahexaenoic acid supplementation in lactating women increases breast milk and plasma docosahexaenoic acid concentrations and alters infant omega 6:3 fatty acid ratio. Prostaglandins Leukot Essent Fatty Acids 2015;95:63–9.
[68] Martin RM, et al. Breastfeeding and cardiovascular mortality: the Boyd Orr cohort and a systematic review with meta-analysis. Eur Heart J 2004;25(9):778–86.
[69] Heinig MJ, et al. Energy and protein intakes of breast-fed and formula-fed infants during the first year of life and their association with growth velocity: the DARLING study. Am J Clin Nutr 1993;58(2):152–61.
[70] Koletzko B, et al. Lower protein in infant formula is associated with lower weight up to age 2 y: a randomized clinical trial. Am J Clin Nutr 2009;89(6):1836–45.
[71] Pico C, et al. Metabolic programming of obesity by energy restriction during the perinatal period: different outcomes depending on gender and period, type and severity of restriction. Front Physiol 2012;3:436.
[72] Badillo-Suarez PA, Rodriguez-Cruz M, Nieves-Morales X. Impact of metabolic hormones secreted in human breast milk on nutritional programming in childhood obesity. J Mammary Gland Biol Neoplasia 2017;22(3):171–91.
[73] Kratzsch J, Bae YJ, Kiess W. Adipokines in human breast milk. Best Pract Res Clin Endocrinol Metabol 2018;32(1):27–38.
[74] Pico C, et al. The intake of physiological doses of leptin during lactation in rats prevents obesity in later life. Int J Obes 2007;31(8):1199–209.
[75] Casabiell X, et al. Presence of leptin in colostrum and/or breast milk from lactating mothers: a potential role in the regulation of neonatal food intake. J Clin Endocrinol Metab 1997;82(12):4270–3.
[76] Sanchez J, et al. Leptin orally supplied to neonate rats is directly uptaken by the immature stomach and may regulate short-term feeding. Endocrinology 2005;146(6):2575–82.
[77] Zhang Y, et al. Positional cloning of the mouse obese gene and its human homologue. Nature 1994;372(6505):425–32.
[78] Ahima RS, et al. Leptin regulation of neuroendocrine systems. Front Neuroendocrinol 2000;21(3):263–307.
[79] Bado A, et al. The stomach is a source of leptin. Nature 1998;394(6695):790–3.

[80] Cinti S, et al. Secretory granules of endocrine and chief cells of human stomach mucosa contain leptin. Int J Obes Relat Metab Disord 2000;24(6):789–93.
[81] Cinti S, et al. Leptin in the human stomach. Gut 2001;49(1):155.
[82] Pico C, et al. Gastric leptin: a putative role in the short-term regulation of food intake. Br J Nutr 2003;90(4):735–41.
[83] Masuzaki H, et al. Nonadipose tissue production of leptin: leptin as a novel placenta-derived hormone in humans. Nat Med 1997;3(9):1029–33.
[84] Houseknecht KL, et al. Leptin is present in human milk and is related to maternal plasma leptin concentration and adiposity. Biochem Biophys Res Commun 1997;240(3):742–7.
[85] Smith-Kirwin SM, et al. Leptin expression in human mammary epithelial cells and breast milk. J Clin Endocrinol Metab 1998;83(5):1810–3.
[86] Bonnet M, et al. Mammary leptin synthesis, milk leptin and their putative physiological roles. Reprod Nutr Dev 2002;42(5):399–413.
[87] Miralles O, et al. A physiological role of breast milk leptin in body weight control in developing infants. Obesity 2006;14(8):1371–7.
[88] Savino F, et al. Evaluation of leptin in breast milk, lactating mothers and their infants. Eur J Clin Nutr 2010;64(9):972–7.
[89] Nozhenko Y, et al. Milk leptin surge and biological rhythms of leptin and other regulatory proteins in breastmilk. PloS One 2015;10(12):e0145376.
[90] Andreas NJ, et al. Effect of maternal body mass index on hormones in breast milk: a systematic review. PloS One 2014;9(12):e115043.
[91] Bouret SG, Draper SJ, Simerly RB. Trophic action of leptin on hypothalamic neurons that regulate feeding. Science 2004;304(5667):108–10.
[92] Pico C, et al. Perinatal programming of body weight control by leptin: putative roles of AMP kinase and muscle thermogenesis. Am J Clin Nutr 2011;94(6 Suppl. l):1830S–7S.
[93] Palou M, et al. Impaired insulin and leptin sensitivity in the offspring of moderate caloric-restricted dams during gestation is early programmed. J Nutr Biochem 2012;23(12):1627–39.
[94] Yura S, et al. Role of premature leptin surge in obesity resulting from intrauterine undernutrition. Cell Metabol 2005;1(6):371–8.
[95] Sanchez J, et al. Oral supplementation with physiological doses of leptin during lactation in rats improves insulin sensitivity and affects food preferences later in life. Endocrinology 2008;149(2):733–40.
[96] Priego T, et al. Leptin intake during the suckling period improves the metabolic response of adipose tissue to a high-fat diet. Int J Obes 2010;34(5):809–19.
[97] Vickers MH, et al. The effect of neonatal leptin treatment on postnatal weight gain in male rats is dependent on maternal nutritional status during pregnancy. Endocrinology 2008;149(4):1906–13.
[98] Doneray H, Orbak Z, Yildiz L. The relationship between breast milk leptin and neonatal weight gain. Acta Paediatr 2009;98(4):643–7.
[99] Schuster S, et al. Leptin in maternal serum and breast milk: association with infants' body weight gain in a longitudinal study over 6 months of lactation. Pediatr Res 2011;70(6):633–7.
[100] Fields DA, Demerath EW. Relationship of insulin, glucose, leptin, IL-6 and TNF-alpha in human breast milk with infant growth and body composition. Pediatr Obes 2012;7(4):304–12.
[101] Quinn EA, et al. Maternal characteristics associated with milk leptin content in a sample of Filipino women and associations with infant weight for age. J Hum Lactation 2015;31(2):273–81.

[102] Chan D, et al. Adiponectin, leptin and insulin in breast milk: associations with maternal characteristics and infant body composition in the first year of life. Int J Obes 2018;42(1):36–43.
[103] Weyermann M, Brenner H, Rothenbacher D. Adipokines in human milk and risk of overweight in early childhood: a prospective cohort study. Epidemiology 2007;18(6):722–9.
[104] Kon IY, et al. The study of breast milk IGF-1, leptin, ghrelin and adiponectin levels as possible reasons of high weight gain in breast-fed infants. Ann Nutr Metab 2014;65(4):317–23.
[105] Meyer DM, et al. The relationship between breast milk leptin and adiponectin with child body composition from 3 to 5 years: a follow-up study. Pediatr Obes 2017;12(Suppl. 1):125–9.
[106] Brunner S, et al. Breast milk leptin and adiponectin in relation to infant body composition up to 2 years. Pediatr Obes 2015;10(1):67–73.
[107] Khodabakhshi A, et al. Comparative measurement of ghrelin, leptin, adiponectin, EGF and IGF-1 in breast milk of mothers with overweight/obese and normal-weight infants. Eur J Clin Nutr 2015;69(5):614–8.
[108] Demmelmair H, Koletzko B. Variation of metabolite and hormone contents in human milk. Clin Perinatol 2017;44(1):151–64.
[109] Szostaczuk N, et al. Oral leptin supplementation throughout lactation in rats prevents later metabolic alterations caused by gestational calorie restriction. Int J Obes 2017;41(3):360–71.
[110] Konieczna J, et al. Oral leptin treatment in suckling rats ameliorates detrimental effects in hypothalamic structure and function caused by maternal caloric restriction during gestation. PloS One 2013;8(11):e81906.
[111] Konieczna J, et al. Leptin intake in suckling rats restores altered T3 levels and markers of adipose tissue sympathetic drive and function caused by gestational calorie restriction. Int J Obes 2015;39(6):959–66.
[112] Szostaczuk N, et al. Leptin intake at physiological doses throughout lactation in male wistar rats normalizes the decreased density of tyrosine hydroxylase-immunoreactive fibers in the stomach caused by mild gestational calorie restriction. Front Physiol 2018;9:256.
[113] Woods SC, et al. The evaluation of insulin as a metabolic signal influencing behavior via the brain. Neurosci Biobehav Rev 1996;20(1):139–44.
[114] Jovanovic-Peterson L, et al. Maternal milk and plasma glucose and insulin levels: studies in normal and diabetic subjects. J Am Coll Nutr 1989;8(2):125–31.
[115] Buts JP, De Keyser N, Dive C. Intestinal development in the suckling rat: effect of insulin on the maturation of villus and crypt cell functions. Eur J Clin Invest 1988;18(4):391–8.
[116] Kinouchi T, et al. Milk-borne insulin with trypsin inhibitor in milk induces pancreatic amylase development at the onset of weaning in rats. J Pediatr Gastroenterol Nutr 2000;30(5):515–21.
[117] Whitmore TJ, et al. Analysis of insulin in human breast milk in mothers with type 1 and type 2 diabetes mellitus. Internet J Endocrinol 2012;2012:296368.
[118] Georgiev IP, et al. Insulin-like growth factor and insulin receptors in intestinal mucosa of neonatal calves. J Endocrinol 2003;176(1):121–32.
[119] Shulman RJ, et al. Effect of oral insulin on lactase activity, mRNA, and post-transcriptional processing in the newborn pig. J Pediatr Gastroenterol Nutr 1992;14(2):166–72.
[120] Lemas DJ, et al. Alterations in human milk leptin and insulin are associated with early changes in the infant intestinal microbiome. Am J Clin Nutr 2016;103(5):1291–300.

[121] Ley SH, et al. Associations of prenatal metabolic abnormalities with insulin and adiponectin concentrations in human milk. Am J Clin Nutr 2012;95(4):867–74.
[122] Yu X, et al. Associations of breast milk adiponectin, leptin, insulin and ghrelin with maternal characteristics and early infant growth: a longitudinal study. Br J Nutr 2018:1–8.
[123] Ahuja S, et al. Glucose and insulin levels are increased in obese and overweight mothers' breast-milk. Food Nutr Sci 2011;2(3):201–6.
[124] Shehadeh N, et al. Insulin in human milk: postpartum changes and effect of gestational age. Arch Dis Child Fetal Neonatal Ed 2003;88(3):F214–6.
[125] Achari AE, Jain SK. Adiponectin, a therapeutic target for obesity, diabetes, and endothelial dysfunction. Int J Mol Sci 2017;18(6).
[126] Frankenberg ADV, Reis AF, Gerchman F. Relationships between adiponectin levels, the metabolic syndrome, and type 2 diabetes: a literature review. Arch Endocrinol Metab 2017;61(6):614–22.
[127] Scherer PE, et al. A novel serum protein similar to C1q, produced exclusively in adipocytes. J Biol Chem 1995;270(45):26746–9.
[128] Bronsky J, et al. Adiponectin, adipocyte fatty acid binding protein, and epidermal fatty acid binding protein: proteins newly identified in human breast milk. Clin Chem 2006;52(9):1763–70.
[129] Cnop M, et al. Relationship of adiponectin to body fat distribution, insulin sensitivity and plasma lipoproteins: evidence for independent roles of age and sex. Diabetologia 2003;46(4):459–69.
[130] Martin LJ, et al. Adiponectin is present in human milk and is associated with maternal factors. Am J Clin Nutr 2006;83(5):1106–11.
[131] Castro H, et al. Offspring predisposition to obesity due to maternal-diet-induced obesity in rats is preventable by dietary normalization before mating. Mol Nutr Food Res 2017;61(3).
[132] Woo JG, et al. Human milk adiponectin is associated with infant growth in two independent cohorts. Breastfeed Med 2009;4(2):101–9.
[133] Woo JG, et al. Human milk adiponectin affects infant weight trajectory during the second year of life. J Pediatr Gastroenterol Nutr 2012;54(4):532–9.
[134] Kojima M, et al. Ghrelin is a growth-hormone-releasing acylated peptide from stomach. Nature 1999;402(6762):656–60.
[135] Kojima M, Kangawa K. Ghrelin: structure and function. Physiol Rev 2005;85(2):495–522.
[136] Gortan Cappellari G, Barazzoni R. Ghrelin forms in the modulation of energy balance and metabolism. Eat Weight Disord 2018.
[137] Aydin S, et al. Ghrelin is present in human colostrum, transitional and mature milk. Peptides 2006;27(4):878–82.
[138] Kierson JA, et al. Ghrelin and cholecystokinin in term and preterm human breast milk. Acta Paediatr 2006;95(8):991–5.
[139] Cesur G, et al. The relationship between ghrelin and adiponectin levels in breast milk and infant serum and growth of infants during early postnatal life. J Physiol Sci 2012;62(3):185–90.
[140] Ilcol YO, Hizli B. Active and total ghrelin concentrations increase in breast milk during lactation. Acta Paediatr 2007;96(11):1632–9.
[141] Aydin S, et al. Presence of obestatin in breast milk: relationship among obestatin, ghrelin, and leptin in lactating women. Nutrition 2008;24(7–8):689–93.

CHAPTER 3

Feeding practices of infants

I. Iglesia[1,2,3,4] L.A. Moreno[1,2,3,5], G. Rodríguez-Martínez[1,2,3,4,6,7]
[1]Growth, Exercise, Nutrition and Development (GENUD) Research Group, Departamento de Fisiatría y Enfermería, Facultad de Ciencias de la Salud, Universidad de Zaragoza, Zaragoza, España; [2]Instituto Agroalimentario de Aragón (IA2), Universidad de Zaragoza, Zaragoza, España; [3]Fundación del Instituto de Investigación Sanitaria Aragón (IIS Aragón), Zaragoza, España; [4]Red de Salud Materno Infantil y del Desarrollo (SAMID), Red de Salud Materno Infantil y del Desarrollo (SAMID), Instituto de Salud Carlos III, Madrid, España; [5]Centro de Investigación Biomédica en Red de Fisiopatología de la Obesidad y Nutrición (CIBERObn), Instituto de Salud Carlos III, Madrid, España; [6]Departamento de Pediatría, Radiología y Medicina Física, Universidad de Zaragoza, Zaragoza, España; [7]Hospital Clínico Universitario "Lozano Blesa", Zaragoza, España

Contents

Introduction

Nutrition-related disorders in children and adolescents are highly prevalent. Feeding practices develop in early infancy and determine future eating habits [1], and interventions that promote adequate infant feeding practices are among the most effective at improving child health, both in the short and long term [2]. Appropriate nutrition behaviors during infancy are

Molecular Nutrition
ISBN 978-0-12-813862-5
https://doi.org/10.1016/B978-0-12-813862-5.00003-7

crucial for physical growth, mental development, and a healthy immune system, and when healthy habits and preferences are kept from childhood to adulthood, the likelihood of high productivity, health, and well-being increase and the risk of infectious and chronic diseases decrease [3]. The first years of life also provide a unique opportunity to ensure children's appropriate growth and development and future health through optimal feeding practices [4]. For this reason, the objective of this chapter was to review the main topics relating to nutrition practices during this important period of life.

The digestive organs of infants progressively mature, but during the first few months of life, their organs are adapted to milk. In terms of the physiology of the digestive system, there are some remarkable aspects that are specific to this period [5]:

- Little digestion occurs in the mouth as the milk only remains there for a few seconds. The main function of the mouth is suction and swallowing until the real chewing begins at around 6 months.
- The functional immaturity of the esophagus cardiotuberosity region during the first few months of life favors postprandial regurgitation.
- The peristaltic movements of the stomach are weak and this becomes more evident with the introduction of supplementary feeding. The enzymes and acids that aid in digestion do not work at an adult level until at least 3 months of age. The digestion of breast milk usually takes two and a half hours, while digestion of formula takes three and a half hours. For this reason, the recommended intervals between feeds vary from 3 to 4 h.
- The transition time through the small intestine is rapid due to the frequent peristaltic movements and the digestion of the gastric chyme is continued here by the pancreatic and intestinal enzymes and by bile. Regarding intestinal absorption, the proteins are efficiently broken down into amino acids and peptides and carbohydrates are also broken down. Lactose is an exception as it is not fully hydrolyzed to lactic acid form to serve as chemical and bacteriological barrier against infection. Regarding fats, infants have a physiological steatorrhea, to a lesser extent in natural lactation than in artificial (80% of the ingested fat is only absorbed in regular conditions).
- Powerful peristaltic contractions displace the feces in a caudal direction. Food intake is the main stimulus of the motility of the colon. With breast milk, stools are more numerous and tend to be softer, golden yellow in color, and aromatic, whereas with formula milk, they are scarcer and tend to be harder, paler, and foul smelling.

Gold standard: breastfeeding

The World Health Organization (WHO) [6] states that breastfeeding within the first hour of birth is the recommended best practice due to the nutritional and immunological benefits that help reduce neonatal mortality and morbidity [7,8]. In addition, there is a large body of evidence that shows that breastfeeding surpasses formula feeding nutritionally, immunologically, and emotionally [9] and that human milk might also serve birth control strategy [10]. Breastfeeding represents the optimal stimuli for the infant's development because it allows the infant to establish a unique emotional link with its mother during a critical period.

Breastfeeding is considered the gold standard for infant feeding [11]; however, some mothers worry that low growth rates in their newborns may be due to inadequate maternal milk supply or poor breast milk quality [12]. These worries may then contribute to the early replacement of breast milk with formula or other breast milk substitutes to try to encourage the infants' growth and development [12]. Apart from the cases where there is a health complication, however, mothers are normally able to sufficiently nourish their children [13,14].

Milk secretion is triggered by the combined action of two hormones: prolactin (PRL) and oxytocin. Prolactin increases during pregnancy and stimulates the growth and development of the mammary tissue in preparation for the production of milk by the alveoli. Milk secretion is blocked before delivery, however, by the high levels of progesterone and estrogen. After delivery, these levels fall rapidly, activating the prolactin and the start of milk secretion [15].

The baby suckling on the nipple also has an important role in this process as this produces sensory impulses that pass from the nipple to the brain. The anterior lobe of the pituitary gland subsequently secretes prolactin and the posterior lobe secretes oxytocin [16]. The oxytocin released into the bloodstream is then responsible for the milk being ejected by the mammary gland [10]. The mammary gland constitutes together with supporting connective tissue and fat, blood and lymphatic vessels, and nerves, the inner part of mammary tissue, while the nipple surrounded by the circular pigmented areola supposed the external part of breast [16]. The Montgomery glands secrete an oil to protect the skin of the nipple and the areola during lactation and this oil also holds the mother's individual scent, which attracts her baby to her breast. The milk ducts beneath the areola become wider during feeding when the oxytocin reflex is active [16] (Fig. 3.1).

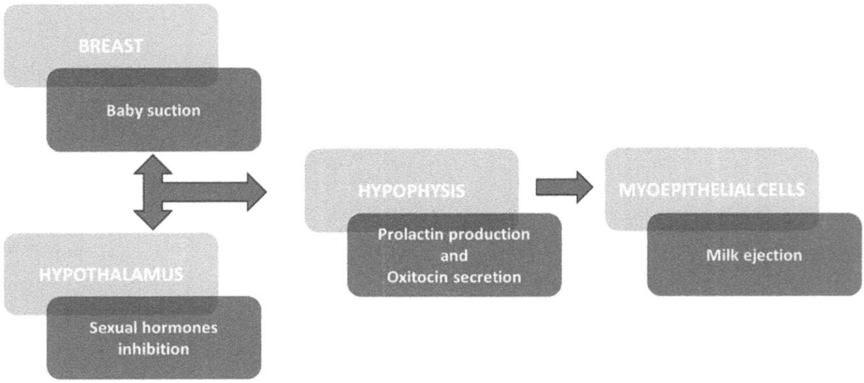

Figure 3.1 Physiology of milk secretion.

Mother's milk is a unique natural food for newborn mammals and its nutritional composition is adapted to the postnatal growth velocity of the specific species [10]. Infancy is a vulnerable lifespan period from a nutritional point of view and restriction of growth may result in permanent stunting [17] and/or long-lasting impairment of neurological function [18].

Despite efforts to define how the growth trajectories during prenatal and postnatal periods affect lifelong health in contemporary populations, there is still a knowledge gap, even though significant advances have been made in determining infant growth standards in the last decade. Indeed, data published by the WHO in 2006 [19] that used longitudinal standardized measurements of healthy infants belonging to six different countries (Brazil, Ghana, India, Norway, Oman, and the United States) showed that infants raised in supportive (without constraints to growth, such as maternal smoking before or after delivery) but diverse environments had similar early growth patterns (length/height for age, weight for age, weight for length/height, and BMI for age) from birth to 24 months [20].

Breastfeeding plays the role of the first vaccine for infants and can be considered as the best source of nutrition. Also, by increasing the rates of breastfeeding, a country's prosperity can improve due to lower healthcare costs. Unfortunately, there is no country that meets the minimum requirements for fully supporting breastfeeding. For example, fewer than 44% of countries reported mothers breastfeeding their infants within the first hour of birth [21]. Similarly, only 23 countries reported exclusive breastfeeding (EBF) rates above 60% at 6 months of age and these countries were mainly in developing areas: Bolivia; Burundi; Cabo Verde; Cambodia;

Democratic People's Republic of Korea; Eritrea; Kenya; Kiribati; Lesotho; Malawi; Micronesia; Federated States of Nauru; Nepal; Peru; Rwanda; São Tome and Principe; Solomon Islands; Sri Lanka; Swaziland; Timor-Leste; Uganda; Vanuatu; and Zambia. This is in contrast with the 49% reported in the United States and the 34% reported in the United Kingdom [22]. The Global Breastfeeding Collective has developed an action strategy to try and improve this situation by 2030 that involves policymakers around the world [21].

There are only a few conditions under which breastfeeding may not be recommended. For example, the main contraindication to breastfeeding is maternal human immunodeficiency virus (HIV) infection. To reduce the risk of HIV transmission, the WHO recommends that "when replacement feeding is acceptable, feasible, affordable, sustainable and safe, avoidance of all breast-feeding by HIV-infected mothers is recommended, otherwise, exclusive breast-feeding is preferred rather than mixed breast feeding, during the first months of life" [23]. There is a considerable risk of mother-to-child transmission of HIV during the second and third trimesters of pregnancy, during delivery (15%—25%), and at any point during breast-feeding (which increases the risk by 5%—20% to a total of 20%—45% as it is cumulative). This risk can be reduced to under 2% by a combination of antiretroviral prophylaxis during pregnancy and delivery and by elective caesarean section and avoidance of breastfeeding [24].

Breastfeeding is also contraindicated in mothers who are human T-cell lymphotropic virus (HTLV) type I- or II-positive, in mothers who have herpes simplex lesions on a breast [25], and in mothers infected by cytomegalovirus in the case of preterm infants [26]. Other inborn metabolism disorders, such as long-chain fatty acid oxidation disorders and congenital lactase deficiency, also represent contraindications for breastfeeding. Mothers receiving diagnostic or therapeutic radioactive isotopes or those exposed to radioactive materials and/or specific medications are also contraindicated to give breast milk.

Even though drugs and environmental chemicals are likely to be transferred into human milk, the health benefits still outweigh the risks [27]. Medications only appear in breast milk in subclinical amounts and no adverse effect has been clinically or epidemiologically demonstrated to be associated with the consumption of human milk containing background levels of environmental chemicals [27]. If drugs are required, consultation between the pediatrician and the mother's physician can help determine which option to choose [28].

Composition of human milk

Milk is the only natural food for newborn mammals. Its nutritional composition (Fig. 3.2) is adapted to mammal species and growth velocity of the postnatal infants [10] when it is known to be the greatest in infancy [29]. Infants are vulnerable and it is well known that inadequate nutrition during this period followed by a restriction of growth may result in permanent stunting [17] or long-lasting impairment in neurological function [18].

Human milk is not a uniform body fluid but a secretion of the mammary gland that changes its composition with time of day, during the course of lactation, and even under specific conditions of necessity (for instance, preterm infants) [30]. In terms of macronutrients, the mature milk is estimated to consist of approximately 0.9–1.2 g/dL of protein, 3.2–3.6 g/dL of fat, and 6.7–7.8 g/dL of lactose. The energy provided ranges from 65 to 70 kcal/dL and is highly correlated with the fat content [31]. The most abundant proteins are casein, α-lactalbumin, lactoferrin, secretory immunoglobulin IgA, lysozyme, and serum albumin [32]. Nonprotein nitrogen-containing compounds include urea, uric acid, creatine, creatinine, amino acids, and nucleotides. The protein content is significantly higher in mothers who deliver preterm in comparison to those who deliver at term [32].

Human milk is characterized by a high content of palmitic and oleic acids. Fat is its most highly variable macronutrient and the amount of fat varies across a feed (the last milk of a feed may contain two to three times more fat than the milk at the beginning [33]), throughout the day (milk has lower fat content in the morning and at night compared to the rest of the day [34]), and depending on the maternal diet, particularly regarding the long-chain polyunsaturated fatty acids [31].

The concentration of lactose (the principal sugar of human milk) is the least variable of the macronutrients, but it seems to be positively correlated with the total production of milk [35]. Other significant carbohydrates of human milk include the oligosaccharides, which comprise approximately 1 g/dL of human milk depending on the stage of lactation and maternal genetic factors [36].

Human milk also contains micronutrients and trace elements, as well as numerous immune-related components such as IgA, leukocytes, oligosaccharides, lysozyme, lactoferrin, interferon-γ, nucleotides, and cytokines. The essential fatty acids, enzymes, hormones, growth factors, polyamines, and other biologically active compounds found in breast milk may also play an important role in the health benefits associated with breastfeeding. Human milk provides the normative standard for infant nutrition in terms of micronutrient supply [31].

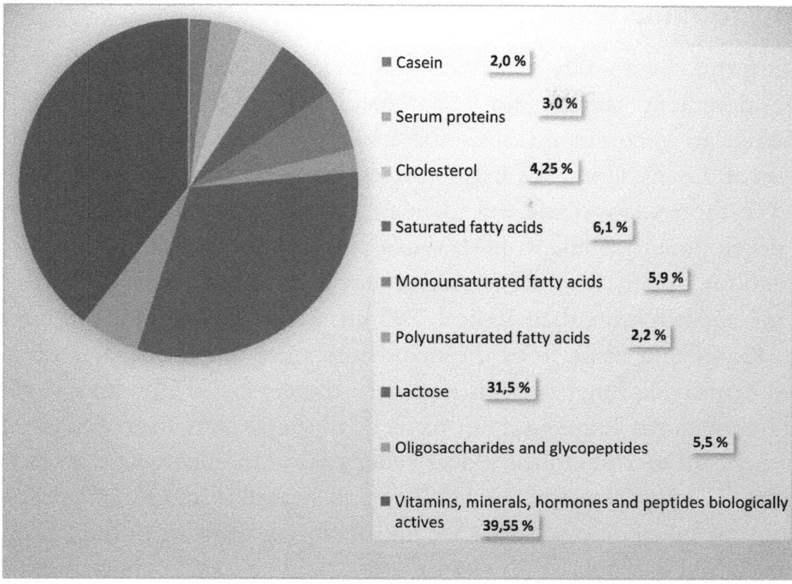

Figure 3.2 Composition of mature human milk in % [10] after excluding the 80% water.

Maternal diet and storage determines the production and/or composition of human milk. In fact, if the mother is malnourished or eats an unusually restrictive diet, she produces less milk [37]. Also some important components such as vitamin B12 might be affected in case of vegan mothers [38]. This is why the European Society for Paediatric Gastroenterology Hepatology and Nutrition (ESPGHAN) Committee of Nutrition recommends supplementing breastfed infants (or their breastfeeding mothers) with vitamin B12 if the lactating mothers follow a vegan diet or with vitamin D as its contents in breast milk is often inadequate due to the limited use of vitamin D supplemented cows' milk and dairy products or because of a lack of sunshine [39]. Vitamin K is another micronutrient that may be inadequate in breastfed infants and European pediatric societies recommend giving a vitamin K supplement during the first weeks or months of life to breastfed infants or sometimes to all infants [85]. Fluoride and iron are also key micronutrients during this period [40].

Infant formula feeding

Infant formula is a product based on the milk of animals (mainly cows) and other ingredients suitable for infant feeding [41]. In 2005, ESPGHAN published its recommendations for infant formulas based on scientific analysis and considering the existing scientific reports on the subject. They stated that formula was safe and adequate for supporting the normal growth and development of infants [41]. Once prepared following manufacturer's instructions, infant formula should contain at least 60 kcal (250 kJ) per 100 mL and not more than 70 kcal (295 kJ), which is very similar to human milk. Ingredients apart from the mandatory ones (see Table 3.1) may be added to provide other benefits similar to those provided by human milk. The International Expert Group formed by the experts from ESPGHAN and its related societies in the global Federation of International Societies on Pediatric Gastroenterology, Hepatology and Nutrition did not support the addition of any additional substance just because it was part of human milk, however, and stated that the extra benefit should be specifically proven [41].

Formula for young children

Young children formula (YCF) refers to milk-based drinks or plant protein used to partially satisfy the nutritional requirements of children aged from 1 to 3 years [42]. YCFs have been available in Europe for more than two decades and their use is increasing [43]. In 2013, the EFSA reported that there are hundreds of YCFs present on the European Union (EU) market, with France, Spain, and Italy having the highest amount and Scandinavian countries the lowest [42]. There is also a huge difference between European countries in terms of their classification of these foods [42], as well as the recommendations from the relevant pediatric and/or nutritional societies throughout Europe. For instance, in 2014, the German Federal Institute for Risk Assessment concluded that after 1 year of age, there is no need to use YCFs as young children should adapt to a diverse diet within the family [44]. In contrast, the medical community in France approves the consumption of 500 mL per day of YCF for 12- to 36-month-olds [45] and more recently, the German Society of Paediatrics and Adolescent Medicine sustained by the ESPGHAN, stated that YCF may contribute to the supply of iron, vitamin D, and iodine.

An additional problem is the lack of compositional guidelines for YCFs, leading some groups [46,47] to publish their recommendations for this. In

Table 3.1 Global standard for the composition of infant formula by the ESPGHAN Coordinated International Expert Group (2005) [41].

Nutrients	Recommendations minimum–maximum
Energy	60.0–70.0 kcal/100 mL
Proteins	
Cows' milk protein	1.8–3.0 g/100 kcal
Soy protein isolates	2.25–3.0 g/100 kcal
Hydrolyzed cows' milk protein	1.8†–3.0 g/100 kcal
Lipids	
Total fat	4.4–6.0 g/100 kcal
Linoleic acid	0.3–1.2 g/100 kcal
a-linolenic acid	50.0–NS mg/100 kcal
Ratio linoleic/a-linolenic acids	5:1–15:1
Lauric + myristic acids	NS–20.0% of fat
Trans fatty acids	NS–3.0% of fat
Erucic acid	NS–1.0% of fat
Carbohydrates	
Total carbohydrates	9.0–14.0 g/100 kcal
Vitamins	
Vitamin A (preformed retinol)	60.0–180.0 μg RE/ 100 kcal§
Vitamin D3	1.0–2.5 μg/100 kcal
Vitamin E	0.5–5.0 mg α-TE/ 100 kcal ∞
Vitamin K	4.0–25.0 μg/100 kcal
Thiamin	60.0–300.0 μg/100 kcal
Riboflavin	80.0–400.0 μg/100 kcal
Niacin (preformed)	300.0–1500.0 μg/100 kcal
Vitamin B6	35.0–175.0 μg/100 kcal
Vitamin B12	0.1–0.5 μg/100 kcal
Pantothenic acid	400.0–2000.0 μg/100 kcal
Folic acid	10.0–50.0 μg/100 kcal
Vitamin C	10.0–30.0 μg/100 kcal
Biotin	1.5–7.5 μg/100 kcal
Minerals and trace elements	–
Iron (cows' milk protein and protein hydrolysate)	0.3–1.3 mg/100 kcal
Iron (soy protein isolate)	0.45–2.0 mg/100 kcal

Continued

Table 3.1 Global standard for the composition of infant formula by the ESPGHAN Coordinated International Expert Group (2005) [41].—cont'd

Nutrients	Recommendations minimum−maximum
Calcium	50.0−140.0 mg/100 kcal
Phosphorus (cows' milk protein and protein hydrolysate)	25.0−90.0 mg/100 kcal
Phosphorus (soy protein isolate)	30.0−100.0 mg/100 kcal
Magnesium	5.0−15.0 mg/100 kcal
Sodium	20.0−60.0 mg/100 kcal
Chloride	50.0−160.0 mg/100 kcal
Potassium	60.0−160.0 mg/100 kcal
Manganese	1.0−50.0 mg/100 kcal
Fluoride	NS−60.0 mg/100 kcal
Iodine	10.0−50.0 mg/100 kcal
Selenium	1.0−9.0 mg/100 kcal
Copper	35.0−80.0 mg/100 kcal
Zinc	0.5−1.5 mg/100 kcal
Other	
Choline	7.0−50.0 mg/100 kcal
Myo-inositol	4.0−40.0 mg/100 kcal
L-carnitine	1.2−NS mg/100 kcal

NS, Not specified; *RE*, Retinol equivalent; *TE*, Tocopherol equivalent.
§1 mg RE = 1 mg all-trans retinol = 3.33 IU vitamin A.
∞1 mg α-TE (α-tocopherol equivalent) = 1 mg D-α-tocopherol (should be at least 0.5 mg α-TE per g polyunsaturated fatty acids).

this respect, the EFSA concluded that even if YCFs represent an adequate choice for increasing the intake of some nutrients, such as iron or omega-3 polyunsaturated fatty acids (n-3 PUFA), the fortification of cows' milk and cereal-based foods, supplements, or the early introduction of meat and fish may also be considered efficient alternatives [42,48].

There is no evidence on the side effects associated with YCF; however, they are some notable disadvantages. For example, they can lead to a preference for liquids over other regular food groups, which can affect control of satiety. Also, parents and caregivers may have the impression that manufactured foods are the best choice to meet the nutritional requirements of young children and this may increase the family's financial burden [43,49]. In a systematic review that included over 1000 infants and compared breastfed and formula-fed infants over 1 year of age, formula-fed infants were found to have higher fat-free mass throughout the first year of life than breastfed infants [50]. Due to the heterogeneity of tissues encompassing fat-free mass, such as bone, muscle, organs, and connective tissue, the biological implications are still uncertain [50]. In contrast, formula feeding has not showed special risk in the development of infant allergies in the literature [51].

With all these limitations, the ESPGHAN Committee of Nutrition provided some recommendations in relation to YCF [46] and stated that breastfeeding was the best choice even after the first year of life if it is mutually desired by the mother and the child. It was concluded that there was no need for the routine use of YCF in children aged between 1 and 3 years, even if it can be used as part of a strategy to increase the intake of iron, vitamin D, and n-3 PUFA and to decrease the intake of protein compared to unfortified cow's milk. Further investigations are needed, however, to unify terms around YCF; to look for other strategies to optimize nutritional intake, including the promotion of a healthy varied diet, the use of fortified foods, and the use of supplements; and to investigate the role of YCF in the diets of young children. Meanwhile, there is a need for the regulation of YCF to avoid inappropriate composition and for a clearer statement on the packaging to differentiate between follow-on formula and infant formula [46].

Complementary feeding

The WHO defined complementary feeding (CF) as "the process starting when breast milk alone is no longer sufficient to meet the nutritional requirements of infants," so that "other foods and liquids are needed, along with breast milk" [52]. These other foods and liquids are necessary for nutrition and development and also for social reasons as the period in which they are introduced represents the transition to family foods and eating as a social event [40].

In its last statement in 2017, the ESPGHAN [40] recommended that complementary foods (solids and liquids other than breast milk or infant formula) should not be introduced before 4 months of age and should not be delayed beyond 6 months of age. They also stated that exclusive or full breastfeeding should be promoted for at least 4 months after birth and that exclusive or predominant breastfeeding should be promoted for approximately 6 months after birth. The WHO agreed that breast milk can provide half or more of a child's energy needs between 6 and 12 months of age and one-third of energy needs and other high-quality nutrients between 12 and 24 months of age [53,54].

The Pediatric Spanish Association (AEP) [55] recently provided a flexible calendar for introducing the different food groups to babies and argued that no rigid instructions should be given and that family preferences and habits must be considered [56]. Food rich in iron and zinc should be a priority, however, and the different foods should be introduced one at a time with intervals of a few days to observe tolerance and acceptance. Also, salt, sugar, and sweeteners must be avoided so the baby can get used to the natural taste of food [40]. Between 6 and 12 months of age, cereals, fruits, vegetables, legumes, eggs, meat, chicken, fish, and olive oil can be introduced. From 12 to 24 months, dairy products such as yogurt, cow's milk, and cheese can be included. After 2 years of age, all solids that have a choking risk (e.g., nuts, apple, raw carrots, etc.) can be incorporated, as well as superfluous foods like cold cuts, pastries, cakes, and cookies [55]. Several aspects of the ESPGHAN's recommendations are summarized below.

Physiological and neurological maturation

It is important to make sure foods are the correct consistency and delivered by a method appropriate to the infant's age and development [40]. The physiological maturation of both renal and gastrointestinal function necessary to metabolize foods other than milk occurs at 4 months of age, while the skills required for an infant to safely accept and swallow pureed food from a spoon typically appears between 4 and 6 months. The ability to self-feed or to eat semisolid foods appears at the end of the first year [52]. The available literature does not specify whether spoon feeding is more or less adequate than self-feeding, and parents should be advised on how to recognize their infant's hunger and satiety cues and adopt the style that is best for their child [40].

Nutritional adequacy of exclusive breastfeeding

The current recommendations regarding the nutrient intake in infants aged 6 months are based on the requirements of typically growing and term infants who are breastfed by well-nourished mothers [52,57]. The EFSA noticed, however, that there is no a concrete age in which EBF might provide insufficient energy, so the introduction of CF needs to be decided individually. Even though those infants grew normally according to WHO growth charts [40], other studies also reported normal growth with fewer months of EBF [58,59]. Indeed, there is also evidence regarding the advantages of CF at 4 months of age for infant iron stores as this is when infants experience rapid growth [60–63].

Iron stores depend on a number of factors, however, and can be optimized by methods other than the earlier introduction of CF, such as delayed umbilical cord clamping [64] and iron supplementation in at-risk infants (e.g., preterm infants or those with a low birth weight). Due to the differences in the composition and health effects of breast milk and infant formula, it may seem logical to give different recommendations for CF; however, this can lead to practical problems and may cause confusion among caregivers [40].

Development of taste and food preferences

Infants' innate preference for sugar and salt and their dislike of bitter tastes are not susceptible to modification; however, avoiding complementary foods with added sugars and salt and introducing a variety of flavors, including bitter green vegetables, can modify subsequent preferences [40].

Health outcomes

It is important to consider the increased risk of infections, allergies, celiac disease, Type 1 diabetes, adiposity, and anemia when introducing CF [40] and the ESPGHAN provides the following recommendations:

- Prolonged EBF leads to a lower risk of gastrointestinal and respiratory infections [65].
- There is an increased risk of allergy when solids are introduced before 3 to 4 months of age, but there is no evidence of any benefit to delaying the introduction of allergenic foods beyond 4 months [66].
- Concerning body composition, the introduction of CF before 4 months may be associated with increased adiposity later on in life. Moreover, a high protein intake (more than 15% of the total daily energy intake) during CF may increase the risk of being overweight or obese, especially in predisposed individuals. Finally, a higher intake of cows' milk means a higher intake of energy, protein, and fat and a lower intake of iron.
- Gluten may be introduced into the infant's diet during CF at any time between 4 and 12 months of age, but large quantities should be avoided during the first few weeks after introduction and during infancy in general to prevent celiac disease [67].

- Iron requirements increase during periods of rapid growth and development and these requirements must be assured, particularly in breastfed infants [68].
- Appropriate supplements for vegan diets may be necessary for normal growth and development to avoid irreversible cognitive impairment and death [69].

Infant feeding and tissue maturation

Growth factors

Human milk contains specific growth factors that have wide-ranging effects on different body systems [31]. For instance, the epidermal growth factor (EGF) found in both amniotic fluid and breast milk is responsible for intestinal maturation and healing [70]. Apart from the involvement of the EGF in the stimulation of the enterocyte to increase deoxyribonucleic acid (DNA) synthesis, cell division, absorption of water and glucose, and protein synthesis, it is critical for the maturation and healing of the intestinal mucosa [71]. EGF helps inhibit cell death and corrects alterations induced by proinflammatory tumor necrosis factor-α in intestinal and liver tight junction proteins [72]. The EGF concentrations in breast milk depend on the infants' requirements and are highest in early infancy and in early milk, especially for preterm infants, and decrease throughout lactation [73].

Besides the immaturity of the newborn intestine, the enteral nervous system also requires the brain-derived neurotrophic factor (BDNF) to enhance peristalsis and the glial cell line—derived neurotrophic factor (GDNF) for its development [74]. Both BDNF and GDNF are present in human milk up to 90 days after birth [75].

Insulin-like growth factor (IGF) superfamily components are also required for tissue growth. These are also found in human milk and their concentrations are the highest in the colostrum and decline throughout the course of lactation [76]. There are no significant differences between preterm and term milk, however [77]. IGF components can be taken up in a bioactive form by the intestine and transported into the blood [78], but its function in such cases remains unclear [79].

Human milk also contains components linked with the regulation of the vascular system and concentrations of vascular endothelial growth factor (which regulates the angiogenesis process) are the highest in the colostrum in both preterm and term human milk [80]. Significant quantities of erythropoietin (Epo), the main hormone responsible for increasing red blood cell count, are also found in human milk. Some studies suggest that administration of Epo may prevent anemia of prematurity [81] as it is safer than transfusions, it is immunologically and biologically indistinguishable from the natural hormone, and its efficacy has been proven in adults [82]. In addition, Epo is an important trophic factor and tightens intestinal junctions [83].

Finally, other hormones important for growth, metabolism, and body composition development are found in considerable quantities in human milk, e.g., calcitonin, its precursor procalcitonin [84], and adiponectin [85]. Adiponectin is a multifunctional hormone that actively regulates metabolism, suppresses inflammation, and which is supposed to modify infant metabolism [85,86]. Its concentration in breast milk also inversely correlates with infant BMI when exclusively breastfeeding and might therefore be linked to the reduction of obesity later in life [85]. Other metabolism-regulating hormones found in effective quantities in human milk are leptin, resistin, and ghrelin, which are related to energy conversion, appetite control, and body composition [87–89].

Immunological factors

Human milk contains immune factors that protect against infections and inflammation [90] and help ensure infant survival [91]. These components are so numerous and multifunctional that understanding them is a challenge for the human milk and breastfeeding research [31]. These components include newly identified families of bioactive lipid mediators synthesized from essential fatty acids that actively stimulate the resolution of inflammation [92]. Collectively, these are called "specialized proresolving mediators" [92] and include lipoxins derived from arachidonic acid, resolvins derived from eicosapentaenoic acid, and resolvins derived from docosahexaenoic acid, protectins, and maresins. All these have recently been found in human milk [93] and are involved in antiinflammation (e.g., limiting further neutrophil inflammation), proresolution (e.g., enhancing macrophage clearance of apoptotic cells, debris, and bacteria), pain reduction, and wound healing [92,93].

Other immunological components present in human milk include macrophages, T cells, stem cells, and lymphocytes [94–100], which provide broad, powerful protection against pathogens while stimulating the development of the infant's immune system [31]. In women infected with HIV-1 and HTLV-1, however, the activity of the macrophages in human milk enables mother-to-infant viral transmission [31]. Stem cells have also been identified in human milk [95], but their specific function is still under investigation [31].

Cytokines are multifunctional peptides found in human milk that induce movement of other cells, influence immune activity, and reduce inflammation. Finally, the antigens and antibodies in human milk also provide significant protection against infection. The concentration of these molecules is typically higher in the colostrum and decreases throughout lactation [31].

Nutritional programming

The concept of nutritional programming was introduced almost 30 years ago by Barker et al. [101] and Hales et al. [102], who found that the prevalence of cardiovascular disease (CVD) and Type 2 diabetes (T2D) was higher in UK men who had a lower birth weight and lower weight at 1 year of age than those who had a normal birth weight. The men with lower birth weights also had the highest rate of death from ischemic heart disease [101]. These results were also observed in women in the United Kingdom [103,104]. These findings led the authors to propose the Thrifty Phenotype Hypothesis [105], which suggests that the fetus adapts under conditions of suboptimal nutrition in utero to ensure its survival. This adaptation involves extra protection of vital organs in detriment of more secondarily organs such as the pancreas, heart, kidney, and skeletal muscle. Simultaneously, metabolic programming allows nutrient storage in conditions of poor postnatal nutrition to enhance survival. Paradoxically, these adaptations can lead to glucose intolerance, T2D, CVD, and hypertension in conditions of adequate nutrition or overnutrition after birth. This hypothesis has been corroborated by various epidemiological studies around the world [106].

Nutrition in the earliest stages of infancy is mainly based on milk that is either provided naturally by the mother or made from formula. There is a large amount of evidence suggesting that disease risk is determined during this period, for example, breastfeeding appears to protect against some immune-related diseases later in life, such as Type 1 diabetes [107] and inflammatory bowel disease [108] due to the antiinfection properties and other bioactive constituents present in human milk. There is a number of methodological concerns regarding these studies, however, as they strongly depend on self-report and the results may be influenced by several confounding factors, such as maternal education level [109].

Environmental behaviors like diet, physical activity, and sleep habits determine a person's health throughout life, including the early postnatal period [110]. The sum of the interactions between the genotype and nutritional or nonnutritional factors across the lifespan influences disease risk. In general, the literature favors the idea that nutritional programming provides a layer of risk modification between the genotype and later lifestyle behaviors. For example, some studies have reported that birth weight modulates the normally observed relationships between specific gene polymorphisms and diseases [111–113].

The persistence of early life factors as influences upon the response to nutritional challenges in adulthood is a testament to early life's impact on the development of organs and systems [110]. The mechanisms related to epigenetic regulation are not yet fully understood and it is speculated that the window for nutritional programming extends even further into infancy [110]. Epigenetics include a variety of processes that cause mitotically and meiotically heritable changes in gene expression without modifying the DNA sequence, being the DNA methylation, histone modification, and noncoding RNA, the main underlying mechanisms [114].

In this sense, the so-called "1000 days period" from conception to the second birthday of the baby is when epigenetic DNA imprinting activity is the most active [115]. The epigenetic changes occurring in this time can play a key role in developmental programming and may consequently influence an individual's susceptibility to the later progress to diseases and noncommunicable chronic conditions [114]. This means that maternal factors also influence these epigenetic changes. For instance, in the Dutch Winter Study, it was shown that famine during early and midgestation can lead to metabolic dysregulation in children later on life, specifically hyperglycemia, higher incidence of coronary heart disease, a more atherogenic lipid profile, disturbed blood coagulation, increased stress responsiveness, and obesity [116].

The progress made in this field has been possible due to integrated analyses from studies of human cohorts, animal models, and cell systems. A current major challenge is to identify individuals at risk of disease due to early factors and to improve public health through appropriate recommendations for pregnant and lactating women. This will have a strong impact on combating the major healthcare issues of the 21st century, such as T2D and CVD [106].

Early influences on the development of food preferences

Childhood is a critical period of rapid growth and development in which food preferences start to be established [117]. The eating habits of infants and children are influenced by both intrinsic (genetics, age, and gender) and environmental (family, peers, community, and society) factors [118]. For instance, intrauterine exposure and breastfeeding have been associated with flavor stimulation and could decrease the risk of obesity [119,120]. CF is also important in terms of taste preferences and infants' attitudes toward food and during this period, parents teach their children about their cultural and familial beliefs and the practices surrounding food and eating [121].

The process of recognizing flavors involves a number of chemosensory sensations, primarily the senses of taste and smell, and begins in the prenatal period [122]. Children usually have a preference for food high in sugar or salt rather than food that is sour or bitter. These preferences can be modified, however, through repeated exposure to flavors in amniotic fluid, the mother's milk, and solid foods during CF [123]. Children are also predisposed to prefer high-energy foods due to a genetic adaptation to the scarcity of such products over thousands of years and because of these foods' higher palatability [124]. Children also tend to reject new foods as an adaptive behavior that ensures they only consume foods that are familiar and safe [125] and to learn associations between food flavors and the digestive consequences of eating [126].

Gustatory and olfactory systems emerge during the first intrauterine trimester and are functionally mature before birth. This prepares the fetus to want foods that are safe and available later on in the postnatal period. Tastes and smells are transferred into the amniotic fluid, where they are able to be detected by the fetus and their repeated exposure influences behavioral responses after birth [127]. For instance, children usually have preference for foods high in sugar or salt over those sour and bitter, such as some vegetables; but these preferences might be modified early through repeated exposure of flavors in amniotic fluid, mother's milk, and solid foods during CF [123].

Only PROP (6-n-propylthiouracil) tasters are likely to accept bitter foods, such as cruciferous vegetables. Children who are unable to taste PROP (the majority of children), like and consume more dietary fat, and are prone to obesity [128]. Consequently, the genetic ability to taste bitter compounds may have important implications for determining dietary patterns and later chronic health in children [129].

The flavor experience of formula-fed infants is remarkably different from those that are breastfed as the former do not receive the flavor profile from breast milk. Also, the flavor experience is more homogenous without the variability introduced by the flavors of the foods in the mother's diet. There are considerable differences in flavors among the different types and brands of formulas and formula-fed infants are more prone to prefer the flavors of the formula they are fed and foods containing these flavors [130]. This should be considered when evaluating the effect of diet composition on growth and health outcomes as composition differences between infant formulas may affect growth and flavor development [131].

Learning about flavors continues during the CF period. The introduction of solids and exposure to a variety of new foods helps infants learn about the perception (texture, taste, and flavor) and nutritional properties (energy density) of the foods that will eventually compose their diet [132]. It is recommended that infants be exposed to a variety of foods during the first year of life to help their acceptance of new foods as exposure in the second year of life may have a more limited impact [133]. Children exhibit heightened levels of food neophobia during the second year of life, which is interpreted as an adaptive mechanism to select foods they know are safe [125].

A study by Maier et al. [134] showed that children who liked a certain food straightaway continued to like it and even increased their preference for it through exposure. Interestingly, those who disliked a food straightaway started to like it after being repeatedly exposed to it and eventually liked it as much as those children who had liked it straightaway. After the age of 2 years, children become more willing to taste new foods if adults are also consuming them [135] or if their peers declare that they like them [136].

Early nutrition and its influence on microbiota

Humans have evolved with microbial symbionts [137]; however, our current lifestyle and declining biodiversity have diminished our exposure to microbes [138]. This means that our microbial communities differ substantially from those of our ancestors [138]. They also have a determinant influence on the immune system shaping homeostasis [139]. This might lead to a dysbiosis, which has been proposed to be a major factor in abnormal postnatal immune maturation [140]. In 1976, Gerrard et al. [141] suggested that allergic diseases are caused by our relative freedom from diseases caused by viruses, bacteria, and helminths. This idea was based on the observation of low allergy prevalence in indigenous populations in

Northern Canada, where helminth infection and untreated viral and bacterial diseases were common.

Decades later, this idea was named the "microbial deprivation hypothesis" [142] after it was found that other immune-mediated diseases such as Type 1 diabetes, multiple sclerosis, and Crohn's disease also showed higher incidences in developed countries [143]. Most of the studies looking at underlying immunomodulatory mechanisms have focused on postnatal microbial exposure [144]; however, there is now evidence that the maternal microbiome during pregnancy is also important for childhood immune programming [145]. In fact, recent studies have suggested that the first interactions between the microbiota and the baby may be initiated in utero [146—148] due to intracellular bacteria in the placental basal plate [149]. In addition, bacterial DNA has been detected in amniotic fluid [150], the placenta [150], umbilical cord blood [151], and meconium [150]. Indeed, the neonate's first stool sample and the microbiota of the meconium have features in common with the microbiota observed in paired amniotic fluid and placental samples collected after term caesarean deliveries [150].

The maternal bacterial components transferred to the fetus help the neonatal immune system respond appropriately to the much larger inoculum transferred during vaginal delivery and breastfeeding [152]. This is why appropriate perinatal microbial sensitization may be needed to prevent the pathophysiological process leading to allergies [140]. In this respect, the gut microbiota must be considered as the most important source of microbial sensitization and as vital for the maturation of the immune system [153]. In addition, breastfeeding-induced microbiota have been shown to regulate the expression of genes involved in digestion, barrier function, and angiogenesis and to enhance immunoglobulin-A secretion [156], thus possibly contributing to the prevention of necrotizing enterocolitis. In a recent systematic review, it was found that a longer duration of EBF was associated with reduced diarrhea-related gut microbiota dysbiosis [155]. Therefore, the window of opportunity for intervention of health-promoting microbiotas that could then be maintained throughout the lifespan in microbial sensitization likely begins during the fetal stage [154] by affecting immune regulation, the endocrine system, and the metabolism.

Up until the third year of life, diet plays a key role in generating changes in the microbiome [157] and has a potential impact on infant development and disease risk, such as dermatologic and immune-mediated disorders, diseases of the respiratory tract, and intestinal disorders [158]. The introduction of regular food to a breastfed infant causes a rapid rise in the number of enterobacteria and enterococci, followed by progressive colonization by *Bacteroides* spp., *Clostridium*, and anaerobic *Streptococcus*. In formula-fed infants, however, the evidence indicates that solid food does not have as great an impact on their gastrointestinal flora [159] as they already have a greater variety compared to breastfed infants. As expected, the longer the time since the introduction of the solid food in the diet, the earlier the bacterial flora approaching that of adults [159].

Advances in the understanding of the colonization patterns during infancy and early childhood and the mechanisms related to how the gut microbiota interact with the immune and endocrine systems and the metabolism may help with the development of strategies that promote healthy microbiota composition [157].

Take home messages and future challenges

Early infancy is a critical period in terms of nutrition, not only because of the requirements for growth and development but also because this period may influence later nutrition-related behaviors and future health. Breastfeeding is the gold standard and should be promoted during the first 6 months of life and later if desired by both the mother and the child. Due to its associations with emotional well-being and health benefits in terms of maturation, immunity, growth, development, inflammation, nutritional components, and development of taste and food preferences, human milk has no comparison with any other feeding practice. In fact, infant formula feeding still requires an extra effort in relation to regulation of terminologies and misleading to consumers and there is no clear evidence regarding the possible side effects associated with its use. CF is necessary for nutrition and development and should not be introduced before 4 months or delayed beyond 6 months. Specific care should also be taken in relation to excess protein intake, cows' milk intake, and iron and vitamin B12 deficiency.

References

[1] Gungor NK. Overweight and obesity in children and adolescents. J Clin Res Pediatr Endocrinol September 2014;6(3):129–43.
[2] Moreno Villares JM. Nutrition in early life and the programming of adult disease: the first 1000 days. Nutr Hosp July 12, 2016;33(Suppl. 4):337.
[3] Steinman L, Doescher M, Keppel GA, Pak-Gorstein S, Graham E, Haq A, et al. Understanding infant feeding beliefs, practices and preferred nutrition education and health provider approaches: an exploratory study with Somali mothers in the USA. Matern Child Nutr January 2010;6(1):67–88.

[4] World Bank. Repositioning nutrition as central to development: a strategy for large scale action. Washington DC: The World Bank; 2006.
[5] Gil A. Tratado de Nutrición. Nutrición humana en el estado de salud.3ª edición. Tomo IV. Editorial Panamericana; 2017, ISBN 9788491101932.
[6] World Health Organization. Early initiation of breastfeeding to promote exclusive breastfeeding. 2016. Available from: http://www.who.int/elena/titles/early_breast feeding/en/.
[7] Khan J, Vesel L, Bahl R, Martines JC. Timing of breastfeeding initiation and exclusivity of breastfeeding during the first month of life: effects on neonatal mortality and morbidity–a systematic review and meta-analysis. Matern Child Health J March 2015;19(3):468–79.
[8] NEOVITA Study Group. Timing of initiation, patterns of breastfeeding, and infant survival: prospective analysis of pooled data from three randomised trials. Lancet Glob Health April 2016;4(4):e266–75.
[9] AAP. Breastfeeding and the use of human milk. Pediatrics 2012;129:e827.
[10] Bueno M, Sarría A, Pérez-González JM, editors. Nutrición en pediatría. 3a edición. Madrid: Ergon; 2007.
[11] Ryan AS, Hay Jr WW. Challenges of infant nutrition research: a commentary. Nutr J April 22, 2016;15:42.
[12] Gatti L. Maternal perceptions of insufficient milk supply in breastfeeding. J Nurs Scholarsh 2008;40(4):355–63.
[13] Meedya S, Fahy K, Kable A. Factors that positively influence breastfeeding duration to 6 months: a literature review. Women Birth December 2010;23(4):135–45.
[14] Thulier D, Mercer J. Variables associated with breastfeeding duration. J Obstet Gynecol Neonatal Nurs May-June;38(3):259–68.
[15] Hartmann PE, et al. Breast development and the control of milk synthesis. Food Nutr Bull 1996;17(4):292–302.
[16] Infant and young child feeding: model chapter for textbooks for medical students and allied health professionals. Geneva: World Health Organization; 2009. SESSION 2, The physiological basis of breastfeeding. Available from: https://www.ncbi.nlm.nih.gov/books/NBK148970/.
[17] Scientific Advisory Committee on Nutrition. The influence of maternal, fetal and child nutrition on the development of chronic disease in later life. London: TSO; 2011.
[18] Innis SM. Impact of maternal diet on human milk composition and neurological development of infants. Am J Clin Nutr March 2014;99(3):734S–41S.
[19] WHO Multicentre Growth Reference Study Group. WHO Child Growth Standards based on length/height, weight and age. Acta Paediatr Suppl 2006;450:76–85.
[20] WHO Child Growth Standards based on length/height, weight and age. Acta Paediatr Suppl April 2006;450:76–85.
[21] UNICEF. Breastfeeding. Available from:www.unicef.org/breastfeeding/. Updated 31/7/2017 Accessed 8/4/2018.
[22] Quigley MA, Carson C. Breastfeeding in the 21st century. Lancet May 21, 2016;387(10033):2087–8.
[23] UNICEF-UNAIDS-WHO-UNFPA. HIVand infant feeding. Guidelines for decision-makers. 2003. ISBN 9241591226. Available at: http://www.unfpa.org/upload/lib_pub_file/340_filename_HIV_IF_DM.pdf. [Accessed 8 April 2018].
[24] World Helath Organization (WHO). HIV transmission through breastfeeding : a review of available evidence, ISBN 92-4-156271-4.
[25] Lawrence RM, Lawrence RA. Given the benefits of breastfeeding, what contraindications exist? Pediatr Clin February 2001;48(1):235–51.

[26] Hamprecht K, Maschmann J, Vochem M, Dietz K, Speer CP, Jahn G. Epidemiology of transmission of cytomegalovirus from mother to preterm infant by breastfeeding. Lancet February 17, 2001;357(9255):513–8.
[27] World Health Organization. Biomonitoring of human milk for persistent organic pollutants (POPs). 2008. http://www.who.int/foodsafety/chem/pops/en/. [Accessed 8 April 2018].
[28] Gupta RC, editor. Reproductiveanddevelopmentaltoxicology. SECOND EDITION. ELSEVIER ACADEMIC PRESS; 2017.
[29] Robinson SM. Infant nutrition and lifelong health: current perspectives and future challenges. J Dev Orig Health Dis October 2015;6(5):384–9.
[30] Agostoni C, Braegger C, Decsi T, Kolacek S, Koletzko B, Michaelsen KF, et al. Breast-feeding: a commentary by the ESPGHAN committee on nutrition. J Pediatr Gastroenterol Nutr July 2009;49(1):112–25.
[31] Ballard O, Morrow AL. Human milk composition: nutrients and bioactive factors. Pediatr Clin February 2013;60(1):49–74.
[32] Lonnerdal B. Human milk proteins: key components for the biological activity of human milk. Adv Exp Med Biol 2004;554:11–25.
[33] Saarela T, Kokkonen J, Koivisto M. Macronutrient and energy contents of human milk fractions during the first six months of lactation. Acta Paediatr September 2005;94(9):1176–81.
[34] Kent JC, Mitoulas LR, Cregan MD, Ramsay DT, Doherty DA, Hartmann PE. Volume and frequency of breastfeedings and fat content of breast milk throughout the day. Pediatrics March 2006;117(3):e387–95.
[35] Nommsen LA, Lovelady CA, Heinig MJ, Lonnerdal B, Dewey KG. Determinants of energy, protein, lipid, and lactose concentrations in human milk during the first 12 mo of lactation: the DARLING Study. Am J Clin Nutr February 1991;53(2):457–65.
[36] Gabrielli O, Zampini L, Galeazzi T, Padella L, Santoro L, Peila C, et al. Preterm milk oligosaccharides during the first month of lactation. Pediatrics December 2011;128(6):e1520–31.
[37] Gonzalez-Cossio T, Habicht JP, Rasmussen KM, Delgado HL. Impact of food supplementation during lactation on infant breast-milk intake and on the proportion of infants exclusively breast-fed. J Nutr October 1998;128(10):1692–702.
[38] Roschitz B, Plecko B, Huemer M, Biebl A, Foerster H, Sperl W. Nutritional infantile vitamin B12 deficiency: pathobiochemical considerations in seven patients. Arch Dis Child Fetal Neonatal Ed May 2005;90(3):F281–2.
[39] Gartner LM, Morton J, Lawrence RA, Naylor AJ, O'Hare D, Schanler RJ, et al. Breastfeeding and the use of human milk. Pediatrics February 2005;115(2):496–506.
[40] Fewtrell M, Bronsky J, Campoy C, Domellof M, Embleton N, Fidler Mis N, et al. Complementary feeding: aposition paper by the European society for paediatric Gastroenterology, Hepatology, and nutrition (ESPGHAN) committee on nutrition. J Pediatr Gastroenterol Nutr January 2017;64(1):119–32.
[41] Koletzko B, Baker S, Cleghorn G, Neto UF, Gopalan S, Hernell O, et al. Global standard for the composition of infant formula: recommendations of an ESPGHAN coordinated international expert group. J Pediatr Gastroenterol Nutr November 2005;41(5):584–99.
[42] European Food Safety Authority (EFSA). Report from the commission to the European parliament and the council on young-child formulae. 2016. http://eur-lex.europa.eu/legal-content/EN/TXT/PDF/?uri=CELEX:52016DC0169&from¼EN. [Accessed 6 April 2017].
[43] Przyrembel H, Agostoni C. Growing-up milk: a necessity or marketing? World Rev Nutr Diet 2013;108:49–55.

[44] Bundesinstitut für Risikobewertung. Kindermilch—abschlussbericht. 2014. https://www.google.hr/url?sa=t&rct=j&q=&esrc=s&source=web&cd=1&ved=0ahUKEwjvla7klJ3XAhWCzKQKHUWsC-0QFggn MAA&url=http%3A%2F%2F. [Accessed 6 April 2017].
[45] Bocquet A, Bresson JL, Briend A, Chouraqui JP, Darmaun D, Dupont C, et al. Feeding of infants based on age. Practice guidelines. Arch Pediatr January 2003;10(1):76–81.
[46] Hojsak I, Bronsky J, Campoy C, Domellof M, Embleton N, Fidler Mis N, et al. Young child formula: aposition paper by the ESPGHAN committee on nutrition. J Pediatr Gastroenterol Nutr January 2018;66(1):177–85.
[47] Suthutvoravut U, Abiodun PO, Chomtho S, Chongviriyaphan N, Cruchet S, Davies PS, et al. Composition of follow-up formula for young children aged 12-36 Months: recommendations of an international expert group coordinated by the nutrition association of Thailand and the early nutrition academy. Ann Nutr Metab 2015;67(2):119–32.
[48] European Food Safety Authority (EFSA). Panel on dietetic products, nutrition and allergies.Scientific opinion on nutrient requirements and dietary intakes of infants and young children in the European Union. EFSA J 2013;11:3408.
[49] Vandenplas Y, De Ronne N, Van De Sompel A, Huysentruyt K, Robert M, Rigo J, et al. A Belgian consensus-statement on growing-up milks for children 12-36 months old. Eur J Pediatr October 2014;173(10):1365–71.
[50] Gale C, Logan KM, Santhakumaran S, Parkinson JR, Hyde MJ, Modi N. Effect of breastfeeding compared with formula feeding on infant body composition: a systematic review and meta-analysis. Am J Clin Nutr March 2012;95(3):656–69.
[51] Goldsmith AJ, Koplin JJ, Lowe AJ, Tang ML, Matheson MC, Robinson M, et al. Formula and breast feeding in infant food allergy: a population-based study. J Paediatr Child Health April 2016;52(4):377–84.
[52] WHO (World Health Organization). Complementary feeding. Report of the global consultation. Geneva, 10–13 December 2001. Summary of guiding principles. 2002. http://www.who.int/nutrition/publications/Complementary_Feeding.pdf. [Accessed 11 March 2016].
[53] Dewey KG, Brown KH. Update on technical issues concerning complementary feeding of young children in developing countries and implications for intervention programs. Food Nutr Bull March 2003;24(1):5–28.
[54] World Health Organization (WHO). Infant and young child feeding. Model Chapter for textbooks for medical students and allied health professionals. Geneva, Switzerland: WHO Press; 2009.
[55] Asociación Española de Pediatría (AEP). Recomendaciones de la Asociación Española de Pediatría sobre la alimentación complementaria. 2018.
[56] Organización Panamericana de la Salud. Organización Mundial de la Salud Principios de orientación para la alimentación complementaria del niño amamantado. En: Asociación Española de Pediatría. Consultado el 17/04/2019. Disponible en. https://www.aeped.es/sites/default/files/1-orientacion_para_la_ac.pdf.
[57] Butte NF, Lopez-Alarcon MG, Garza C. Nutrient adequacy of exclusive breastfeeding for the term infant during the first 6 Months of life. Geneva: World Health Organization; 2001.
[58] Jonsdottir OH, Kleinman RE, Wells JC, Fewtrell MS, Hibberd PL, Gunnlaugsson G, et al. Exclusive breastfeeding for 4 versus 6 months and growth in early childhood. Acta Paediatr January 2014;103(1):105–11.
[59] Perkin MR, Logan K, Tseng A, Raji B, Ayis S, Peacock J, et al. Randomized trial of introduction of allergenic foods in breast-fed infants. N Engl J Med May 5, 2016;374(18):1733–43.

[60] Chantry CJ, Howard CR, Auinger P. Full breastfeeding duration and risk for iron deficiency in U.S. infants. Breastfeed Med June 2007;2(2):63–73.
[61] Dube K, Schwartz J, Mueller MJ, Kalhoff H, Kersting M. Iron intake and iron status in breastfed infants during the first year of life. Clin Nutr December 2010;29(6):773–8.
[62] Dube K, Schwartz J, Mueller MJ, Kalhoff H, Kersting M. Complementary food with low (8%) or high (12%) meat content as source of dietary iron: a double-blinded randomized controlled trial. Eur J Nutr February 2010;49(1):11–8.
[63] Jonsdottir OH, Thorsdottir I, Hibberd PL, Fewtrell MS, Wells JC, Palsson GI, et al. Timing of the introduction of complementary foods in infancy: a randomized controlled trial. Pediatrics December 2012;130(6):1038–45.
[64] Domellof M, Braegger C, Campoy C, Colomb V, Decsi T, Fewtrell M, et al., ESPGHAN Committee on Nutrition. Iron requirements of infants and toddlers. J Pediatr Gastroenterol Nutr January 2014;58(1):119–29.
[65] Kramer MS, Guo T, Platt RW, Sevkovskaya Z, Dzikovich I, Collet JP, et al. Infant growth and health outcomes associated with 3 compared with 6 mo of exclusive breastfeeding. Am J Clin Nutr August 2003;78(2):291–5.
[66] Muraro A, Dreborg S, Halken S, Host A, Niggemann B, Aalberse R, et al. Dietary prevention of allergic diseases in infants and small children. Part III: critical review of published peer-reviewed observational and interventional studies and final recommendations. Pediatr Allergy Immunol August 2004;15(4):291–307.
[67] Akobeng AK, Ramanan AV, Buchan I, Heller RF. Effect of breast feeding on risk of coeliac disease: a systematic review and meta-analysis of observational studies. Arch Dis Child January 2006;91(1):39–43.
[68] Aggett PJ, Agostoni C, Axelsson I, Bresson JL, Goulet O, Hernell O, et al. Iron metabolism and requirements in early childhood: do we know enough?: a commentary by the ESPGHAN Committee on Nutrition. J Pediatr Gastroenterol Nutr April 2002;34(4):337–45.
[69] Dagnelie PC, van Staveren WA. Macrobiotic nutrition and child health: results of a population-based, mixed-longitudinal cohort study in The Netherlands. Am J Clin Nutr May 1994;59(5 Suppl. l):1187S–96S.
[70] Wagner CL, Taylor SN, Johnson D. Host factors in amniotic fluid and breast milk that contribute to gut maturation. Clin Rev Allergy Immunol April 2008;34(2):191–204.
[71] Chang CJ, Chao JC. Effect of human milk and epidermal growth factor on growth of human intestinal Caco-2 cells. J Pediatr Gastroenterol Nutr April 2002;34(4):394–401.
[72] Khailova L, Dvorak K, Arganbright KM, Williams CS, Halpern MD, Dvorak B. Changes in hepatic cell junctions structure during experimental necrotizing enterocolitis: effect of EGF treatment. Pediatr Res August 2009;66(2):140–4.
[73] Dvorak B, Fituch CC, Williams CS, Hurst NM, Schanler RJ. Increased epidermal growth factor levels in human milk of mothers with extremely premature infants. Pediatr Res July 2003;54(1):15–9.
[74] Rodrigues DM, Li AY, Nair DG, Blennerhassett MG. Glial cell line-derived neurotrophic factor is a key neurotrophin in the postnatal enteric nervous system. Neuro Gastroenterol Motil February 2011;23(2):e44–56.
[75] Li R, Xia W, Zhang Z, Wu K. S100B protein, brain-derived neurotrophic factor, and glial cell line-derived neurotrophic factor in human milk. PloS One 2011;6(6):e21663.
[76] Milsom SR, Blum WF, Gunn AJ. Temporal changes in insulin-like growth factors I and II and in insulin-like growth factor binding proteins 1, 2, and 3 in human milk. Horm Res 2008;69(5):307–11.

[77] Blum JW, Baumrucker CR. Colostral and milk insulin-like growth factors and related substances: mammary gland and neonatal (intestinal and systemic) targets. Domest Anim Endocrinol July 2002;23(1–2):101–10.
[78] Philipps AF, Dvorak B, Kling PJ, Grille JG, Koldovsky O. Absorption of milk-borne insulin-like growth factor-I into portal blood of suckling rats. J Pediatr Gastroenterol Nutr August 2000;31(2):128–35.
[79] Kling PJ, Taing KM, Dvorak B, Woodward SS, Philipps AF. Insulin-like growth factor-I stimulates erythropoiesis when administered enterally. Growth Factors September 2006;24(3):218–23.
[80] Loui A, Eilers E, Strauss E, Pohl-Schickinger A, Obladen M, Koehne P. Vascular Endothelial Growth Factor (VEGF) and soluble VEGF receptor 1 (sFlt-1) levels in early and mature human milk from mothers of preterm versus term infants. J Hum Lactation November 2012;28(4):522–8.
[81] Carbonell-Estrany X, Figueras-Aloy J, Alvarez E. Erythropoietin and prematurity–where do we stand? J Perinat Med 2005;33(4):277–86.
[82] Goodnough LT, Monk TG, Andriole GL. Erythropoietin therapy. N Engl J Med March 27, 1997;336(13):933–8.
[83] Shiou SR, Yu Y, Chen S, Ciancio MJ, Petrof EO, Sun J, et al. Erythropoietin protects intestinal epithelial barrier function and lowers the incidence of experimental neonatal necrotizing enterocolitis. J Biol Chem April 8, 2011;286(14):12123–32.
[84] Struck J, de Almeida P, Bergmann A, Morgenthaler NG. High concentrations of procalcitonin but not mature calcitonin in normal human milk. Horm Metab Res August 2002;34(8):460–5.
[85] Newburg DS, Woo JG, Morrow AL. Characteristics and potential functions of human milk adiponectin. J Pediatr February 2010;156(2 Suppl. l):S41–6.
[86] Martin LJ, Woo JG, Geraghty SR, Altaye M, Davidson BS, Banach W, et al. Adiponectin is present in human milk and is associated with maternal factors. Am J Clin Nutr May 2006;83(5):1106–11.
[87] Palou A, Sanchez J, Pico C. Nutrient-gene interactions in early life programming: leptin in breast milk prevents obesity later on in life. Adv Exp Med Biol 2009;646:95–104.
[88] Savino F, Liguori SA. Update on breast milk hormones: leptin, ghrelin and adiponectin. Clin Nutr February 2008;27(1):42–7.
[89] Savino F, Sorrenti M, Benetti S, Lupica MM, Liguori SA, Oggero R. Resistin and leptin in breast milk and infants in early life. Early Hum Dev October 2012;88(10):779–82.
[90] Goldman AS. Modulation of the gastrointestinal tract of infants by human milk.Interfaces and interactions.An evolutionary perspective. J Nutr February 2000;130(2S Suppl. l):426S–31S.
[91] Gao X, McMahon RJ, Woo JG, Davidson BS, Morrow AL, Zhang Q. Temporal changes in milk proteomes reveal developing milk functions. J Proteome Res July 6, 2012;11(7):3897–907.
[92] Serhan CN. Pro-resolving lipid mediators are leads for resolution physiology. Nature June 5, 2014;510(7503):92–101.
[93] Arnardottir H, Orr SK, Dalli J, Serhan CN. Human milk proresolving mediators stimulate resolution of acute inflammation. Mucosal Immunol May 2016;9(3):757–66.
[94] Ichikawa M, Sugita M, Takahashi M, Satomi M, Takeshita T, Araki T, et al. Breast milk macrophages spontaneously produce granulocyte-macrophage colony-stimulating factor and differentiate into dendritic cells in the presence of exogenous interleukin-4 alone. Immunology February 2003;108(2):189–95.

[95] Indumathi S, Dhanasekaran M, Rajkumar JS, Sudarsanam D. Exploring the stem cell and non-stem cell constituents of human breast milk. Cytotechnology May 2012;65(3):385–93.
[96] Jarvinen KM, Suomalainen H. Leucocytes in human milk and lymphocyte subsets in cow's milk-allergic infants. Pediatr Allergy Immunol August 2002;13(4):243–54.
[97] Patki S, Kadam S, Chandra V, Bhonde R. Human breast milk is a rich source of multipotent mesenchymal stem cells. Hum Cell May 2010;23(2):35–40.
[98] Riskin A, Almog M, Peri R, Halasz K, Srugo I, Kessel A. Changes in immunomodulatory constituents of human milk in response to active infection in the nursing infant. Pediatr Res February 2012;71(2):220–5.
[99] Sabbaj S, Ibegbu CC, Kourtis AP. Cellular immunity in breast milk: implications for postnatal transmission of HIV-1 to the infant. Adv Exp Med Biol 2012;743:161–9.
[100] Yagi Y, Watanabe E, Watari E, Shinya E, Satomi M, Takeshita T, et al. Inhibition of DC-SIGN-mediated transmission of human immunodeficiency virus type 1 by Toll-like receptor 3 signalling in breast milk macrophages. Immunology August 2010;130(4):597–607.
[101] Barker DJ, Winter PD, Osmond C, Margetts B, Simmonds SJ. Weight in infancy and death from ischaemic heart disease. Lancet September 9, 1989;2(8663):577–80.
[102] Hales CN, Barker DJ, Clark PM, Cox LJ, Fall C, Osmond C, et al. Fetal and infant growth and impaired glucose tolerance at age 64. BMJ October 26, 1991;303(6809):1019–22.
[103] Barker DJ, Hales CN, Fall CH, Osmond C, Phipps K, Clark PM. Type 2 (non-insulin-dependent) diabetes mellitus, hypertension and hyperlipidaemia (syndrome X): relation to reduced fetal growth. Diabetologia January 1993;36(1):62–7.
[104] Phipps K, Barker DJ, Hales CN, Fall CH, Osmond C, Clark PM. Fetal growth and impaired glucose tolerance in men and women. Diabetologia March 1993;36(3):225–8.
[105] Hales CN, Barker DJ. The thrifty phenotype hypothesis. Br Med Bull 2001;60:5–20.
[106] Tarry-Adkins JL, Ozanne SE. Mechanisms of early life programming: current knowledge and future directions. Am J Clin Nutr December 2011;94(6 Suppl. l):1765S–71S.
[107] Pereira PF, Alfenas Rde C, Araujo RM. Does breastfeeding influence the risk of developing diabetes mellitus in children? A review of current evidence. J Pediatr 2014 ;90(1):7–15.
[108] Klement E, Cohen RV, Boxman J, Joseph A, Reif S. Breastfeeding and risk of inflammatory bowel disease: a systematic review with meta-analysis. Am J Clin Nutr November 2004;80(5):1342–52.
[109] Schack-Nielsen L, Michaelsen KF. Advances in our understanding of the biology of human milk and its effects on the offspring. J Nutr February 2007;137(2):503S–10S.
[110] Langley-Evans SC. Nutrition in early life and the programming of adult disease: a review. J Hum Nutr Diet 2015;28(Suppl. 1):1–14.
[111] de Rooij SR, Painter RC, Roseboom TJ, Phillips DI, Osmond C, Barker DJ, et al. Glucose tolerance at age 58 and the decline of glucose tolerance in comparison with age 50 in people prenatally exposed to the Dutch famine. Diabetologia April 2006;49(4):637–43.
[112] Eriksson JG, Lindi V, Uusitupa M, Forsen TJ, Laakso M, Osmond C, et al. The effects of the Pro12Ala polymorphism of the peroxisome proliferator-activated receptor-gamma2 gene on insulin sensitivity and insulin metabolism interact with size at birth. Diabetes July 2002;51(7):2321–4.
[113] Labayen I, Ruiz JR, Vicente-Rodriguez G, Turck D, Rodriguez G, Meirhaeghe A, et al. Early life programming of abdominal adiposity in adolescents: the HELENA Study. Diabetes Care November 2009;32(11):2120–2.

[114] Indrio F, Martini S, Francavilla R, Corvaglia L, Cristofori F, Mastrolia SA, et al. Epigenetic matters: the link between early nutrition, microbiome, and long-term health development. Front Pediatr 2017;5:178.
[115] Bhutta ZA, Das JK, Rizvi A, Gaffey MF, Walker N, Horton S, et al. Evidence-based interventions for improvement of maternal and child nutrition: what can be done and at what cost? Lancet August 3, 2013;382(9890):452−77.
[116] Roseboom T, de Rooij S, Painter R. The Dutch famine and its long-term consequences for adult health. Early Hum Dev August 2006;82(8):485−91.
[117] Alles MS, Eussen SR, van der Beek EM. Nutritional challenges and opportunities during the weaning period and in young childhood. Ann Nutr Metab 2014;64(3−4):284−93.
[118] Bellows LL, Johnson SL, Davies PL, Anderson J, Gavin WJ, Boles RE. The Colorado LEAP study: rationale and design of a study to assess the short term longitudinal effectiveness of a preschool nutrition and physical activity program. BMC Publ Health December 9, 2013;13:1146.
[119] Arenz S, Ruckerl R, Koletzko B, von Kries R. Breast-feeding and childhood obesity−a systematic review. Int J Obes Relat Metab Disord October 2004;28(10):1247−56.
[120] Owen CG, Martin RM, Whincup PH, Smith GD, Cook DG. Effect of infant feeding on the risk of obesity across the life course: a quantitative review of published evidence. Pediatrics May 2005;115(5):1367−77.
[121] Birch LL, Fisher JO. Development of eating behaviours among children and adolescents. Pediatrics March 1998;101(3 Pt 2):539−49.
[122] Robinson S, Fall C. Infant nutrition and later health: a review of current evidence. Nutrients August 2012;4(8):859−74.
[123] Forestell CA. The development of flavor perception and acceptance: the roles of nature and nurture. Nestle Nutr Inst Workshop Ser 2016;85:135−43.
[124] Vandeweghe L, Vervoort L, Verbeken S, Moens E, Braet C. Food approach and food avoidance in young children: relation with reward sensitivity and punishment sensitivity. Front Psychol 2016;7:928.
[125] Ventura AK, Worobey J. Early influences on the development of food preferences. Curr Biol May 6, 2013;23(9):R401−8.
[126] Hetherington MM, Schwartz C, Madrelle J, Croden F, Nekitsing C, Vereijken CM, et al. A step-by-step introduction to vegetables at the beginning of complementary feeding.The effects of early and repeated exposure. Appetite January 2015;84:280−90.
[127] Anzman-Frasca S, Ventura AK, Ehrenberg S, Myers KP. Promoting healthy food preferences from the start: a narrative review of food preference learning from the prenatal period through early childhood. Obes Rev April 2018;19(4):576−604.
[128] Keller KL, Adise S. Variation in the ability to taste bitter thiourea compounds: implications for food acceptance, dietary intake, and obesity risk in children. Annu Rev Nutr July 17, 2016;36:157−82.
[129] De Cosmi V, Scaglioni S, Agostoni C. Early taste experiences and later food choices. Nutrients February 4, 2017;9(2).
[130] Mennella JA. Ontogeny of taste preferences: basic biology and implications for health. Am J Clin Nutr March 2014;99(3):704S−11S.
[131] Trabulsi JC, Mennella JA. Diet, sensitive periods in flavour learning, and growth. Int Rev Psychiatr June 2012;24(3):219−30.
[132] Nicklaus S. The role of food experiences during early childhood in food pleasure learning. Appetite September 1, 2016;104:3−9.
[133] Bouhlal S, Issanchou S, Chabanet C, Nicklaus S. Just a pinch of salt'. An experimental comparison of the effect of repeated exposure and flavor-flavor learning with salt or spice on vegetable acceptance in toddlers. Appetite December 2014;83:209−17.

[134] Maier A, Chabanet C, Schaal B, Issanchou S, Leathwood P. Effects of repeated exposure on acceptance of initially disliked vegetables in 7-month old infants. Food Qual Prefer 2007;18(8):1023–32.
[135] Addessi E, Galloway AT, Visalberghi E, Birch LL. Specific social influences on the acceptance of novel foods in 2-5-year-old children. Appetite 2005;45(3):264–71.
[136] Greenhalgh J, Dowey AJ, Horne PJ, Fergus Lowe C, Griffiths JH, Whitaker CJ. Positive- and negative peer modelling effects on young children's consumption of novel blue foods. Appetite June 2009;52(3):646–53.
[137] Rosenberg E, Zilber-Rosenberg I. Microbes drive evolution of animals and plants: the hologenome concept. mBio March 31, 2016;7(2):e01395.
[138] Moeller AH. The shrinking human gut microbiome. Curr Opin Microbiol August 2017;38:30–5.
[139] Honda K, Littman DR. The microbiota in adaptive immune homeostasis and disease. Nature July 7, 2016;535(7610):75–84.
[140] Gollwitzer ES, Marsland BJ. Impact of early-life exposures on immune maturation and susceptibility to disease. Trends Immunol November 2015;36(11):684–96.
[141] Gerrard JW, Geddes CA, Reggin PL, Gerrard CD, Horne S. Serum IgE levels in white and metis communities in Saskatchewan. Ann Allergy August 1976;37(2):91–100.
[142] Bjorksten B. Effects of intestinal microflora and the environment on the development of asthma and allergy. Springer Semin Immunopathol February 2004;25(3–4):257–70.
[143] Torow N, Hornef MW. The neonatal window of opportunity: setting the stage for life-long host-microbial interaction and immune homeostasis. J Immunol January 15, 2017;198(2):557–63.
[144] Hansel TT, Johnston SL, Openshaw PJ. Microbes and mucosal immune responses in asthma. Lancet March 9, 2013;381(9869):861–73.
[145] Macpherson AJ, de Aguero MG, Ganal-Vonarburg SC. How nutrition and the maternal microbiota shape the neonatal immune system. Nat Rev Immunol August 2017;17(8):508–17.
[146] Gomez-Arango LF, Barrett HL, McIntyre HD, Callaway LK, Morrison M, Nitert MD. Contributions of the maternal oral and gut microbiome to placental microbial colonization in overweight and obese pregnant women. Sci Rep June 6, 2017;7(1):2860.
[147] Mor G, Aldo P, Alvero AB. The unique immunological and microbial aspects of pregnancy. Nat Rev Immunol August 2017;17(8):469–82.
[148] Stinson LF, Payne MS, Keelan JA. Planting the seed: origins, composition, and postnatal health significance of the fetal gastrointestinal microbiota. Crit Rev Microbiol May 2017;43(3):352–69.
[149] Stout MJ, Conlon B, Landeau M, Lee I, Bower C, Zhao Q, et al. Identification of intracellular bacteria in the basal plate of the human placenta in term and preterm gestations. Am J Obstet Gynecol March 2013;208(3):226 e1–7.
[150] Collado MC, Rautava S, Aakko J, Isolauri E, Salminen S. Human gut colonisation may be initiated in utero by distinct microbial communities in the placenta and amniotic fluid. Sci Rep 2016;6:23129.
[151] Jimenez E, Fernandez L, Marin ML, Martin R, Odriozola JM, Nueno-Palop C, et al. Isolation of commensal bacteria from umbilical cord blood of healthy neonates born by cesarean section. Curr Microbiol October 2005;51(4):270–4.
[152] Martin R, Makino H, Cetinyurek Yavuz A, Ben-Amor K, Roelofs M, Ishikawa E, et al. Early-life events, including mode of delivery and type of feeding, siblings and gender, shape the developing gut microbiota. PloS One 2016;11(6):e0158498.

[153] West CE, Jenmalm MC, Prescott SL. The gut microbiota and its role in the development of allergic disease: a wider perspective. Clin Exp Allergy January 2015;45(1):43–53.
[154] Jenmalm MC. The mother-offspring dyad: microbial transmission, immune interactions and allergy development. J Intern Med December 2017;282(6):484–95.
[155] Ho NT, Li F, Lee-Sarwar KA, Tun HM, Brown BP, Pannaraj PS, et al. Meta-analysis of effects of exclusive breastfeeding on infant gut microbiota across populations. Nat Commun October 9, 2018;9(1):4169.
[156] Hooper LV, Wong MH, Thelin A, Hansson L, Falk PG, Gordon JI. Molecular analysis of commensal host-microbial relationships in the intestine. Science February 2, 2001;291(5505):881–4.
[157] Koenig JE, Spor A, Scalfone N, Fricker AD, Stombaugh J, Knight R, et al. Succession of microbial consortia in the developing infant gut microbiome. Proc Natl Acad Sci USA March 15, 2011;108(Suppl. 1):4578–85.
[158] Johnson CL, Versalovic J. The human microbiome and its potential importance to pediatrics. Pediatrics May 2012;129(5):950–60.
[159] Stark PL, Lee A. The microbial ecology of the large bowel of breast-fed and formula-fed infants during the first year of life. J Med Microbiol May 1982;15(2):189–203.

CHAPTER 4

Maternal undernutrition and antenatal and postnatal growth trajectories—Epidemiology and pathophysiology

Julie Bienertova-Vasku
RECETOX, Faculty of Sciences, Masaryk University, Brno, Czech Republic

Contents

Epidemiology

Maternal malnutrition represents a critical public health problem in developing countries. Poor maternal nutrition status is of a prime health concern as it not only has major health risks for the mother and subsequent pregnancy and birth outcomes but goes beyond to impact child growth and cognitive development in their future life. This leads to grave consequences for not only the individual or a family but the society as a whole and

Molecular Nutrition
ISBN 978-0-12-813862-5
https://doi.org/10.1016/B978-0-12-813862-5.00004-9

impedes the economic growth and development of the whole populations. On the other hand, with the rising prevalence of high calorie diets and subsequent overweight and obesity issues in developed countries, the impact of this overnutrition situation upon pregnancy outcome is highlighted as a contributing factor for adverse metabolic outcomes in offspring later in life [1]. Both human and animal studies now provide sufficient evidence that undernutrition, overnutrition, and diet composition negatively impact fetoplacental growth and metabolic patterns, having adverse later life metabolic effects for the offspring. Maternal malnutrition during or before pregnancy affects the growth of the child as well as its cognitive development[2], increases susceptibility to adverse health outcomes, mainly infections, and massively increases child's morbidity and mortality.

According to WHO, the total of 1.9 billion adults worldwide are overweight or obese as of 2018, while approximately 462 million are underweight, the total of 52 million children under 5 years of age are wasted, 17 million are severely wasted, and 155 million are stunted, on the other hand, 41 million are overweight or obese [3]. In a very recent study based on 2009 population-based studies, with measurements of height and weight in more than 112 million adults, reporting national, regional, and global trends in mean body mass index (BMI) segregated by place of residence (a rural or urban area) from 1985 to 2017, it was shown that contrary to the prevailing beliefs, more than 55% of the global rise in mean BMI from 1985 to 2017—and more than 80% in some low- and middle-income regions—was due to increases in BMI in rural areas [4]. Such huge contribution stems from the fact that, except for women in sub-Saharan Africa, BMI is increasing at the same rate or faster in rural areas than in cities in low- and middle-income regions [4]. These observations emphasize the fact that the distribution of BMI geographically changes in a highly complex manner in a strong relationship to socioeconomic status of the investigated individuals and populations.

This chapter primarily deals with the maternal undernutrition as a risk factor and the growth of the offspring as the endpoint variable.

Maternal malnutrition/undernutrition

This chapter card primarily uses the term undernutrition, defined as the outcome of insufficient food intake (hunger), often associated with repeated or severe infectious diseases, such as AIDS. The term "undernutrition" covers either being underweight for one's age or too short for one's age (i.e., stunted), or extremely thin (wasted) and/or deficient in vitamins and minerals while having low, normal, or high body mass (which is a condition called micronutrient malnutrition). The term malnutrition refers generally to both undernutrition and overnutrition in all their forms and comprises undernutrition (wasting, stunting, underweight) [5], inadequate vitamins or minerals intake, overweight or obesity, and associated noncommunicable diseases. While wasting is usually associated with a heavy weight loss due to largely insufficient caloric intake and/or concomitant infectious diseases, stunting represents a long-term problem in growth and development of children as a result of repeated illnesses and insufficient nutrition (although with sufficient caloric intake) [3]. Stunting in the early life of the child (especially during the first 1000 days after conception (the so-called first 1000 d; www.thousanddays.org) may have detrimental consequences not only for growth and overall health of the child but also for the cognitive development and educational performance later in life, which may constitute a huge burden for the whole society [5].

Maternal undernutrition causes

A key factor underlying most of the determinants of undernutrition is the socioeconomic status; hence, the lower socioeconomic status and rural dwelling with bad access to infrastructure are indirectly associated with undernutrition [6]. Not surprisingly, the access to drinkable water is a major factor associated with maternal undernutrition, among other factors being the size of the household, parity, the timing of pregnancies, seasonality (harvest period vs. other parts of the year), maternal education, completion of immunization scheme, stunted growth of the mother herself, and infectious diseases in the area [7].

However, there is a strong influence of the socioeconomic status on all these variables that are intensely intercorrelated (e.g., mothers with lower socioeconomic status tend to suffer more from infectious diseases, have a rapid succession of pregnancies, larger family sizes). Although the maternal educational level is very often associated with stunting, the causal mechanism is not known; this variable may be a proxy for socioeconomic status or a determinant of the maternal–infant interaction, use of health services, or maternal diet [8].

Millennium declaration

In 2000, the Millennium Declaration by The United Nations commits world leaders to combat poverty, hunger, disease, illiteracy, environmental degradation, and discrimination against women. The Millennium Declaration identified fundamental values essential to international relations (A/RES/55/2). The Millennium Development Goals (MDGs) were defined as eight international development goals to be achieved by 2015 addressing poverty, hunger, maternal and child mortality, communicable disease, education, gender inequality, environmental damage, and the global partnership [9]. The "**hunger**" component of the first MDG aimed to reduce the proportion of people who suffer from hunger by half between 1990 and 2015 [9]. The preparation of this goal was specifically based on the understanding that undernutrition which includes fetal growth restriction, stunting, wasting, and deficiencies of vitamin A and zinc, along with suboptimal breastfeeding, represents the crucial underlying cause of death in an estimated 45% of all deaths among children under 5 years of age.[9] The proportion of underweight children in developing countries has declined from 28% to 17% between 1990 and 2013 [10]. This rate of progress is close to the rate required to meet the MDG target; however, the improvements have been unevenly distributed between and within different regions [10]. While many countries are successfully engaged in reducing poverty, only less than a quarter of developing countries really achieved the goal of halving undernutrition.

The global burden of undernutrition remains high with surprisingly little evidence of change in many countries despite economic growth, in fact, the positive trend in stunting and wasting prevalence toward a decline in incidence/prevalence has been reversed and the actual numbers of affected children are again on the rise [11]. Nearly half of all deaths in children under 5 worldwide are attributable to mal/undernutrition; the main reason being that undernutrition increases mortality of children due to infectious disease as well as the frequency and severity of such infections, and significantly compromises recovery [11]. The vicious interplay between undernutrition and infection that strongly correlate together can create a potentially lethal cycle of worsening illness and deteriorating nutritional status in a given population. As mentioned previously, poor nutrition in the first 1000 days of a child's life can also lead to stunted growth, which is associated with impaired cognitive ability and reduced educational and occupational performance.

While the 2019 edition of the joint malnutrition estimates in a report by UNICEF, WHO, and World Bank group shows that stunting prevalence has been declining since the year 2000, nearly one in four—149 million children under 5—were stunted in 2018, and over 49 million suffered from wasting [11]. Meanwhile, the number of overweight children worldwide has remained stagnant for more than a decade. In the Post-2015 Development Era, estimates of child malnutrition should determine whether the world is on track to achieve the Sustainable Development Goals—particularly, Goal 2 to "end hunger, achieve food security and improved nutrition, and promote sustainable agriculture."

To spur further action and monitor progress, WHO Global Nutrition Targets were established for six malnutrition indicators to be achieved by 2025 [12]. These indicators include stunting (the goal of 40% reduction in the number of children under 5 who are stunted), anemia (the goal is the 50% reduction of anemia in women of reproductive age), low birth weight (LBW) (the goal is the 30% reduction in LBW), childhood overweight (the goal is no further increase in childhood overweight), breastfeeding (the goal is the increase in the rate of exclusive breastfeeding in the first 6 months up to at least 50%), and wasting (reduce and maintain childhood wasting to less than 5%). A WHO and UNICEF review in 2018 concluded that the goal of eliminating all forms of malnutrition by 2030 is unfortunately not achievable and, on the basis of trends so far, and recommended targets for the malnutrition indicators up to 2030 [13].

Maternal undernutrition and pregnancy

Out of all perinatal conditions associated with restriction of the fetal growth, maternal undernutrition is the most common one. Even though the phenotype of aberrant fetal growth is highly complex, several diagnostic categories can be used to roughly describe fetal growth, of which the LBW, intrauterine growth restriction (IUGR), and small for gestational age (SGA) are the most common. Low birth is generally defined as birth weight under 2500 g [14]. IUGR can be then vaguely defined as a rate of fetal growth that is less than normal in light of the growth potential of that specific infant [15]. The "normal" infant is the one whose birth weight is between the 10th and 90th percentile as per the gestational age, gender, and race with no clinical signs of malnutrition and/or growth retardation. The term IUGR has been often interchangeably used together with "small for gestational age" (SGA) in medical literature, which is not entirely methodologically correct [15]. The SGA definition is based on the cross-sectional evaluation (either prenatal or postnatal), and this term is used for those neonates whose birth weight is less than the 10th percentile for given gestational age or two standard deviations below the cut-off values on growth charts for a given population. The definition for SGA, therefore, considers only the birth weight without any consideration of the in utero growth and physical characteristics at birth. IUGR, on the contrary, is a clinical definition and should apply to all neonates born with clinical features of malnutrition and in utero growth retardation, irrespective of their birth weight percentile.

Based on the anthropometric and clinical feature, three types of IUGR, asymmetrical IUGR (malnourished babies), symmetrical IUGR (hypoplastic small for date), and mixed IUGR, can be distinguished [16]. IUGR has a complex etiology and occurs as a result of complex interplay between the maternal, placental, fetal, and environmental factors. Among the most common maternal factors predisposing to IUGR are maternal age, high altitude and hypoxia, low socioeconomic status, race and ethnicity, maternal substance abuse, maternal medication, parity, assisted reproduction techniques, and history of IUGR in a previous pregnancy. Among the most often placental factors predisposing to IUGR are placental weight, abnormal uteroplacental vasculature, confined placental mosaicism, placental dysfunction, thrombophilia-associated placental complications, multiple infarctions, syncytial knots, and many others. Among the most common fetal factors are constitutionally small (50%–70% of SGAs), chromosomal abnormalities, genetic syndromes, major congenital defects, multiple gestations, congenital infections, metabolic disorders, and poor nutrition during embryonic and/or fetal phase of development [15].

There is a huge difference in the distribution of causes of LBW between the developed and developing countries. While in developing countries the majority of LBW cases are due to IUGR, the most common cause of LBW in developed countries is the preterm birth and inborn defects of the fetus. In the developing countries, the major prognostic factor for IUGR development is maternal undernutrition and IUGR has been reported to be more frequent in women who are underweight or stunted before conception or who did not have sufficient weight gain during pregnancy. Among other factors that strongly impair fetal growth in utero are infections, both acute and chronic, and cigarette smoking. In the developed countries, on the contrary, cigarette smoking is the leading factor for IUGR development, followed by maternal undernutrition, preeclampsia, genetics, and substance abuse.

The prevalence of LBW in 2015 was 14.6% (uncertainty range [UR] 12.4–17.1) compared with 17.5% (14.1–2.3) in 2000 (average annual reduction rate [AARR] 1.23%) [14]. It has been reported that in 2015, an estimated 20.5 million (UR 17·4–24·0 million) livebirths fulfilled the criteria for the LBW, whereas 91% of these cases originated from low- and middle-income countries, mainly southern Asia (48%) and sub-Saharan Africa (24%) [14].

Pathophysiology of IUGR with respect to maternal nutrition

The placenta of mammals is a unique structure as it represents a highly efficient multifunctional interface that integrates signals from the mother as well as the child to match the demands of the fetus with the maternal supply of nutrients and oxygen. Moreover, it simultaneously ensures that fetal waste products are transferred back to the mother and further eliminated from the body. Aberrant structure or function of placenta, i.e., anomalies in its size, histopathological morphology, blood supply and vasculature, as well as transport capacity for individual nutrients, may contribute to altered nutrient supply and is critically important for the prenatal growth trajectory of the fetus and are intercorrelated with birth weight [17].

The placenta, therefore, exists as an interface between the maternal—fetal circulations and as such is critical for fetal nutrition and oxygenation. Physiologically, the placenta undergoes during ongoing pregnancy a variety of physiological changes tightly regulated by maternal as well as fetal hormones, nutrient-sensing genes, as well as other factors, regulating, e.g., angiogenesis, to maximize efficiency for a steadily increasing demand for nutrients. Perturbations in the maternal environment resulting in maternal undernutrition may adversely alter these changes [17].

Generally, maternal undernutrition can be associated with i) altered placental size, ii) altered histomorphological picture, iii) changes in vascularization and angiogenesis, iv) modification of capacity for transfer of nutrients as well as with v) modified endocrine reactions of the fetus, and vi) aberrant growth of the fetus.

Effects of maternal undernutrition on the fetus

Animal studies

Outcomes of fetal programming have been studied epidemiologically in humans, but specific cause and effect changes have been largely determined with the use of murine, nonhuman primate, porcine, and ovine models [18]. As such, these models facilitated understanding of important mechanisms explaining the relationship between maternal nutrition and fetal/postnatal growth.

First, ovine research has shown that preconception is a critical period in which nutritional insult has adverse consequences for offspring [19]. Studies with sheep show that diet intervention in early pregnancy can largely overcome prepregnancy obesity [20]. In this study, ovine ewes that were over- or underfed before conception (resulting in obese or malnourished states) had the offspring that each had deleterious metabolic phenotypes. The design of this study was based on assignment to one of four groups: control—control group fed at 100% maintenance energy requirements for at least 5 months, control-restricted group that was fed 100% MER for 4 months and 70% MER for 1 month, high—high group fed ad libitum (170%—190% MER) for 5 months, or high-restricted group that was fed ad libitum for 4 months and 70% for 1 month. The authors of this study conclude that the exposure to maternal overnutrition in the periconceptional period alone results in an increased body fat mass in the offspring and that recovery is possible after a relatively short period of time.

Second, the research on cattle has shown specific biological effects behind the compromised ability to achieve and maintain pregnancy, if extreme energy malnutrition occurs preconception. It has been reported that high-yielding dairy cows are experiencing a substantial decline in fertility of decades of intense breeding [21]. The decrease in fertility has been observed for the long periods of time, whereas factors such as farm management, feed ratios, breed of the cattle, and genetics are being considered the underlying causes. The impact on oocyte and embryo quality is compromised in relation to the severity of energy malnutrition [22].

Third, porcine research has provided structure for pregnancy-stage nutrition priorities to optimally support subsequent lactation and fetal and infant growth. From a global health perspective, unless adequate energy and quality protein intake (containing adequate essential amino acids) are provided to young, first-time (e.g., teenage) mothers in late pregnancy continuing through lactation, then small maternal body mass (from which to draw energy and amino acids) and mammary growth will be inadequate to support optimal milk production. Decreased maternal body mass and decreased milk secretion could limit postnatal infant growth and may complicate the plight of infants born to young mothers who presumably (as with dairy cows and pigs) may also provide less immune protection[18].

Fourth, there is enormous amount of evidence from mice that describe the direct effect of maternal malnutrition on the offspring in mice [23]. The explanation of these observations goes to the periconceptional period with the combination of metabolic, mitochondrial, and chromosomal alterations in oocytes and embryos resulting in specific proobesogenic phenotypes of the offspring later in life [24]. It has been reported in murine models that obese mothers have smaller fetuses and pups which subsequently develop overgrowth, adiposity, and glucose intolerance after birth [25]. Using this murine model of diet-induced obesity, it has been suggested that pre- and periconceptional aberrations in maternal glucose metabolism have adverse effects on oocytes and embryos that carry on to the fetus and may results in an adverse phenotype, such as obesity and metabolic syndrome, later in life. In another study on Naval Medical Research Institute (NMRI) mice that had artificially induced preconceptional and gestational obesity, the periconceptional obesogenic exposure was sufficient to shape offspring gene expression patterns as well as consequent health outcomes indicating varying developmental vulnerabilities between sexes toward metabolic disease in response to maternal overnutrition [26]. This is taken even further into the preconceptional period by the studies from Sasson et al. who describe that the pregestational exposure to a maternal HFD (HFD/control) impaired fetal and placental growth in mice despite an otherwise normal gestational milieu [27]. The mechanisms underlying these observations are still under investigation and include a vast majority of processes involved in conception/gestation, including placenta formation [28].

The main strength of the animal studies lies in the fact that these studies demonstrated the important distinction between maternal nutrition, fetal nutrition, and fetal growth. The general picture that the animal studies provide is that of the fetus growing at the end of a long supply line, depending not only on maternal nutrition but also on uterine and umbilical blood flows, placental transport, and placental and fetal metabolism that are carefully orchestrated to provide adequate nutrition to the fetus at any time. Considering these highly complex mechanisms, the changes in maternal nutrition do not always result in altered fetal nutrition, as there may be sufficient adaptation reserve in the fetal supply line. However, once significant, the changes in maternal nutrition can affect long-term health independent of size at birth.

Effects of undernutrition on fetal health in humans

The effects of the fetal health can originate in different time periods and mechanisms and can be divided to (i) preconceptional (the period before the first pregnancy, any postpartum phase (6 wk after delivery), and the interpregnancy intervals (IPIs)), (ii) periconceptional (14 weeks before conception till 10 weeks after conception), (iii) early and late pregnancy (these terms are ubiquitously used without being strictly defined), and (iv) postnatal period associated with breastfeeding quality/quantity (from the birth till the complete weaning). It has been also suggested to define the periconceptional period as the key events broadly covering the completion of meiotic maturation and differentiation of gametes, fertilization, and resumption of mitotic cell cycles in the zygote [29]. From the perspective of nutrients, the maternal nutritional factor influencing the fetal health can be seen as (i) acute, associated with the actual composition of maternal nutrition, and (ii) long-term, associated with maternal long-term nutritional status. There is an ongoing discussion on which of these time periods/mechanisms is the most critical one; however, it seems that the adverse outcomes stem most probably from various combinations of the aforementioned factors and their timelines.

Based on currently available evidence, it seems likely that the fetal growth is most susceptible to adverse effects of maternal undernutrition during the preimplantation period and in the very early stages of development of placenta. This has potential critically important consequences for the health outcomes of children from artificial reproduction as many manipulations, including nutritional ones, are being performed during these highly sensitive stages of development. The disruptions of development can at these stages result both in morphological anomalies, aberrant development, and function of placenta and altered placental transcriptome that has unknown consequences for the future health of the offspring.

Even though the pathogenesis of the restriction of the fetal growth seems from this perspective extremely complex, there are mechanisms that are undoubtedly associated with maternal undernutrition and IUGR risk.

The altered placental permeability/barrier function and transplacental transfer

To explain the relationships between placental permeability and nutritional status of the mother, there are currently two models available that do not exclude each other. In the placental nutrient-sensing model, it is assumed that placenta responds to the maternal demands, which can lead to downregulation of placental signaling pathways in response to decreased availability of nutrients in undernutrition or restriction of blood flow. There are a multitude of signals that provide information with respect to the ability of the maternal supply line to support pregnancy, with oxygen having a paramount importance and circulating maternal levels of nutrients and metabolic hormones such as cortisol, insulin, leptin, and IGF-I being other core metabolic signals informing the placenta about the nutritional status of the mother [22]. In placental nutrient-sensing model, the IUGR develops as a consequence of the availability of the nutrients. The other model of regulating placental permeability/functions comes from the animal studies and presumes that placental function is primarily controlled not by availability of the nutrients via mother but by the fetal demands. Based on these animal studies, it is proposed that the fetus signals the placenta to regulate growth and nutrient transport from the mother to the child [30]. This model in fact represents a classical homeostatic mechanism by which the fetus compensates for changes in the nutrient availability by regulating nutrient supply (i.e., placental transport) in the opposite direction, hence by increasing demands in the setting of decreased availability.

These two models do not logically exclude each other and it is highly likely that the resulting phenotype of the pregnancy (i.e., with IUGR or without it) is a consequence of multiple interaction pathways involving both model situations. A multitude of nutrient-sensing pathways have been already identified in the syncytiotrophoblast that could participate in the integration of maternal and fetal signals and the regulation of the nutrient availability to the fetus.

Alteration in the maternal endocrine system

Another possible explanation of maternally driven IUGR comes from the human as well as animal endocrinology. There is no doubt that undernutrition has huge effects on the maternal endocrine setting. The animal experiments show that insulin-like growth factor binding protein 2 (IGFBP2) is independently associated with obesity and diabetes risk in an experiment where Smith et al. examined the IGF-IGFBP axis in male rat offspring following either maternal UN or maternal obesity [31]. In another study in pregnant ewes, prenatal maternal undernutrition was found to be associated with unexpected endocrine responses of leptin, IGF1, and cortisol during fasting (lack of or the opposite response compared with the controls) in 2-year-old offspring [32]. In a recent paper, it was suggested that due to an increase in hepatic gluconeogenesis enzymes in IUGR offspring, the aberrant intrauterine milieu may lead to impaired unfolded protein response signaling in hepatic tissues; these alterations early in life might contribute to the predisposition of IUGR fetuses to adult metabolic disorders [33]. In a in vitro study on rat adipocytes, metabolic dysregulation in offspring of undernourished mothers was mediated by increased adipocyte size and reduced insulin responsiveness in samples of both subcutaneous and retroperitoneal adipose tissue. Moreover, these functional and morphological changes in adipocytes were followed by impaired activity of the insulin signaling cascade highlighting the important role of different adipose tissue depots [34].

Altered organ structure

Further understanding of the maternally driven IUGR associated with malnutrition comes with an understanding of the effects of altered organ structure/function associated with undernutrition. Early nutrient restriction may cause irreversible changes in the structure/physiology of the body that may from the long-term perspective contribute to enhanced risks further in life. The capacity of the body to compensate for the loss and/or underdevelopment of certain structures is reduced after birth. e.g., the total adult number of nephrons is set very early on during nephrogenesis suggesting that maternal undernutrition affects the staged development of nephrons in as yet unknown manner [35]. Reduced nephron reserve may further on increase the risk of hypertension in the offspring. A low protein maternal diet during gestation has been reported to decrease the activity of placental 11β-hydroxysteroid dehydrogenase, therefore exposing the fetus to maternal glucocorticoids and modifying the hypothalamic–pituitary–adrenal axis in the offspring [36].

Effect of maternal undernutrition on growth trajectories of the child

It has been estimated that 20% of linear growth faltering occurs already in utero [37]. Although there is a wide variation between countries, 11%–16% of newborns in developing countries are born with LBW (i.e., birth weight <2500 g), and 27% of newborns are SGA, which is defined as being <10th percentile in weight for infant gestational age and sex [16]. Distribution of the in utero growth faltering is heterogeneous—the analyses of cross-sectional data from 54 countries have shown that the mean length-for-age z score in Africa and Asia is below the WHO standard median at birth and progressively declines through 24 months of age with little to no recovery thereafter [38].

Only a few studies have been performed so far that has grouped infants according to their individual linear growth [39]. One of such studies used pooled height and weight data from five nationally representative longitudinal studies totaling 176,720 observations from 41,567 children and adults to estimate the risk of adult obesity at the age of 35 years for the current population of children in the United States [40]. The authors of this study concluded that using this methodology, the majority of today's US children (57.3%; 95% uncertainly interval [UI], 55.2 to 60.0) will be obese at the age of 35 years, and roughly half of the projected prevalence will occur during childhood [40]. In another study, the total of four trajectory groups of linear growth was identified. When comparing the group with the optimum growth trajectory, the subjects in the group with the slowest growth trajectory were shorter already at birth (mean: 45.4 compared with 49.7 cm; $P = .003$) and their birth weight was lower (mean: 2.59 compared with 3.49 kg; $P < .001$) [41]. However, this study did not give any specifics on maternal determinants of fetal growth, hence the interpretation of the findings is difficult.

In another study on a large, HIV-unexposed, urban birth cohort from Zimbabwe who was followed from birth through 2 y of age, a total of four patterns of postnatal linear growth were identified [8]. The following five antenatal factors explained the probability of infant membership in any given group: maternal height and education and infant birth length, birth weight, and sex. Analyses of multicountry data have shown 2.90-times greater odds (95% CI: 2.56, 3.33) of stunting in 12- to 60-month-old children who were born with LBW than in children with normal birth weight [37]. These results show the importance of focusing on multisectoral interventions to improve the education, health, and nutritional status of females before pregnancy to improve transgenerational effects on infant growth.

Effects of maternal undernutrition on health of the offspring later in life

Important evidence for the largely epigenetic and transgenerational nature of the effects of undernutrition is the existence of intergenerational cycle of growth failure. This cycle was first described in 1992 in the Second report on the world nutrition situation [42]. Basically, the intergenerational cycle of growth failure describes how poor nutrition perpetuates itself across multiple generations of females. The young girls suffering from stunting become subsequently stunted women that are more likely to give birth to low birth weight children. If these infants are of female gender, they further continue in the cycle till the adulthood. The main presumption of the whole concepts, therefore, is that adult women who are shorter are more

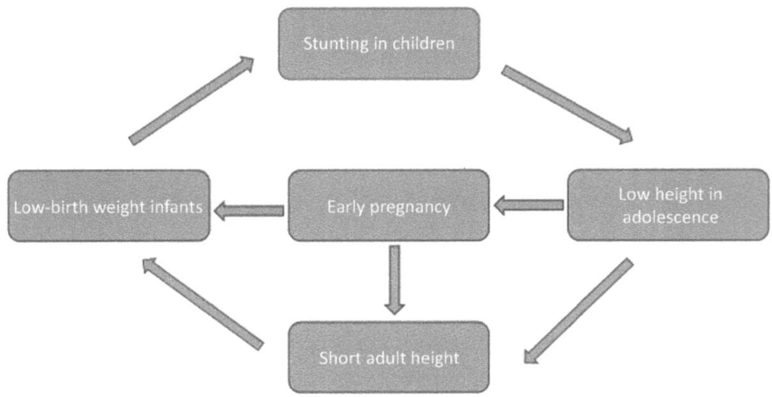

Figure 4.1 Transmission of growth failure across generations through female population.

likely to have low birth weight infants, as maternal size and birth weight are strongly intercorrelated. Also, it is known that children born with the LBW have a higher probability of displaying growth failure during childhood. Small girls therefore tend to turn into smaller women who have higher probability of having a child with LBW. It seems logical to base the interventions on breaking the cycle through improving the birth weights of the children as it is substantially easier than influencing the socioeconomic factors associated with stunted growth in later childhood and adolescence. This cycle therefore explains how growth failure is transmitted across generations through the mothers (Fig. 4.1).

The developmental origins of adult disease hypothesis—initially proposed by Dr. Barker—states that environmental influences, including nutrition, can in the early life "program" the risks of complex diseases later in life [43]. The mechanisms for this are largely unknown, although it may seem logical that maternal nutrition during pregnancy can program adult disease susceptibility through epigenetic changes of the fetal genome that program for the adult genotype and phenotype (Fig. 4.2).

A link between epigenetics and prenatal programming has recently started to emerge in multiple humans studies. Epigenetic alterations, such as DNA methylation, histone modification, chromatin packing, and microRNA expression, are emerging as key mediators of developmental programming [44]. As the known epigenetic mechanisms are highly flexible in their nature and can accumulate over time, developmental insults can have profound effect on this process, leading to altered gene expression and development of disease phenotypes further in life [45].

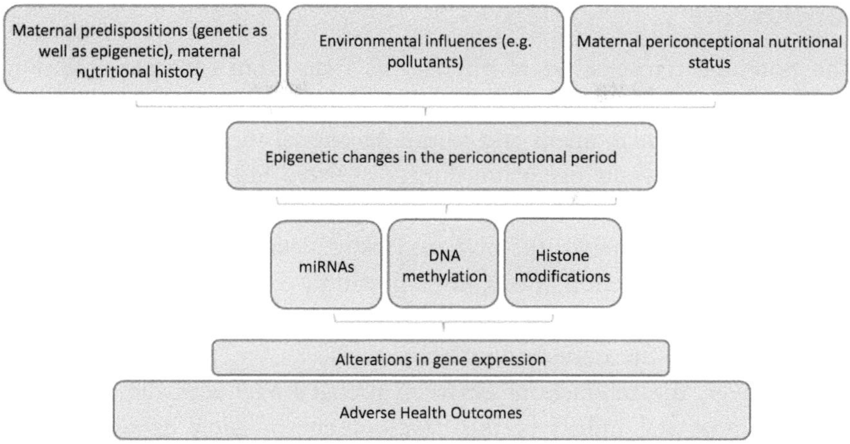

Figure 4.2 Epigenetic processes leading toward fetal adverse health outcomes.

Evidence comes from, e.g., one of the classical studies in the field that describe that individuals who were prenatally exposed to famine during the Dutch Hunger Winter in 1944–45 had six decades later less DNA methylation of the imprinted IGF2 gene compared with their unexposed, same-sex siblings [46]. Additionally, a higher risk of insulin resistance was found in the daughters of women exposed to the Dutch Hunger Winter, suggesting that programming might be transmitted to the following generations [47]. An evidence comes, e.g., from a recent study of the methylation of the leptin promoter in a cohort of children at birth, at 12 months, and at 4 years. Methylation at a specific site (cg19594666) of the leptin promoter at 12 months was inversely associated with 4-year weight ($r = -0.11$, $P = .02$) and BMI ($r = -0.13$, $P = .007$), which persisted following adjustment for weight at birth and at 12 months [48]. In another study on adult offspring of women with gestational diabetes, the offspring of women with diabetes in pregnancy exhibited increased *ADIPOQ* DNA methylation and decreased *ADIPOQ* and *RETN* gene expression in SAT [49]. In a study that followed GF2 DMR methylation in 120 children aged 17 months of whom 86 mothers had used and 34 had not used folic acid periconceptionally, the periconceptional use of folic acid was associated with significant epigenetic changes in IGF2 in the child that can be involved in the intrauterine programming of growth and development with currently unknown consequences for health and disease throughout life [50].

Conclusions

The potential transmission of phenotypic traits from one generation to another constitutes a very promising field of research. Epidemiological data obtained both from humans and studies in animal models clearly indicate that a plenty of events occurring during in utero life may impact on the offspring's long-term health, with the dietary signals being the major players in the game. Nevertheless, the obvious lack of detailed information on the maternal/fetal interaction throughout gestation following such events as well as the low number of longitudinal studies in humans hinder the understanding of the underlying mechanisms.

Moreover, the interactions between prenatal events including dietary ones and postnatal milieu in the development of adult diseases remain poorly understood. Even though the animal models of perinatal programming currently serve as a critical research tool to study the impact of developmental insults on the offspring's health, novel approaches are needed to follow the trajectories of related health outcomes in humans.

Acknowledgment

This paper was supported by the CETOCOEN PLUS (CZ.02.1.01/0.0/0.0/15_003/0000469) project of the Ministry of Education, Youth and Sports of the Czech Republic. The project was also supported by the RECETOX Research Infrastructure (LM2015051 and CZ.02.1.01/0.0/0.0/16_013/0001761).

References

[1] Morrison JL, Regnault TRH. Nutrition in pregnancy: optimisingmaternal diet and fetal adaptations to altered nutrient supply. Nutrients 2016;8.

[2] Borge TC, Aase H, Brantsæter AL, Biele G. The importance of maternal diet quality during pregnancy on cognitive and behavioural outcomes in children: a systematic review and meta-analysis. BMJ Open 2017;7:e016777.

[3] Malnutrition. https://www.who.int/news-room/fact-sheets/detail/malnutrition.

[4] NCD Risk Factor Collaboration (NCD-RisC). Rising rural body-mass index is the main driver of the global obesity epidemic in adults. Nature 2019;569:260–4.

[5] UNICEF - Progress for Children - What is undernutrition?. https://www.unicef.org/progressforchildren/2006n4/index_undernutrition.html.

[6] Owoaje E, Onifade O, Desmennu A. Family and socioeconomic risk factors for undernutrition among children aged 6 to 23 Months in Ibadan, Nigeria. Pan Afr. Med. J. 2014;17:161.

[7] Ravaoarisoa L, et al. Socioeconomic determinants of malnutrition among mothers in the Amoron'i Mania region of Madagascar: a cross-sectional study. BMC Nutr 2018;4:6.

[8] Gough EK, et al. Linear growth trajectories in Zimbabwean infants. Am JClinNutr 2016;104:1616–27.
[9] Lomazzi M, Borisch B, Laaser U. The Millennium Development Goals: experiences, achievements and what's next. GlobHealth Action 2014;7.
[10] Millennium Development Goals (MDGs). https://www.who.int/news-room/fact-sheets/detail/millennium-development-goals-(mdgs).
[11] Malnutrition in Children. UNICEF DATA, https://data.unicef.org/topic/nutrition/malnutrition/.
[12] WHO | Global Targets 2025. WHO, http://www.who.int/nutrition/global-target-2025/en/.
[13] Branca F, Grummer-Strawn L, Borghi E, Blössner M, Onis M de. Extension of the WHO maternal, infant and young child nutrition targets to 2030. SCN News 2015:55–8.
[14] Blencowe H, et al. National, regional, and worldwide estimates of low birthweight in 2015, with trends from 2000: a systematic analysis. Lancet Glob.Health 2019;7:e849–60.
[15] Sharma D, Shastri S, Sharma P. Intrauterine growth restriction: antenatal and postnatal aspects. ClinMed Insights Pediatr 2016;10:67–83.
[16] Priante E, et al. Intrauterine growth restriction: new insight from the metabolomicapproach. Metabolites 2019;9.
[17] Belkacemi L, Nelson DM, Desai M, Ross MG. Maternal undernutrition influences placental-fetal development. BiolReprod 2010;83:325–31.
[18] Odle J, et al. The potential impact of animal science research on global maternal and child nutrition and health: alandscape Review12. Adv. Nutr. 2017;8:362–81.
[19] Ford SP, Tuersunjiang N. Maternal obesity: how big an impact does it have on offspring prenatally and during postnatal life? Expet Rev Endocrinol Metabol 2013;8:261–73.
[20] Rattanatray L, et al. Impact of maternal periconceptionalovernutrition on fat mass and expression of adipogenic and lipogenic genes in visceral and subcutaneous fat depots in the postnatal lamb. Endocrinology 2010;151:5195–205.
[21] Crowe MA, Hostens M, Opsomer G. Reproductive management in dairy cows - the future. Ir Vet J 2018;71.
[22] Leroy JLMR, et al. Nutrition and maternal metabolic health in relation to oocyte and embryo quality: critical views on what we learned from the dairy cow model. ReprodFertilDev 2015;27:693–703.
[23] Fleming TP, Eckert JJ, Denisenko O. The role of maternal nutrition during the periconceptional period and its effect on offspring phenotype. Adv Exp Med Biol 2017;1014:87–105.
[24] Fleming T, et al. Origins of lifetime health around the time of conception: causes and consequences. Lancet Lond.Engl. 2018;391:1842–52.
[25] Jungheim ES, et al. Diet-induced obesity model: abnormal oocytes and persistent growth abnormalities in the offspring. Endocrinology 2010;151:4039–46.
[26] Dahlhoff M, et al. Peri-conceptional obesogenic exposure induces sex-specific programming of disease susceptibilities in adult mouse offspring. BiochimBiophysActa 1842:304–17. 2014.
[27] Sasson IE, Vitins AP, Mainigi MA, Moley KH, Simmons RA. Pre-gestational vs gestational exposure to maternal obesity differentially programs the offspring in mice. Diabetologia 2015;58:615–24.
[28] Connor KL, et al. Maternal malnutrition impacts placental morphology and transporter expression: an origin for poor offspring growth. J. NutrBiochem 2020;78:108329.

[29] Bedzhov I, Graham SJL, Leung CY, Zernicka-Goetz M. Developmental plasticity, cell fate specification and morphogenesis in the early mouse embryo. Philos. Trans. R. Soc. B Biol. Sci. 2014;369.
[30] Sibley CP, Brownbill P, Dilworth M, Glazier JD. Review: adaptation in placental nutrient supply to meet fetal growth demand: implications for programming. Placenta 2010;31(Suppl. l):S70–4.
[31] Smith T, Sloboda DM, Saffery R, Joo E, Vickers MH. Maternal nutritional history modulates the hepatic IGF-IGFBP axis in adult male rat offspring. Endocrine 2014;46:70–82.
[32] Kongsted AH, et al. Pre- and postnatal nutrition in sheep affects β-cell secretion and hypothalamic control. JEndocrinol 2013;219:159–71.
[33] Liu X, Wang J, Gao L, Jiao Y, Liu C. Maternal proteinrestriction induces alterations in hepatic unfolded protein response-related molecules in adult rat offspring. FrontEndocrinol 2018;9:676.
[34] Thompson N, et al. Metabolic programming of adipose tissue structure and function in male rat offspring by prenatal undernutrition. NutrMetab 2014;11:50.
[35] Tafti SA, et al. Maternal undernutrition upregulates apoptosis in offspring nephrogenesis. J. Dev. Orig. Health Dis. 2011;2:226–35.
[36] Mesquita FF, Gontijo JaR, Boer PA. Maternal undernutrition and the offspring kidney: from fetal to adult life. Braz. J. Med. Biol. Res. Rev. Bras. Pesqui.Medicas E Biol. 2010;43:1010–8.
[37] Christian P, et al. Risk of childhood undernutrition related to small-for-gestational age and preterm birth in low- and middle-income countries. Int J. Epidemiol 2013;42:1340–55.
[38] Victora CG, de Onis M, Hallal PC, Blössner M, Shrimpton R. Worldwide timing of growth faltering: revisiting implications for interventions. Pediatrics 2010;125:e473–480.
[39] MON A, CABANA M, Halpern-Felsher B, Meyerhoff DJ. Human linear growth trajectory defined. Am. J. Hum. Biol. Off. J. Hum. Biol. Counc. 2013;25:666–72.
[40] Ward ZJ, et al. Simulation of growth trajectories of childhood obesity into adulthood. N Engl J Med 2017;377:2145–53.
[41] Martins C, et al. Diverse physical growth trajectories in institutionalized Portuguese children below age 3: relation to child, family, and institutional factors. J. PediatrPsychol 2013;38:438–48.
[42] Martorell R, Zongrone A. Intergenerational influences on child growth and undernutrition. PaediatrPerinatEpidemiol 2012;26(Suppl. 1):302–14.
[43] Wadhwa PD, Buss C, Entringer S, Swanson JM. Developmental origins of health and disease: brief history of the approach and current focus on epigenetic mechanisms. SeminReprodMed 2009;27:358–68.
[44] Silveira PP, Portella AK, Goldani MZ, Barbieri MA. Developmental origins of health and disease (DOHaD). JPediatr(Rio J) 2007;83:494–504.
[45] Jirtle RL, Skinner MK. Environmental epigenomics and disease susceptibility. Nat Rev Genet 2007;8:253–62.
[46] Heijmans BT, et al. Persistent epigenetic differences associated with prenatal exposure to famine in humans. Proc Natl Acad Sci USA 2008;105:17046–9.
[47] Stein AD, Lumey LH. The relationship between maternal and offspring birth weights after maternal prenatal famine exposure: the Dutch Famine Birth Cohort Study. HumBiol 2000;72:641–54.

[48] Mansell T, et al. Methylation of the LEP gene promoter in blood at 12 months and BMI at 4 years of age-a population-based cohort study. Int J. Obes 2005. https://doi.org/10.1038/s41366-020-0553-3. 2020.
[49] Houshmand-Oeregaard A, et al. Differential adipokine DNA methylation and gene expression in subcutaneous adipose tissue from adult offspring of women with diabetes in pregnancy. Clin Epigenet 2017;9:37.
[50] Steegers-Theunissen RP, et al. Periconceptional maternal folic acid use of 400 microg per day is related to increased methylation of the IGF2 gene in the very young child. PloS One 2009;4:e7845.

CHAPTER 5

Vitamin status in pregnancy and newborns

Emily C. Keats[1], Rehana A. Salam[2], Kimberly D. Charbonneau[1], Zulfiqar A. Bhutta[1,2]

[1]Centre for Global Child Health, the Hospital for Sick Children, Toronto, ON, Canada; [2]Center of Excellence in Women and Child Health, Aga Khan University, Karachi, Pakistan

Contents

Molecular Nutrition
ISBN 978-0-12-813862-5
https://doi.org/10.1016/B978-0-12-813862-5.00005-0

Maternal vitamin status

Background and global burden of maternal vitamin deficiencies

Maternal nutritional status is closely associated with fetal development and newborn health. Undernutrition during pregnancy, including vitamin deficiencies, does not only inflict major health risks on the mother and fetus through poor pregnancy and birth outcomes, but goes beyond parturition to impact child growth and development [1,2]. Inadequate dietary intakes are a major cause of vitamin deficiencies, but general infections, chronic diseases, malaria, and helminths infestation can also contribute to undernutrition through directly inhibiting absorption of nutrients [3,4].

Pregnancy is a state of special nutrient needs because the body is providing for the developing fetus. As such, vitamin deficiencies can be exacerbated during this time. However, assessment of vitamin and mineral status during pregnancy is difficult and there is a general lack of pregnancy-specific laboratory indexes for nutritional evaluation. Furthermore, assessment of vitamin status can be challenging due to alterations in vitamin and mineral concentrations during pregnancy. This occurs because of the physiological increase in blood volume and subsequent hemodilution that results in decreased plasma levels of certain vitamins, while others are unaffected due to increases in carrier proteins [5]. The role of confounding factors, like infections, remains uncertain and are poorly quantified, making it difficult to estimate the actual number of subclinical deficiencies.

The World Health Organization (WHO) estimates that over two billion people are at risk of vitamin A, iodine and/or iron deficiency globally [2]. Other vitamin and micronutrient deficiencies of public health concern include zinc, vitamin D, and the B vitamins. Anemia, one of the major global nutrition concerns, can be caused by deficiency of iron in the diet but is also associated with vitamin deficiencies like vitamin A, B6, B12, riboflavin (vitamin B2), and folate (vitamin B9), making it challenging to discern the primary deficiency. The vast majority of women and children with vitamin deficiencies reside in low and middle-income countries (LMICs), where diets are often insufficient to meet daily requirements. However, these deficiencies can occur in some population groups in high-income settings as well. In 1995, the WHO estimated the global distribution of vitamin A deficiency (VAD), finding that about three million children in over 60 countries had some form of xerophthalmia (a progressive eye disease caused by VAD), and that subclinical

VAD was considered a problem for at least 251 million people including school-age children and pregnant women [6–8]. In 2005, night blindness, which is an indicator of VAD, was estimated to affect 9.7 million women, while about 19.1 million pregnant women had deficient serum retinol concentrations. VAD is a public health problem particularly in Africa and South-East Asia. In contrast to VAD, the global prevalence of other vitamin deficiencies, like folate (vitamin B9), have not been estimated because of the scarcity of suitable population-based data [6,8]. The majority of data on folate deficiencies are based on small, local surveys, but they suggest that this type of deficiency may be a public health problem affecting millions of people globally. Although few nationally representative surveys exist for vitamin D status, people residing in diverse geographical areas, and many in LMICs in Asia, might be vitamin D insufficient or deficient. Thiamine (vitamin B1) and vitamin B6 deficiencies have been observed in diverse populations globally while pellagra, which occurs due to insufficient vitamin B3, exists endemically in poorer areas of Africa, China, and India [6].

Much of what we know about vitamin deficiencies during pregnancy is based on observational studies and intervention trials in which low or high maternal intakes are associated with negative or positive pregnancy outcomes. Vitamins play a key role in maternal health and fetal growth and development. Folate and B12 deficiencies during pregnancy are associated with adverse congenital and pregnancy outcomes including neural tube defects (NTDs), low birth weight (LBW), and preterm birth [9,10]. Deficiencies of vitamins other than folate have also been associated with complications of pregnancy and abnormal fetal development. There is some evidence suggesting that low maternal vitamin D levels in pregnancy might be associated with an increased risk of preeclampsia, gestational diabetes (GDM), preterm birth, and small for gestational age (SGA); along with several disorders of calcium metabolism in both the mother and her infant, including neonatal hypocalcemia and tetany, infant hypoplasia of tooth enamel, and maternal osteomalacia [11]. In addition, low maternal vitamin A status has been associated with intrauterine growth retardation in communities at risk for vitamin A deficiency [5]. These observational studies and intervention trials have given rise to speculation about the biological pathways of action of vitamins during pregnancy, especially for folate and vitamin B6, where adverse outcomes are commonly reported. For example, folates play a critical role in cellular metabolism, including for amino acids and other compounds that are needed for nucleic acid synthesis [12].

As such, folate deficiency in early pregnancy could lead to impaired cell growth and division, resulting in fetal malformations. Vitamin B6 is also required for metabolism, and is involved in hormonal, immune, and erythrocyte functions [12]. The physiologically active form of vitamin B6 is involved in over 100 known chemical reactions that are needed to synthesize nonessential amino acids and other important compounds including histamine, dopamine, serotonin, aminobutyric acid, and heme [12]. Though these functions are undoubtedly essential for normal physiological processes during pregnancy, studies have been unable to convincingly link vitamin B6 supplements with improved pregnancy outcomes [12]. In general, more research into the mechanistic actions of vitamins during pregnancy is warranted.

The role of vitamins during pregnancy

Vitamin A

Vitamin A (retinol) is important in small amounts for visual health, immune function, and fetal growth and development. Women are susceptible to VAD throughout pregnancy; however, susceptibility is at its highest during the third trimester of pregnancy due to accelerated fetal development and the physiological increase in blood volume during this period. VAD during gestation can lead to fetal wastage, although high doses of vitamin A in early pregnancy can be teratogenic as well [13]. Maternal night blindness, a symptom of VAD, has been associated with LBW and infant mortality [14,15].

B vitamins

A substantial proportion of NTDs are related to inadequate maternal consumption of folic acid around the time of conception, and can also be associated with genetic factors that increase the need for dietary folic acid in some populations. Risk of NTDs increases 10-fold as maternal folate status goes from adequate to poor. Between days 21 and 27 postconception, the fetal neural plate closes to form what will eventually be the spinal cord and cranium; NTDs result from improper closure of the spinal cord and cranium, and are the most common congenital abnormalities associated with folate deficiency. Folate and vitamin B12 deficiencies are also associated with adverse pregnancy outcomes, including LBW and preterm birth. Thiamine, vitamin B6 and B12 deficiencies are of unknown importance for pregnancy outcomes, but associations have been previously made with abnormal fetal development [16]. Vitamin B6 plays a vital role in numerous metabolic processes in the human body, such as nervous system development and functioning. Deficiency of riboflavin and B6 almost invariably occur in combination with deficiencies of other B-complex vitamins.

Vitamin C and E

Oxidative stress occurs when there is an imbalance in the number of free radicals circulating in the body and antioxidants to counter the free radicals [16]. Links have been made between oxidative stress during pregnancy and the development of preeclampsia, increased risk of intrauterine growth restriction, and preterm rupture of membranes (PROM). Oxidative stress has also been implicated in many disorders common to preterm infants including chronic lung disease, necrotizing enterocolitis, and others [6]. As antioxidants, vitamins E and C act synergistically to help prevent oxidative stress, and thus supplementation with vitamins E and C is often concurrent. Deficiencies in vitamins C and E have been associated with pregnancy complications, but further research is required to determine the true relationship [16]. One trial in women at risk of preeclampsia found that provision of vitamins C and E during pregnancy resulted in a 60% lower rate of preeclampsia [1,17].

Vitamin D

Vitamin D is a fat-soluble vitamin which is generated in the body primarily through exposure to sunlight. It is found naturally in only a few foods, such as fish-liver oils, fatty fish, mushrooms, egg yolks, and liver. Vitamin D is required to maintain normal blood levels of calcium and phosphate, which are in turn needed for the normal mineralization of bone, muscle contraction, nerve conduction, and general cellular function in all cells of the body. Vitamin D also possesses immunomodulatory properties that may alter responses to infections *in vivo* [6]. Vitamin D has an essential role in fetal development, ensuring the fetal supply of calcium for bone development, enabling the immunological adaptation required to maintain normal pregnancy, preventing miscarriage, and promoting normal brain development [18]. Poor maternal vitamin D status has been associated with severe preeclampsia, in turn leading to an increased risk of perinatal morbidity and mortality [19]. Maternal vitamin D deficiency, especially in early pregnancy, has been associated with an increased risk of preeclampsia, preterm birth, and infants born SGA [11].

Vitamin K

Vitamin K is an essential fat-soluble vitamin needed for a unique post-translational chemical modification in a small group of proteins with calcium-binding properties, collectively known as vitamin K-dependent or Gla proteins. Specifically, vitamin K acts as a cofactor in a carboxylation reaction that converts selective glutamate (Glu) residues to γ-carboxyglutamate (Gla) residues that then bind with the protein prothrombin for coagulation. Thus far, the only unequivocal role of vitamin K in health is in the maintenance of normal coagulation [6]. Its role during pregnancy is not yet clear; however, vitamin K deficiency can cause bleeding in an infant in the first weeks of life, known as hemorrhagic disease of the newborn.

Vitamin requirements during pregnancy

Table 5.1 below summarizes the vitamin requirements during pregnancy and lactation, based on the Institute of Medicine guidelines and other sources [20–22].

Strategies for the prevention of maternal vitamin deficiencies

Pregnant women should especially be encouraged to maintain adequate nutrition, which is best achieved through consumption of a healthy, balanced diet. However, in many settings, this isn't feasible and multiple deficiencies coexist, suggesting the need for simple approaches that address multiple micronutrient and vitamin deficiencies at once [23]. Several strategies have been employed to prevent and manage these deficiencies among pregnant women, including education, dietary modification, food provision, agricultural interventions, and supplementation and fortification, either alone or in combination [24].

Supplementation is the most widely practiced intervention and is currently in place to combat iron, folate, and vitamin A deficiencies among high-risk populations. Daily oral iron and folic acid (a synthetic form of folate) supplementation is recommended as part of routine antenatal care to reduce the risk of LBW, anemia, and iron deficiency [25]. Two systematic reviews examining the effects of folic acid supplementation during pregnancy identified a 69% reduction in the risk of NTDs, but no important impact on the reduction of preterm births, stillbirths, neonatal deaths, LBW babies, or pre-delivery maternal anemia [9,26]. Vitamin A supplementation

Table 5.1 Vitamin requirements during pregnancy and lactation.

Vitamins	Unit	RDA*			Institute of medicine RDA for Pregnancy			Institute of medicine RDA for Lactation		
		PP	P	L	14–18 years	19–30 years	31–50 years	14–18 years	19–30 years	31–50 years
Vitamin A (retinol)	μg	700	770	1300	750	770	770	1200	1300	1300
Vitamin B1 (thiamin)	Mg	1.1	1.4	1.4	1.4	1.4	1.4	1.4	1.4	1.4
Vitamin B2 (riboflavin)	Mg	1.1	1.4	1.6	1.4	1.4	1.4	1.6	1.6	1.6
Vitamin B3 (niacin)	Mg	14	18	17	18	18	18	17	17	17
Vitamin B5 (pantothenic acid)	Mg	5	6	7	*6*	*6*	*6*	7	7	7
Vitamin B6 (pyridoxine)	Mg	1.3	1.9	2.0	1.9	1.9	1.9	2.0	2.0	2.0
Vitamin B7 (biotin)	μg	30	30	35	*30*	*30*	*30*	*35*	*35*	*35*
Vitamin B9 (folate)	μg	400	600	500	600	600	600	500	500	500
Vitamin B12 (cobalamin)	μg	2.4	2.6	2.8	2.6	2.6	2.6	2.8	2.8	2.8
Vitamin C (ascorbate)	Mg	75	85	120	80	85	85	115	120	120
Vitamin D (cholecalciferol)	IU	600	600	600	15	15	15	15	15	15
Vitamin E (tocopherol acetate)	Mg	15	15	19	15	15	15	19	19	19
Vitamin K (phytomenadione)	μg	90	90	90	*75*	*90*	*90*	*75*	*90*	*90*

Note: adequate intakes are in *italics*. *L*, lactation; *P*, pregnancy; *PP*, pre-pregnancy; *RDA*, recommended dietary allowance.

is only recommended for pregnant women in areas where vitamin A deficiency is a severe public health problem (i.e., if $\geq$ 5% of women in a population have a history of night blindness in their most recent pregnancy in the previous 3–5 years that ended in a live birth, or if $\geq$ 20% of pregnant women have a serum retinol level <0.70 μmol/L) [27]. Two systematic reviews of vitamin D supplementation in pregnancy showed an overall reduction, of borderline significance, in LBW. The impact of vitamin D supplementation in pregnancy on long-term growth and developmental outcomes of children has not been sufficiently evaluated, and the current evidence base is too poor to support definite clinical recommendations regarding vitamin D supplementation in pregnancy [28,29]. However, there is modest evidence to support a relationship between maternal vitamin D status and offspring birthweight, bone mass, and serum calcium concentrations, but these findings are limited by their observational nature and low quality of the included studies [28,30,31]. Vitamin D supplementation during pregnancy has been associated with improved maternal vitamin D status, which may have a direct influence on the fetal and neonatal supply of vitamin D [29,32–34], and may be necessary to ensure adequate concentrations of vitamin D in breast milk during lactation [35]. Existing data do not support routine vitamin C or vitamin E supplementation, alone or in combination with other supplements, for the prevention of fetal or neonatal death, poor fetal growth, preterm birth, or preeclampsia [36], and the WHO does not currently recommend vitamin E and C supplementation for pregnant women to improve maternal and perinatal outcomes. The existing review on vitamin B6 supplementation found very few trials that met the inclusion criteria; of them, many possessed unclear trial methodology, reported few clinical outcomes, and had inadequate follow-up, suggesting that there is not enough evidence to understand the potential clinical benefits of vitamin B6 supplementation in pregnancy and/or during labor, other than one trial suggesting protection against dental decay [37].

Food fortification is a cost-effective public health intervention that targets a larger population through a single strategy [38,39]. A recent systematic review on the real world effectiveness of food fortification strategies suggests that iron fortification of staple foods led to a significant increase in serum ferritin (iron stores) and reduction in anemia among pregnant women and women of reproductive age [40]. Folate fortification significantly reduced the incidence of congenital abnormalities, such as NTDs, without increasing the incidence of twinning. The number of studies pooled for zinc and multiple micronutrients for women were few, though the evidence suggested some benefit. Overall, these reviews have pointed to a dearth of evidence for the impact of fortification strategies on morbidity (i.e., diarrhea, pneumonia, malaria, urinary tract infections (UTI), and fever) and mortality outcomes in women and children [40,41]. In addition, the evidence of effectiveness studies from developing countries, where vitamin deficiencies are highly prevalent, is scarce when compared to studies in high-income settings. Key challenges when ensuring a sustainable fortification program include identifying the right food vehicle (considering bioavailability, interaction with other foods, availability, acceptability, and cost) and target population, as well as ensuring the quality of product along with population-level consumption of the fortified food in sufficient quantities [41].

In the last decade, point-of-use, or home, fortification of maternal and child foods consumed in the household has emerged to tackle widespread micronutrient deficiencies. Multiple micronutrient powders (MNPs), sometimes termed Sprinkles, are powdered, encapsulated vitamins and minerals that can be added to prepared foods with little change to the foods' taste or texture. MNPs are designed to provide the recommended daily nutrient intake of two or more vitamins and minerals to their target populations. The use of MNPs has been tested for effectiveness in children; however, its effectiveness in improving micronutrient status among pregnant and lactating women is yet to be explored outside emergency settings [42].

Table 5.2 below summarizes the efficacy of vitamin supplementation interventions during pregnancy on key maternal and child health outcomes. Effect estimates are based on the most recent Cochrane review of the intervention [9,15,26,29,33,36,37,43].

Newborn vitamin status

Vitamins play critical roles relating to growth, metabolism, prevention of disease, and maintenance of health. They are obtained from the diet and, consequently, vitamin deficiencies among women and children are common where consumption of food is in insufficient quantities or diets are not diverse enough to provide the recommended daily dietary intake. Vitamin deficiencies can also occur from inhibited absorption of nutrients due to infections, inflammation, or chronic disease. Considering the rapid physiological changes that take place as a neonate matures into a child, any

Table 5.2 Known effects of vitamin supplementation interventions during pregnancy on key maternal, birth, and child survival outcomes.

	Maternal anemia	Maternal mortality	Miscarriage	Low birthweight	Small-for-gestational age	Preterm	Stillbirth	Perinatal mortality	Neonatal mortality	Other
Vitamin B9 (folate)	– (RR = 0.62, 95% CI: 0.35 to 1.10)	Insufficient evidence	– (RR = 1.10, 95% CI: 0.94 to 1.28)	– (RR = 0.83, 95% CI: 0.66−1.04)	Insufficient evidence	– (RR = 1.01, 95% CI: 0.73 to 1.38)	Pooled with neonatal mortality to get perinatal mortality	– (RR = 1.33, 95% CI: 0.96 −1.85)	Pooled with stillbirth to get perinatal mortality	Neural tube defects: ⬇ RR = 0.31 (95% CI: 0.17 to 0.58)
Vitamin A (retinol)	⬇ (RR = 0.64, 95% CI: 0.43 to 0.94)	– (RR = 0.88, 95% CI: 0.65 to 1.20)	Insufficient evidence	– (RR = 1.02, 95% CI: 0.89 to 1.16)	Insufficient evidence	– (RR = 0.98, 95% CI: 0.94 to 1.01)	– (RR = 1.04, 95% CI: 0.98 to 1.10)	– (RR = 1.01, 95% CI: 0.95 to 1.07)	– (RR = 0.97, 95% CI: 0.90 to 1.05)	Maternal night blindness:(this should have a downward arrow) (RR = 0.79, 95% CI: 0.64 to 0.98)
Vitamin D (cholecalciferol)	Insufficient evidence	Insufficient evidence	Insufficient evidence	⬇ (RR = 0.55, 95% CI: 0.35 to 0.87)	Insufficient evidence	– (RR = 0.66, 95% CI: 0.34 to 1.30)	– (RR = 0.35, 95% CI: 0.06 to 1.98)	Insufficient evidence	– (RR = 0.27, 95% CI 0.04 to 1.67)	Preeclampsia:(this should have a downward arrow) (RR = 0.48, 95% CI: 0.30 to 0.79)
Vitamin E (tocopherol acetate)	Insufficient evidence	– (RR = 0.60, 95% CI: 0.14 to 2.51)	Insufficient evidence	Insufficient evidence	Insufficient evidence	– (RR = 0.98, 95% CI: 0.88 to 1.09)	– (RR = 1.17, 95% CI: 0.88 to 1.56)	Insufficient evidence	– (RR = 0.81, 95% CI: 0.58 to 1.13)	Placental abruption: ⬇ (RR = 0.64, 95% CI: 0.44 to 0.93)
Vitamin C (ascorbate)	Insufficient evidence	– (RR = 0.60; 95% CI: 0.14 to 2.51)	Insufficient evidence	Insufficient evidence	Insufficient evidence	– (RR = 0.99, 95% CI: 0.90 to 1.10)	– (RR = 1.15, 95% CI: 0.89 to 1.49)	– (RR = 1.07, 95% CI: 0.77 to 1.49)	– (RR = 0.79, 95% CI: 0.58 to 1.08)	Placental abruption: ⬇ (RR = 0.64, 95% CI: 0.44 to 0.92)

–, no statistically significant effect of the intervention;

⬇, intervention significantly reduces outcome; *CI*, confidence interval; *RR*, relative risk.

vitamin deficiencies relating to the mother or the offspring themselves can have severely detrimental consequences on newborn growth and development [6].

A newborn will have acquired most of its store of vitamins from the mother when it was in the womb. Water-soluble vitamins (B-complex vitamins and vitamin C) are actively transported across the placenta throughout pregnancy whereas fat-soluble vitamins (vitamins A, D, and E) are delivered toward the end of gestation [44]. The exception to this is vitamin K, another fat-soluble vitamin, that is transferred in very minimal amounts to the fetus [45]. Breast milk from mothers with adequate nutritional status will provide sufficient levels of vitamins to newborns, with the exception of vitamins K and D. Infants that are not supplemented with vitamin K postnatally will rely on its synthesis by gut bacteria. Vitamin D is acquired antenatally, but is also synthesized in the skin from UV sunlight [45].

Recommended nutrient intakes (RNIs) are set at 2 standard deviations around the estimated average requirement (EAR), which is based on the average intake of healthy, exclusively breastfed infants. However, there are several factors that can influence the vitamin and mineral requirements of a newborn. For example, those with darker skin or those who are not exposed to adequate amounts of sunlight, either for geographical or cultural reasons, are at risk of vitamin D deficiency. Additionally, genetic variability and maternal nutritional status can play a significant role. Higher reference values are used for recommended intakes in order to capture these at-risk populations. RNIs for infants aged 0–6 months are found in Table 5.3. Information on specific vitamins is summarized below.

Vitamin A

Infants up to 6 months of age who are exclusively breastfed will have adequate amounts of vitamin A to maintain optimal growth and development and build up proper stores of retinol in the liver. Retinol is the main circulating form of vitamin A in the blood. The recommended intake is 180 μg retinol equivalents (RE)/day, with a tolerable upper limit of 375 μg RE/day [6].

Vitamin A deficiencies can occur in infants who are not fed breast milk or where maternal retinol levels are low. Infections have been shown to lower serum retinol concentrations by as much as 25% [6], and other

Table 5.3 Recommended nutrient intakes (RNI) for infants 0–6 months [6]

RNI (0–6 months)	Recommended nutrient intakes (RNI) by WHO	Adequate intakes (AIs) by IOM
Water-soluble vitamins		
Vitamin C (ascorbate) (mg/day)	25	40
Vitamin B1(thiamine) (mg/day)	0.2	0.2
Vitamin B2 (riboflavin) (mg/day)	0.3	0.3
Vitamin B3 (niacin[a]) (mg NE/day)	2	2
Vitamin B6 (pyridoxine) (mg/day)	0.1	0.1
Vitamin B5 (pantothenic acid) (mg/day)	1.7	1.7
Vitamin B7 (biotin) (μg/day)	5	5
Vitamin B12 (cobalamin) (μg/day)	0.4	0.4
Vitamin B9 (folate) (μg DFE/day)	80	65
Fat-soluble vitamins		
Vitamin A (retinol) (μg RE/day)	375	400
Vitamin D (cholecalciferol) (μg/day)	5	10
Vitamin E (tocopherol) (mg α-TE/day)	2.7	4
Vitamin K (phytomenadione) (μg/day)	5	2.0

[a]preformed niacin; *IOM*, Institute of Medicine; *WHO*, World Health Organization.

micronutrient deficiencies can also inhibit levels. For example, zinc is required for the synthesis of retinol-binding protein (RBP), thus deficiencies in zinc will lead to low levels of RBP, which is the carrier protein for circulating retinol [46]. Children with protein-energy malnutrition or those who are malnourished will also produce lower levels of RBP, which leads to reduced serum retinol [47]. Consequences of vitamin A deficiency in infants are visual impairments, including blindness, anemia, and increased risk and severity of infections including measles and diarrhea [48]. For at-risk infants (i.e., those residing in vitamin A-deficient populations), the recommended intake is increased to 190 μg RE/day, with a safe upper intake level of 400 μg RE/day [6].

Vitamin D

Due to low levels in breast milk, the vitamin D that has been acquired by the fetus at the time of parturition is used throughout the first few months of infancy. If a mother has poor vitamin D status during pregnancy, low levels of vitamin D will be seen in her infant as well [49]. Vitamin D plays many important roles throughout the neonatal period relating to bone development, growth, and maturation of tissues, largely through the regulation of calcium and phosphate homeostasis. It's also thought to play a regulatory role within the immune system. Consequently, vitamin D deficiency in infants can lead to the development of rickets, or the softening and weakening of bones, and to seizures, and respiratory problems [50].

Neonates are particularly vulnerable to vitamin D insufficiency due to their increased needs during rapid skeletal growth, coupled with low levels of vitamin D that are obtained from human breast milk. This indicates that exclusively breastfed infants are a particularly high-risk population [6]. Infants that are not exposed to adequate amounts of sunlight because of cultural, seasonal (i.e., born in the winter months), or latitudinal reasons are at additional risk because of their inability to synthesize vitamin D in the skin from UV light [51].

Vitamin E

Vitamin E is a fat-soluble vitamin that is comprised of eight biologically active tocopherols (of which alpha-tocopherol has the highest antioxidant activity) that work to scavenge free radicals and prevent oxidative damage. Though there is some transport of vitamin E while the infant is in utero, neonates are relatively deficient in this vitamin at birth. Plasma levels rise rapidly among breastfed term infants, but are slower to rise in those that do not receive breast milk or are born preterm (<37 weeks gestation) or very low birth weight (<1500 g) [52]. There is evidence to show that, among these populations, insufficient body stores of vitamin E can result in oxidative stress and negative health outcomes, including retinopathy of prematurity, edema, thrombocytosis, and hemolytic anemia [53].

Vitamin K

As noted above, vitamin K (phylloquinone) is transported in minimal amounts to the fetus in utero and, consequently, infants must obtain their vitamin K through other means. The recommended nutrient intake of vitamin K for infants 0–6 months is 5 μg/day; an intake that cannot be met by breastfeeding alone. Vitamin K deficiency can have extreme consequences for neonates and infants up to 6 months of age, manifesting as vitamin K deficiency bleeding (VKDB) syndrome, a type of hemorrhagic disease. VKDB syndrome is classified based on its timing of onset: early (0–24 h after birth), classic (1–7 days), and late (1–12 weeks). However, there is no available screening for VKDB [6]. There are two major risk factors for classic and late VKDB: exclusive breastfeeding and lack of vitamin K prophylaxis [54,55]. Late VKDB is particularly problematic because it can be associated with brain damage and death [6]. The incidence of late VKDB varies depending on geography and can range from 4.4/100,000 births in the UK to 72/100,000 births in Thailand [56]. Based on the fact that mothers of infants with late VKDB appear to have normal vitamin K concentrations in their breast milk, other factors, such as reduced absorption efficiency, can contribute to the development of this condition [55].

Vitamin C

For infants aged 0–6 months, the RNI for vitamin C is set arbitrarily at 25 mg/day. Vitamin C deficiency manifests as scurvy and, in infants, this mostly affects sites of active bone growth. Characteristic signs of scurvy in infants include pseudoparalysis of limbs caused by pain associated with movement and swelling and hemorrhages of the gums and periosteum (connective tissue surrounding the bones). To prevent signs of scurvy in infants, only 8 mg/day of maternal vitamin C is needed [6].

B-complex vitamins

It is assumed that exclusively breastfed infants are receiving adequate amounts of B-complex vitamins, therefore recommendations for intakes are largely based on quantities found in breast milk. However, if a mother is deficient in one or more B-complex vitamin, then this deficiency will also arise in the infant. For example, a maternal deficiency in thiamine will result in beriberi developing in the breastfed infant. There are other situations that can precipitate a B-complex vitamin deficiency in infants as well. For example, infants receiving phototherapy for the treatment of neonatal jaundice are at risk of developing riboflavin deficiency. Subsequently, the infant may be at risk for developing a deficiency in vitamin B6 because of the role that riboflavin plays in the formation of the functional enzyme, pyridoxal 5′-phosphate (PLP). Because PLP is involved in the metabolism of amino acids, infants that are deficient in vitamin B6 can experience epileptic-form convulsions and immune dysfunction. Riboflavin and vitamin B6 also have a biochemical relationship to niacin because of their role in the conversion of L-tryptophan to niacin equivalents [6].

Importance of breast milk

Breast milk contains all the essential nutrients required for healthy growth and development in an infant's first 6 months of life, with continued nutritional benefits seen beyond 1 year. Serving as a significant source of energy and key nutrients, breast milk is important in the protection against many common childhood illnesses, such as diarrhea and pneumonia. Continued, frequent breastfeeding, particularly in developing countries, has proven to aid in greater linear growth [57], reduced risk for overweight or obesity in childhood and adolescence [57–59], and reduced risk of child morbidity and mortality [57,60]. Accordingly, to ensure optimal growth, development, and health, the WHO recommends that all infants be exclusively breastfed for the first 6 months of life, after which nutritionally adequate complementary foods should be incorporated with continued breastfeeding for up to 2 years or beyond [57]. The WHO additionally recommends early initiation of breastfeeding, within 1 hour of delivery, as it further reduces the risk for neonatal morbidity and mortality, as colostrum (i.e., the first milk) is rich in protective effects [61–63].

Breast milk vitamin concentrations

For newborns, EARs are based on the average intake of healthy, exclusively breastfed infants. Retinol concentrations in breast milk vary by country, ranging from 0.70 to 2.45 μmol/L. As infants consume on average 750 mL of breast milk per day during the first 6 months, exclusively breastfed infants will consume about 375 μg RE each day, which is well above the recommended value [6]. The average intake of vitamin K from breast milk is < 1 μg/day, which is approximately 100 times lower than intake of phylloquinone from infant formula. However, in the case of classic VKDB, studies have suggested that it is the low intake of breast milk, as opposed to a lower than normal concentration of vitamin K in the milk, which is important [54,55]. A German study concluded that a minimum daily intake of 100 mL colostral milk (0.2–0.3 μg phylloquinone) is sufficient for hemostasis during the early neonatal period [54], highlighting the importance of early breastfeeding practices. Similarly, high concentrations of vitamin E can be found in breast milk, particularly colostrum, with average concentrations of 3.28 mg/dL. When term infants are exclusively breastfed, serum vitamin E levels comparable to those of adults can be seen within 4 to 6 days [64]. Infants who are breastfed should receive adequate amounts of vitamin C, as breast milk contains a mean of 40 mg/L vitamin C, and the RNI is 25 mg/day. Contrarily, breast milk contains low levels of vitamin D and infants are not provided with their required dose through breast milk alone, with many infants relying on vitamin D stores acquired in utero [6]. Mean breast milk contents of B-complex vitamins for an average intake of 0.75 L per day are summarized in Table 5.4. It is assumed that exclusively breastfed infants are receiving adequate amounts of B-complex vitamins [6].

Infant formula

When breastfeeding is not feasible, infant formula is often used as a substitute. Cow milk or soymilk are most commonly used for infant formulas, with supplemental ingredients added to closely align the nutrient content with that of human breast milk [65]. For instance, the concentration of vitamin E in human milk is approximately 0.32 mg/100 mL milk, and thus formula milk is required to contain at least 0.3 mg α-TE/100 mL of reconstituted feed and not less than 0.4 mg α-TE/g polyunsaturated fatty acid (PUFA). Similarly, infant formulas are enriched with 6 −15 mg of

Table 5.4 The mean content of B-complex vitamins found in human breast milk

Vitamin	Breast milk content (/0.75 L secreted milk per day)
Vitamin B1 (thiamine)	0.16 mg
Vitamin B2 (riboflavin)	0.26 mg
Vitamin B3 (niacin[a])	4 mg
Vitamin B_6 (pyridoxine)	0.1 mg
Vitamin B5 (pantothenic acid)	1.7 mg
Vitamin B7 (biotin)	5 μg
Vitamin B12 (cobalamin)	0.3 μg
Vitamin B9 (folate)	80 μg

[a]niacin equivalents.

vitamin D in order to prevent rickets. Phylloquinone concentrations are about 50 μg/L in most fortified formulas and infants solely fed on formula have plasma levels 10 times higher than the adult average of about 1.0 nmol/L (0.5 μg/L), greatly reducing their risk for VKDB [6].

In some environments, infants who are fed formula can be at an increased health risk due to the high cost of infant formula, lack of clean water, difficulties associated with reading or following mixing instructions, and poor hygiene. Particularly, risks with formula use have arisen due to the use of unsafe water and unsterilized equipment during preparation and the potential presence of contaminants such as bacteria in some powdered formulas. Malnutrition may also result from the overdilution of formula, usually done to make one's supplies last longer, especially by people without proper education.

With the high cost of formula, supply may become unavailable, and a return to breastfeeding may not be possible due to diminished breast milk production, further putting an infant at risk of malnutrition [66,67]. In light of the risks involved with improper use of breast-milk substitutes such as infant formulas, an International Code of Marketing of Breast-milk Substitutes was implemented to prohibit the promotion of breast-milk substitutes to the general public. This code states that usual marketing practices are unsuitable for these products and the marketing of breast-milk substitutes requires special treatment. According to the WHO, the decision on whether to use infant formula, which product, and how should not depend upon the effectiveness of commercial advertising but instead on informed decision-making based on objective and consistent advice, and appropriate supervision [66]. It is WHO's hope that implementation of this code will improve breastfeeding practices, as the production and promotion of manufactured breast-milk substitutes has resulted in a decline in breastfeeding, with only 38% of infants being exclusively breastfed during their first 6 months [67].

Global burden of newborn vitamin deficiencies

There remains a dearth of data on the prevalence of vitamin deficiencies in many countries, especially for newborns, making it difficult to quantify deficiencies across the globe. The more common worldwide micronutrient deficiencies, such as vitamin A, are highlighted in a larger number of studies, allowing for estimations of prevalence to be made. Though data on the prevalence rates for a number of vitamin deficiencies are not readily available, it is certain that vitamin deficiencies exist in the poorer regions of the world where undernutrition, food shortages, and undiversified diets persist [68].

Vitamin A

While the prevalence of VAD is more commonly reported than other types of deficiencies, particularly in regards to LMICs, no studies have specifically looked at deficiency prevalence in newborns. A pooled analysis of 138 LMICs analyzed the trends in VAD, defined as a serum retinol concentration lower than 0·70 μmol/L, in children aged 6–59 months between 1991 and 2013 [69]. In 1991, approximately 39% of children aged 6–59 months were vitamin-A deficient, with prevalence rates ranging from 40% in sub-Saharan Africa, East and Southeast Asia and Oceania, and South Asia, to under 25% in Latin America and the Caribbean, Central Asia, the Middle East, and North Africa. From 1991 to 2013, there was a small improvement in VAD worldwide, decreasing to 29% prevalence. The prevalence of VAD decreased to 6% in East and Southeast Asia and Oceania, to 11% in Latin American and the Caribbean, Central Asia, the Middle East, and North Africa. However, little change occurred in sub-Saharan Africa and South Asia, with both maintaining prevalence rates above 40% [69].

Vitamin D

Fewer studies have reported the prevalence of vitamin D deficiency in LMICs, and no study assessed prevalence rates in newborns. The level at which to determine vitamin D deficiency is not clearly defined, with many professionals debating the cut-off as less than 75 nmol/L or less than 50 nmol/L [70]. A 2013 systematic review utilized both definitions to assess global vitamin D status in infants. When assessing the prevalence of vitamin D levels below 75 nmol/L, vitamin D deficiency prevalence ranged from 31% to 98%. Specifically, the prevalence of infants with vitamin D levels below 75 nmol/L was 31% in Alaska, 34% in China, 47% of black infants and 56% of white infants in the United States, 56% in Tanzania, 64% in Argentina, 88% in Pakistan, and 98% in Turkey. When looking at vitamin D levels below 50 nmol/L, prevalence rates remained high among infants in certain geographies: 5% in China, 9% in Tanzania, 11% in Alaska, 24% in Argentina, 10% of white infants and 46% of black infants in the United States, 40% in Australia, 69% in Germany, 71% in Pakistan, 90% in Turkey,

93% in Iran, 96% in Kuwait, and 99% in India [70]. A number of studies included in the review additionally assessed vitamin D levels below 30 nmol/L, finding prevalence rates of 0.4% in China, 3% in Argentina, 11% in Australia, 33% in Pakistan, 51% in Turkey, 61% in India, 66% in Kuwait, and 86% in Iran [70]. The data available demonstrates the high prevalence of low vitamin D status across the globe, with higher prevalence rates seen in the Middle East. Based on the limited number of countries with data available, this review also highlights the need for more studies within this area to further understand the issue of vitamin D deficiency across the globe [70].

Multiple micronutrient deficiencies

Many infants in LMICs are deficient in more than one micronutrient. Multiple micronutrient deficiencies often involve a combination of vitamins and minerals, with the most common deficiencies being vitamin A, iodine, iron, and zinc. These deficiencies can result from a lack of breastfeeding and low consumption of micronutrient-rich foods such as fruits, vegetables, animal products, and fortified foods [68,71–73]. The presence of disease also plays a significant role in multiple micronutrient deficiencies. For instance, diarrhea in infants has been associated with VAD [74], vitamin D deficiency [75], as well as vitamin K deficiency due to decreased nutrient absorption from the intestinal tract and reduced synthesis as a result of a shift in the bacterial flora [76]. Additionally, malaria has been associated with reduced levels of vitamin E [77] and vitamin A [77,78].

Strategies for newborn vitamin deficiencies

Vitamin A

Guidance from the WHO indicates that supplementation with vitamin A is not recommended for neonates (0–28 days). It is, however, recommended for children 6–59 months to reduce morbidity and mortality where VAD is a public health problem [48]. The degree of public health problem is established using population prevalence of low serum retinol ($\leq$0.70 μmol/L) for infants 6–71 months of age, where 2%–9% indicates a mild problem, 10%–19% indicates a moderate problem, and $\geq$20% indicates a severe public health problem [79]. Interest in vitamin A supplementation for neonates was explored through randomized controlled trials conducted in populations with varying levels of vitamin A deficiency. A subsequent Cochrane review (2017) synthesized results from 12 trials and found no significant reduction in infant death at 6 or 12 months following supplementation [80]. There has been some evidence to suggest an increased risk of bulging fontanelles in infants less than 6 months of age who were given two or more doses of 7500 μg or 15,000 μg preformed vitamin A in oil [81,82].

Vitamin D

Though there are no WHO guidelines yet, current evidence suggests that vitamin D supplements may be efficacious in preventing rickets, especially among high-risk infants [51]. There are several ongoing systematic reviews that will inform the evidence on the efficacy of vitamin D supplementation for preventing vitamin D deficiency and improving bone health among term babies [83] and among preterm and LBW infants [84].

Vitamin E

A systematic review examining the potential benefits of providing high dose, intravenous vitamin E to preterm or LBW neonates found conflicting results; beneficial effects on severe retinopathy and blindness, but a significantly increased risk of sepsis among supplemented infants [53]. Consequently, the WHO currently does not recommend high-dose vitamin E supplementation for preterm infants.

Vitamin K

The recommended vitamin K intake for infants cannot be met by breastfeeding alone. As such, it has become common practice in most developed and some developing countries to provide vitamin K supplements in the period immediately following parturition [6]. Following a reported epidemiologic association between intramuscular vitamin K and the development of childhood cancer [85], oral supplements are more commonly used now (this is despite the fact that subsequent studies did not support this linkage) [86,87]. However, oral supplements may not be effective for preventing VKDB among infants with poor absorption [88]. National vitamin K prophylactic strategies differ by country and may include a single intramuscular injection or multiple oral doses throughout the neonatal period [6]. A systematic review compared the effects of a 0.2 mg intravenous dose of vitamin K, a 0.2 mg intramuscular dose of vitamin K, and a 0.5 mg intramuscular dose of vitamin K, on vitamin K levels in infants less than 32 weeks' gestation. Infants in all groups had normal or supraphysiologic levels following vitamin K dose administration, with no significant differences found between doses or administration methods. However, limited evidence is available on the most appropriate dose and administration method for preterm infants and further research is needed [89].

Conclusions

We have demonstrated the critical role that both water- and fat-soluble vitamins play in pregnancy and during the neonatal period. Without them, normal physiological processes can be impaired, resulting in adverse consequences for both mother and baby. Vitamins are especially important for growth and developmental processes, and can result in poor long-term outcomes if not available in sufficient amounts during critical windows, both in utero and in infancy. Vitamin deficiencies are more common in LMICs, where women and children may not consume enough diverse foods that will provide adequate daily amounts, though deficiencies have been noted in several population groups in high-income settings as well. Strategies to prevent and manage these deficiencies, such as micronutrient supplementation or fortification, should focus on populations at risk for deficiencies.

References

[1] Black RE. Micronutrients in pregnancy Micronutrients in pregnancy. Br J Nutr 2001;85:S193–7.

[2] Black RE, Victora CG, Walker SP, Bhutta ZA, Christian P, De Onis M, Ezzati M, Grantham-Mcgregor S, Katz J, Martorell R, et al. Maternal and child undernutrition and overweight in low-income and middle-income countries. The Lancet 2013:427–51. Lancet Publishing Group.

[3] Bhutta ZA, Salam RA, Das JK. Meeting the challenges of micronutrient malnutrition in the developing world. Br Med Bull [Internet] 2013;106:7–17 [cited 2019 Sep 18]. Available from, http://www.ncbi.nlm.nih.gov/pubmed/23645843.

[4] Guerrant RL, Lima AA, Davidson F. Micronutrients and infection: interactions and implications with enteric and other infections and future priorities. J Infect Dis Immun 2000;182(Suppl. 1):S134–8 [cited 2019 Sep 18]. Available from, http://www.ncbi.nlm.nih.gov/pubmed/10944495.

[5] Picciano MF. Pregnancy and lactation: physiological adjustments, nutritional requirements and the role of dietary supplements. J Nutr [Internet] 2003;133(6):1997S–2002S [cited 2019 Sep 18]. Available from, http://www.ncbi.nlm.nih.gov/pubmed/12771353.

[6] WHO. WHO | Vitamin and mineral requirements in human nutrition. WHO. World Health Organization; 2005.
[7] McLean E, Cogswell M, Egli I, Wojdyla D, De Benoist B. Worldwide prevalence of anaemia, WHO vitamin and mineral nutrition information system, 1993-2005. Publ Health Nutr 2009;12:444−54.
[8] WHO. WHO | Global prevalence of vitamin A deficiency in populations at risk 1995-2005. WHO. World Health Organization; 2009.
[9] De-Regil LM, Peña-Rosas JP, Fernández-Gaxiola AC, Rayco-Solon P. Effects and safety of periconceptional oral folate supplementation for preventing birth defects. Cochrane Database of Syst Rev 2015;(12). John Wiley and Sons Ltd.
[10] Bhaskaram P. Micronutrient malnutrition, infection, and immunity: an overview. Nutr Rev 2002;60(5):S40−5. Pt. 2, [cited 2019 Sep 18]. Available from, http://www.ncbi.nlm.nih.gov/pubmed/12035857.
[11] Wei S-Q, Qi H-P, Luo Z-C, Fraser WD. Maternal vitamin D status and adverse pregnancy outcomes: a systematic review and meta-analysis. J Matern Fetal Neonatal Med 2013;26(9):889−99 [cited 2019 Sep 18]. Available from: http://www.ncbi.nlm.nih.gov/pubmed/23311886.
[12] Institute of Medicine (US). Committee on nutritional status during pregnancy and lactation. Water-soluble vitamins. Nutrition during pregnancy: Part I weight gain: Part II nutrient supplements [Internet]. Washington, D.C.: National Academies Press (US); 1990. Available from: https://www.ncbi.nlm.nih.gov/books/NBK235220/.
[13] Azaïs-Braesco V, Pascal G. Vitamin A in pregnancy: requirements and safety limits. Am J Clin Nutr 2000;71(Suppl. 5):1325S−33S [cited 2019 Sep 18]. Available from: http://www.ncbi.nlm.nih.gov/pubmed/10799410.
[14] Christian P, West KP, Khatry SK, Katz J, Shrestha SR, Pradhan EK, LeClerq SC, Pokhrel RP. Night blindness of pregnancy in rural Nepal - nutritional and health risks. Int J Epidemiol 1998;27:231−7.
[15] McCauley ME, van den Broek N, Dou L, Othman M. Vitamin A supplementation during pregnancy for maternal and newborn outcomes. Cochrane database Syst Rev [Internet] 2015;(10):CD008666 [cited 2019 Sep 18]. Available from: http://www.ncbi.nlm.nih.gov/pubmed/26503498.
[16] Ramakrishnan U, Manjrekar R, Rivera J, Gonzáles-Cossío T, Martorell R. Micronutrients and pregnancy outcome: a review of the literature. Nutr Res 1999:103−59.
[17] Chappell LC, Seed PT, Briley AL, Kelly FJ, Lee R, Hunt BJ, Parmar K, Bewley SJ, Shennan AH, Steer PJ, et al. Effect of antioxidants on the occurrence of pre-eclampsia in women at increased risk: a randomised trial. Lancet, vol. 354. Elsevier Limited; 1999. p. 810−6.
[18] Wagner CL, Taylor SN, Johnson DD, Hollis BW. The role of vitamin D in pregnancy and lactation: emerging concepts. Women's Health 2012;8:323−40.
[19] Lm D, Palacios C, Ansary A, Kulier R, Jp P. Vitamin D supplementation for women during pregnancy. Cochrane Database Syst Rev 2012;(2).
[20] Institute of Medicine (US). Committee to review dietary reference intakes for vitamin D and calcium. Dietary reference intakes for calcium and vitamin D [internet]. In: Ross AC, Taylor CL, Yaktine AL, Del Valle HB, editors. Dietary reference intakes for calcium and vitamin D. Washington, DC: National Academies Press (US); 2011. p. 1116 [cited 2019 Oct 30] Available from: http://www.ncbi.nlm.nih.gov/pubmed/21796828.
[21] Dietary Reference Intakes for Calcium. Phosphorus, magnesium, Vitamin D, and fluoride. DietAry reference intakes for calcium, phosphorus, magnesium, Vitamin D, and fluoride. National Academies Press; 1997.

[22] Trumbo P, Yates AA, Schlicker S, Poos M. Dietary reference intakes: vitamin A, vitamin K, arsenic, boron, chromium, copper, iodine, iron, manganese, molybdenum, nickel, silicon, vanadium, and zinc. J Am Diet Assoc 2001;101:294–301.
[23] Ramakrishnan U. Prevalence of micronutrient malnutrition worldwide, vol. 60. Nutr Rev. Oxford University Press (OUP); 2002. p. S46–52.
[24] Bhutta ZA, Das JK, Rizvi A, Gaffey MF, Walker N, Horton S, Webb P, Lartey A, Black RE. Evidence-based interventions for improvement of maternal and child nutrition: what can be done and at what cost? The Lancet 2013:452–77. Lancet Publishing Group.
[25] World Health Organization. Guideline. Daily iron and folic acid supplementation in pregnant women. 2012. p. 27.
[26] Lassi ZS, Salam RA, Haider BA, Bhutta ZA. Folic acid supplementation during pregnancy for maternal health and pregnancy outcomes. Cochrane database Syst Rev [Internet] 2013:CD006896 [cited 2019 Sep 18]. Available from: http://www.ncbi.nlm.nih.gov/pubmed/23543547.
[27] WHO UNICEF, IVACG Task Force. Vitamin A supplements: a guide to their use in the treatment and prevention of vitamin A deficiency and xerophthalmia. 1997.
[28] Harvey NC, Holroyd C, Ntani G, Javaid K, Cooper P, Moon R, Cole Z, Tinati T, Godfrey K, Dennison E, et al. Vitamin D supplementation in pregnancy: a systematic review. Health Technol Assess [Internet] 2014;18(45):1–190 [cited 2019 Sep 18]. Available from: http://www.ncbi.nlm.nih.gov/pubmed/25025896.
[29] Palacios C, Kostiuk LK, Peña-Rosas JP. Vitamin D supplementation for women during pregnancy. Cochrane Database Syst Rev [Internet] 2019;(7) [cited 2019 Nov 4]; Available from: http://doi.wiley.com/10.1002/14651858.CD008873.pub4.
[30] Maxwell JD, Ang L, Brooke OG, Brown IR. Vitamin D supplements enhance weight gain and nutritional status in pregnant Asians. Br J Obstet Gynaecol [Internet] 1981;88(10):987–91 [cited 2019 Sep 18]. Available from: http://www.ncbi.nlm.nih.gov/pubmed/6793058.
[31] Thorne-Lyman AL, Fawzi WW. Vitamin A and carotenoids during pregnancy and maternal, neonatal and infant health outcomes: a systematic review and meta-analysis. Paediatr Perinat Epidemiol [Internet] 2012;26(Suppl. 1):36–54 [cited 2019 Sep 18]. Available from: http://doi.wiley.com/10.1111/j.1365-3016.2012.01284.x.
[32] Brooke OG, Carter ND, Brown IRF, Cleeve HJW, Robinson VP, Bone CDM, Maxwell JD, Winder SM. Vitamin D supplements in pregnant Asian women: effects on calcium status and fetal growth. Br Med J 1980;280:751.
[33] Lm D, Palacios C, Ansary A, Kulier R, Jp P. Vitamin D supplementation for women during pregnancy (Review) summary of findings for the main comparison. Cochrane Database Syst Rev 2012;(2).
[34] Yu CKH, Sykes L, Sethi M, Teoh TG, Robinson S. Vitamin D deficiency and supplementation during pregnancy. Clin Endocrinol (Oxf) [Internet] 2009;70(5):685–90 [cited 2019 Sep 18]. Available from: http://www.ncbi.nlm.nih.gov/pubmed/18771564.
[35] Christian P, Khatry SK, Katz J, Pradhan EK, LeClerq SC, Shrestha SR, Adhikari RK, Sommer A, West KP. Effects of alternative maternal micronutrient supplements on low birth weight in rural Nepal: double blind randomised community trial. BMJ [Internet] 2003;326(7389):571 [cited 2019 Sep 18]. Available from: http://www.ncbi.nlm.nih.gov/pubmed/12637400.
[36] Rumbold A, Ota E, Nagata C, Shahrook S, Crowther CA. Vitamin C supplementation in pregnancy. Cochrane Database Syst Rev [Internet] 2015 [cited 2019 Sep 18]; Available from: http://doi.wiley.com/10.1002/14651858.CD004072.pub3.

[37] Salam RA, Zuberi NF, Bhutta ZA. Pyridoxine (vitamin B6) supplementation during pregnancy or labour for maternal and neonatal outcomes. Cochrane Database of Systematic Reviews 2015;(3). John Wiley and Sons Ltd.
[38] World Health Organization. Food and agricultural organization of the united nations. Guidelines on food fortification with micronutrients. WHO. World Health Organization; 2006.
[39] Garrett GS, Matthias D, Keats EC, Mbuya M, Wouabe E. Doubling down on food fortification to fortify the future [Internet]. The Optimist. 2019 [cited 2019 Nov 30]. Available from: https://www.gatesfoundation.org/TheOptimist/Articles/food-fortification-to-fortify-the-future.
[40] Keats EC, Neufeld LM, Garrett GS, Mbuya MNN, Bhutta ZA. Improved micronutrient status and health outcomes in low-and middle-income countries following large-scale fortification: evidence from a systematic review and meta-Analysis. Am J Clin Nutr. Oxford University Press 2019;109:1696–708.
[41] Das JK, Salam RA, Kumar R, Bhutta ZA. Micronutrient fortification of food and its impact on woman and child health: a systematic review. Syst Rev [Internet] 2013;2:67 [cited 2019 Sep 18]. Available from: http://www.ncbi.nlm.nih.gov/pubmed/23971426.
[42] Salam RA, Macphail C, Das JK, Bhutta ZA. Effectiveness of micronutrient powders (MNP) in women and children. BMC Publ Health 2013;(Suppl. 3).
[43] Rumbold A, Ota E, Hori H, Miyazaki C, Crowther CA. Vitamin E supplementation in pregnancy. Cochrane database Syst Rev [Internet] 2015 [cited 2019 Sep 18]; Available from: http://doi.wiley.com/10.1002/14651858.CD004069.pub3.
[44] Leaf AA. Vitamins for babies and young children. Arch Dis Child 2007:160–4.
[45] Powers HJ. Vitamin requirements for term infants: considerations for infant formulae. Nutr Res Rev [Internet] 1997;10(1):1–33 [cited 2019 Sep 16]. Available from: http://www.ncbi.nlm.nih.gov/pubmed/19094256.
[46] Mann J, Truswell AS. Organic and inorganic essential nutrients. Essentials of human nutrition [Internet]. Oxford University Press; 2017. p. 113–269 [cited 2019 Sep 16]. Available from: +J.,+%26+Truswell,+S.+(Eds.).+(2017).+Organic+and+inorganic+essential+nutrients.+En:+Essentials+of+human+nutrition.+pp.113–269++Oxford+University+Press&ots=cr4pA2xTy_&sig=uBfiCI.
[47] Sommer A, Sommer A, World Health Organization. Vitamin A deficiency and its consequences: a field guide to detection and control. World Health Organization; 1995. p. 69.
[48] World Health Organization. Guideline. Neonatal vitamin A supplementation. 2011. p. 21.
[49] Greer FR. 25-Hydroxyvitamin D: functional outcomes in infants and young children. Am J Clin Nutr [Internet] 2008;88:529S–33S [cited 2019 Sep 16]. Available from: http://www.ncbi.nlm.nih.gov/pubmed/18689395.
[50] WHO. WHO | Vitamin D supplementation in infants. WHO. World Health Organization; 2019.
[51] Lerch C, Meissner T. Interventions for the prevention of nutritional rickets in term born children. Cochrane database Syst Rev [Internet] 2007;(4):CD006164 [cited 2019 Sep 16]. Available from: http://www.ncbi.nlm.nih.gov/pubmed/17943890.
[52] Pacifici GM. Effects of vitamin E in neonates and young infants, vol. 4. Mashhad Univ Med Sci. Mashhad University of Medical Sciences; 2016. p. 1745–57.
[53] Brion LP, Bell EF, Raghuveer TS. Vitamin E supplementation for prevention of morbidity and mortality in preterm infants. Cochrane database Syst Rev [Internet] 2003;(4):CD003665 [cited 2019 Sep 16]. Available from: http://www.ncbi.nlm.nih.gov/pubmed/14583988.

[54] von Kries R, Becker A, Göbel U. Vitamin K in the newborn: influence of nutritional factors on acarboxy-prothrombin detectability and factor II and VII clotting activity. Eur J Pediatr [Internet] 1987;146(2):123–7 [cited 2019 Sep 16]. Available from: http://www.ncbi.nlm.nih.gov/pubmed/3569346.
[55] von Kries R, Shearer MJ, Göbel U. Vitamin K in infancy. European J Pediatr 1988:106–12. Springer-Verlag.
[56] von Kries R, Hanawa Y. Neonatal vitamin K prophylaxis. Report of scientific and standardization subcommittee on perinatal haemostasis. Thromb Haemost [Internet] 1993;69(3):293–5 [cited 2019 Sep 16]. Available from: http://www.ncbi.nlm.nih.gov/pubmed/8470054.
[57] WHO. WHO | Continued breastfeeding for healthy growth and development of children. WHO. World Health Organization; 2019.
[58] Horta BL, Loret De Mola C, Victora CG. Long-term consequences of breastfeeding on cholesterol, obesity, systolic blood pressure and type 2 diabetes: a systematic review and meta-analysis. Acta Paediatrica 2015:30–7. Intl J Paediatr. Blackwell Publishing Ltd.
[59] Yan J, Liu L, Zhu Y, Huang G, Wang PP. The association between breastfeeding and childhood obesity: a meta-analysis. BMC Public Health [Internet] 2014;14(1):1267 [cited 2019 Sep 16]. Available from: http://bmcpublichealth.biomedcentral.com/articles/10.1186/1471-2458-14-1267.
[60] Sankar MJ, Sinha B, Chowdhury R, Bhandari N, Taneja S, Martines J, Bahl R. Optimal breastfeeding practices and infant and child mortality: a systematic review and meta-analysis. Acta Paediatrica 2015:3–13. International Journal of Paediatrics. Blackwell Publishing Ltd.
[61] WHO. WHO | Early initiation of breastfeeding to promote exclusive breastfeeding. WHO. World Health Organization; 2019.
[62] Debes AK, Kohli A, Walker N, Edmond K, Mullany LC. Time to initiation of breastfeeding and neonatal mortality and morbidity: a systematic review. BMC Publ Health 2013;(Suppl. 3).
[63] Khan J, Vesel L, Bahl R, Martines JC. Timing of breastfeeding initiation and exclusivity of breastfeeding during the first month of life: effects on neonatal mortality and morbidity–a systematic review and meta-analysis. Matern Child Health J [Internet] 2015;19(3):468–79 [cited 2019 Sep 16]. Available from: http://www.ncbi.nlm.nih.gov/pubmed/24894730.
[64] Ostrea EM, Balun JE, Winkler R, Porter T. Influence of breast-feeding on the restoration of the low serum concentration of vitamin E and β-carotene in the newborn infant. Am J Obstet Gynecol 1986;154:1014–7.
[65] Martin CR, Ling PR, Blackburn GL. Review of infant feeding: key features of breast milk and infant formula. Nutrients. MDPI AG; 2016.
[66] WHO, Nutrition for Health and Development. Infant formula and related trade issues IN the context OF the international code OF marketing OF breast-milk substitutes health implications OF direct advertising OF infant formula. 2001.
[67] WHO. Breastfeeding: only 1 in 5 countries fully implement WHO's infant formula Code. WHO. World Health Organization; 2014.
[68] WHO. WHO | Guidelines on food fortification with micronutrients. WHO. World Health Organization; 2018.
[69] Stevens GA, Bennett JE, Hennocq Q, Lu Y, De-Regil LM, Rogers L, Danaei G, Li G, White RA, Flaxman SR, et al. Trends and mortality effects of vitamin A deficiency in children in 138 low-income and middle-income countries between 1991 and 2013: a pooled analysis of population-based surveys. Lancet Glob Heal [Internet] 2015;3(9):e528–36 [cited 2019 Sep 17]. Available from: http://www.ncbi.nlm.nih.gov/pubmed/26275329.

[70] Palacios C, Gonzalez L. Is vitamin D deficiency a major global public health problem? J Steroid Biochem Mol Biol [Internet] 2014;144(Pt A):138–45 [cited 2019 Sep 17]. Available from: http://www.ncbi.nlm.nih.gov/pubmed/24239505.
[71] WHO. WHO | the world health report 2002 - reducing risks, promoting healthy life. WHO. World Health Organization; 2013.
[72] Imdad A, Bhutta ZA. Global micronutrient deficiencies in childhood and impact on growth and survival: challenges and opportunities. Nestle Nutr Inst Workshop Ser [Internet] 2012;70:1–10 [cited 2019 Sep 18]. Available from: http://www.ncbi.nlm.nih.gov/pubmed/25825289.
[73] Bhutta ZA. Micronutrient needs of malnourished children. Curr Opin Clin Nutr Metab Care [Internet] 2008;11(3):309–14 [cited 2019 Sep 18]. Available from: http://www.ncbi.nlm.nih.gov/pubmed/18403929.
[74] Ahmed FU, Rahman ME, Mahmood CB. Vitamin A deficiency in children with acute diarrhoea: a community-based study in Bangladesh. J Health Popul Nutr [Internet] 2000;18(2):119–22 [cited 2019 Sep 18]. Available from: http://www.ncbi.nlm.nih.gov/pubmed/11057069.
[75] Bucak IH, Ozturk AB, Almis H, Cevik MÖ, Tekin M, Konca Ç, Turgut M, Bulbul M. Is there a relationship between low vitamin D and rotaviral diarrhea. Pediatr Int [Internet] 2016;58(4):270–3 [cited 2019 Sep 18]. Available from: http://www.ncbi.nlm.nih.gov/pubmed/26287796.
[76] Bay A, Oner AF, Celebi V, Uner A. Evaluation of vitamin K deficiency in children with acute and intractable diarrhea. Adv Ther [Internet] 2006;23(3):469–74 [cited 2019 Sep 18]. Available from: http://www.ncbi.nlm.nih.gov/pubmed/16912029.
[77] Adelekan DA, Adeodu OO, Thurnham DI. Comparative effects of malaria and malnutrition on plasma concentrations of antioxidant micronutrients in children. Ann Trop Paediatr [Internet] 1997;17(3):223–7 [cited 2019 Sep 18]. Available from: http://www.ncbi.nlm.nih.gov/pubmed/9425377.
[78] Sanjoaquin MA, Molyneux ME. Malaria and vitamin A deficiency in African children: a vicious circle. Malar J [Internet] 2009;8:134 [cited 2019 Sep 18]. Available from: http://www.ncbi.nlm.nih.gov/pubmed/19534807.
[79] WHO. WHO | Serum retinol concentrations for determining the prevalence of vitamin A deficiency in populations. WHO. World Health Organization; 2018.
[80] Haider BA, Sharma R, Bhutta ZA. Neonatal vitamin A supplementation for the prevention of mortality and morbidity in term neonates in low and middle income countries. Cochrane database Syst Rev [Internet] 2017;2:CD006980 [cited 2019 Sep 16]. Available from: http://www.ncbi.nlm.nih.gov/pubmed/28234402.
[81] Baqui AH, de Francisco A, Arifeen SE, Siddique AK, Sack RB. Bulging fontanelle after supplementation with 25,000 IU of vitamin A in infancy using immunization contacts. Acta Paediatr [Internet] 1995;84(8):863–6 [cited 2019 Sep 16]. Available from: http://www.ncbi.nlm.nih.gov/pubmed/7488807.
[82] de Francisco A, Chakraborty J, Chowdhury HR, Yunus M, Baqui AH, Siddique AK, Sack RB. Acute toxicity of vitamin A given with vaccines in infancy. Lancet (London, England) [Internet] 1993;342(8870):526–7 [cited 2019 Sep 16]. Available from: http://www.ncbi.nlm.nih.gov/pubmed/8102669.
[83] Tan ML, Abrams SA, Osborn DA. Vitamin D supplementation for term breastfed infants to prevent vitamin D deficiency and improve bone health. Cochrane Database Syst Rev 2018;(6). John Wiley and Sons Ltd.
[84] Pharande P, Pammi M, Collins CT, Zhou SJ, Abrams SA. Vitamin D supplementation for prevention of vitamin D deficiency in preterm and low birth weight infants. Cochrane Database Syst Rev 2015:2015. John Wiley and Sons Ltd.

[85] Golding J, Greenwood R, Birmingham K, Mott M. Childhood cancer, intramuscular vitamin K, and pethidine given during labour. BMJ [Internet] 1992;305(6849):341–6 [cited 2019 Sep 16]. Available from: http://www.bmj.com/cgi/doi/10.1136/bmj.305.6849.341.
[86] Draper G, Mcninch A. Vitamin K for neonates: the controversy. BMJ 1994;308:867.
[87] von Kries R. Neonatal vitamin K prophylaxis: the Gordian knot still awaits untying. BMJ [Internet] 1998;316(7126):161–2 [cited 2019 Sep 16]. Available from: http://www.bmj.com/cgi/doi/10.1136/bmj.316.7126.161.
[88] Cornelissen M, von Kries R, Loughnan P, Schubiger G. Prevention of vitamin K deficiency bleeding: efficacy of different multiple oral dose schedules of vitamin K. Eur J Pediatr [Internet] 1997;156(2):126–30 [cited 2019 Sep 16]. Available from: http://www.ncbi.nlm.nih.gov/pubmed/9039517.
[89] Ardell S, Offringa M, Ovelman C, Soll R. Prophylactic vitamin K for the prevention of vitamin K deficiency bleeding in preterm neonates. Cochrane Database of Syst Rev 2018;(2). John Wiley and Sons Ltd.

CHAPTER 6

Fatty acid intake during perinatal periods

Ana Laura de la Garza[1,2], Carolina Treviño-de Alba[1], Robbi Elizabeth Cárdenas-Pérez[3,4], Alberto Camacho[3,4], Myriam Gutierrez-Lopez[1], Heriberto Castro[1]

[1]Universidad Autonoma de Nuevo Leon, Facultad de Salud Pública y Nutrición, Centro de Investigación en Nutrición y Salud Pública, Monterrey, Nuevo León, Mexico; [2]Universidad Autonoma de Nuevo Leon, Unidad de Nutrición, Centro de Investigación y Desarrollo en Ciencias de La Salud, Monterrey, Nuevo León, Mexico; [3]Universidad Autonoma de Nuevo Leon, Facultad de Medicina, Departamento de Bioquimica y Medicina Molecular, Monterrey, Nuevo Leon, Mexico; [4]Universidad Autonoma de Nuevo Leon, Unidad de Neurometabolismo, Centro de Investigación y Desarrollo en Ciencias de La Salud, Monterrey, Nuevo Leon, Mexico

Contents

Introduction

In 1990s, Barker proposed the theory of the developmental origins of health and disease (DOHaD), suggesting that adverse influences on development, particularly during perinatal period, can lead to permanent changes in physiology and metabolism, which results in an increased risk of disease in adulthood [9,10]. This theory was confirmed with two human cohort studies, including the Dutch famine and Överkalix, showing that the effect of famine and food availability during the embryonic development

Molecular Nutrition
ISBN 978-0-12-813862-5
https://doi.org/10.1016/B978-0-12-813862-5.00006-2

affects longevity and health of the descendants, increasing the susceptibility to develop diseases [36]. In order to identify the molecular and cellular effects of DOHaD, several studies in animal models revealed that maternal calorie or protein restriction during pregnancy and lactation affects offspring in their growth, metabolism, and cognition [91]. Also, in the past years, different animal models and human studies have proved that maternal obesity triggers a transgenerational effect related to epigenetic changes leading to obesity in the offspring [32,78].

Obesity is a chronic disease characterized by a deregulation in lipid metabolism leading to hyperlipidemia and hypertriglyceridemia which might affect cellular physiology in relevant metabolic organs. In this context, fatty acids increase during obesity and might accumulate in non-adipose tissues and trigger cell dysfunction, a molecular toxic processes known as lipotoxicity [82]. In fact, lipotoxicity has been related to type 2 diabetes and metabolic syndrome. However, in the context of fatty acids, not all the lipids are potentially toxic, for instance, saturated fatty acids (SFAs), ceramides, or diacylglycerols show potential toxic effect in comparison to unsaturated fatty acids (UFAs).

SFAs are fatty acids that are totally hydrogenated and can be divided into subgroups according to their chain length (short chain saturated fatty acids (SCFA), medium chain saturated fatty acids (MCFA), long chain saturated fatty acids (LCFA), and very long chain saturated fatty acids (VLCFA)) [26]. The SFAs are in solid state at room temperature and diets high in SFAs are associated with chronic diseases and linked to a three to five fold increased risk for infant mortality [48]. SFAs are known to produce endoplasmic reticulum (ER) stress, inflammatory response, reactive oxygen species (ROS) production, and mitochondrial dysfunction in numerous in vitro and in vivo animal models [33,44], and several studies demonstrated that maternal obesity linked to high fat diet (HFD) intake promotes cellular dysfunction in offspring by epigenetic modulation [23,57,78,85,100]. However, during fetal period, all nutrients are important for achieving normal development. Many studies demonstrated that insufficient maternal nutrition leads to impairment in brain development and decreases growth factors which may have long-term effects on cerebral structure function [4].

Therefore, fatty acids, particularly long chain polyunsaturated fatty acids (LC-PUFA) play an important role in the growth and development of the fetus. An imbalanced fatty acid intake during the developmental early period may result in metabolic programming of diseases in adulthood.

Fatty acids

Lipids are small molecules with no affinity for water, which have important functions in our body, such as, the building block of the cell membrane, energy storage, and as precursors for hormone synthesis. Lipids can be classified into several groups such as fatty acids, sterols, phospholipids, among others. Particularly, fatty acids are chains formed of nonaromatic hydrocarbon compounds varying from 2 to 36 carbon atoms that can be either saturated or unsaturated. Fatty acids are important energy substrates which comprise about 30% of the total calories, supplying 9 kcal/g [26].

The most characteristic fatty acid properties are the chain length and the degree of saturation. Chain length can vary from two to six carbon atoms called short chain fatty acid to very long chain fatty acids composed of more than 22 carbon atoms. These carbon atoms chains can be either saturated or unsaturated, meaning they can have a single or double bond, respectively. Since saturated fatty acids are composed of single bonds, they have higher melting points compared to unsaturated fatty acids. Thus, saturated fatty acids require more metabolism energy to break down than unsaturated chains. Also, the length of the hydrocarbon chain influences the melting point, and a smaller chain will need less energy to break down than a longer one [92].

Fatty acids are stored as triacylglycerols (also called triglycerides) in the body. Fat digestion starts in the mouth, and then continues in the stomach (by an acid stable gastric lipase), where lipids of all sorts tend to form large fatty globules. As fat globules enter the duodenum, they are coated with bile salts of hepatic origin. As soon as fatty acids reach the duodenum and jejunum, cholecystokinin is released into the portal circulation and stimulates the pancreas to release triglyceride lipase and co-lipase. Both enzymes hydrolyze triglycerides leading to the formation of monoglycerides and fatty acids. The interaction of fatty acids and monoglycerides with bile salts forms mixed micelles which are necessary to absorb fat-soluble vitamins (D, E, and K). On the other hand, after digestion with pancreatic lipase, fatty acids may form vesicles to begin the process of absorption [17].

Fatty acids are absorbed by passive diffusion, facilitated diffusion, and active transport through the enterocyte. Free fatty acids and monoglycerides are synthesized into new triglyceride molecules and phospholipids, which are transported to the different organs via lipoproteins, especially chylomicrons [6].

Classification

There are several classifications for fatty acids, e.g., according to the carbon chain length, type of chemical bonds. As previously described, fatty acids can be divided as short, medium, long, and very long chain fatty acids. The most abundant fatty acids are the long chain fatty acids, with specifically 16 to 18 carbon atom chain. In addition, several authors subclassified very long chain fatty acids with more than 26 carbon atoms as ultra-very long chain fatty acids. On the other hand, another classification is the type of the carbon chain saturation. Based on the number of chemical bonds in the chain, fatty acids can also be classified as saturated and unsaturated fatty acids [81]. The presence or absence of carbon-carbon double bonds in the hydrocarbon chain is the difference between both groups. Saturated fatty acids do not have double bonds in the hydrocarbon chain and unsaturated fatty acids contain at least one double bond.

Saturated fatty acids

SFAs are hydrocarbon chains with no double bonds. The term *saturated* refers to the concentration of hydrogen atoms in the carbon chain. In this case, the concentration is at its fullest, making it a stable molecule [87].

Unsaturated fatty acids

Contrary to saturated fatty acids, unsaturated fatty acids contain one or more double bonds in the hydrocarbon chain. These type of fatty acids are divided into two more categories based on the number of double bonds present in the carbon chain and because of this, this molecule is characterized for its instability [77].

Monounsaturated fatty acid (MUFA)

As the name implies, monounsaturated means one carbon-carbon double bond. By adding a double bond to the chain the configuration of the molecule changes. There are two types of configuration, *cis* and *trans*, the first depicting two hydrogen atoms at the side of the chain, whereas the latter is characterized by having the same atoms but at opposite sides of the chain. Monounsaturated carbon chains are generally *cis*, which not only changes the shape of the molecule but also confers different biological function [16].

Polyunsaturated fatty acid (PUFA)

PUFAs are characterized by more than one carbon-carbon double bond. Like monounsaturated fatty acids, polyunsaturated can have either *cis* or *trans* configuration in their carbon chain. Within this type of molecule there are two polyunsaturated fatty acids that can't be synthesized by the body and therefore they are essential for the human body [1]. Omega-3 and omega-6, also called α-linolenic acid and linoleic acid, can be obtained from green leaves and different oils such as canola, flaxseed, and fish, respectively. Both essential molecules play important physiological functions, such as maintaining the cell membrane and normal brain function, regulating inflammatory responses, cell growth and division, among others. Several studies have shown their role in preventing chronic diseases such as hypertension and type 2 diabetes [99].

Animal models and diets as a tool to study maternal obesity-offspring development

Animal models are a common and strategic avenue to dissect potential effects of maternal environment on offspring development and postnatal susceptibility to metabolic diseases. Selective diet exposure during maternal programming including pre and postnatal periods might mimic caloric intake of Western human societies, which give us advantage to perform reproducible and selective food intake manipulations for data acquisition and potential clinical interventions [102].

Models of maternal obesity in rodents and nonhuman primates

In the literature, maternal obesity is perhaps the most commonly used model for research when the goal is to identify potential physiological and molecular alterations related to metabolic compromise. At first, mice and rats have a lot of advantage in terms of physiology related with humans that include their gestation and lifespan, but also show cost-effectiveness [2]. In general terms, maternal obesity or maternal overnutrition induces body weight gain and adiposity was increased in both male and female offspring [31,76]. Likewise, hypercaloric maternal diet exposure causes glucose intolerance and hyperinsulinemia in male and female offspring, independent of mother's obesity before gestation [40].

On the other hand, nonprimate models have the advantage of their closer relation to human species and greater similarities in terms of development patterns during gestation, but long gestation periods and increased cost for the maintenance make them less favorable [2]. It is known that in baboons overfeeding during the preweaning stage led to elevated triglyceride levels and increased adiposity in young adult females [45]. In macaques, for instance, hypercaloric maternal diet exposure trigger lipotoxicity in fetal liver and predisposes the offspring to nonalcoholic fatty liver disease [2,55].

Selective diets in animal models to mimic maternal obesity

Intake of hypercaloric diets in humans might be simulated in rodents and nonhuman primates by a cocktail recipe of High Fat Diets (HFD) [50]. Exposure to hypercaloric chronic diets rich in SFAs and sugars reproduce in animals models the metabolic abnormalities found in humans, leading to obesity and susceptibility to the metabolic syndrome [12]. However, the definition of HFD has not been standardized, in part due to kcal percentage of fat present in the HFDs, which exemplifies 20% to 60% energy [12].

Thus, another widely used diet to promote obese-phenotype in animals is the Cafeteria diet, which mimics more accurately highly palatable-energy dense foods in the Western society due to its content of SFAs plus carbohydrates [14,79]. Sampey et al. proposed the Cafeteria diet as a robust model of human metabolic syndrome compared to traditional lard-based HFD. Sampey's Cafeteria diet food schedule proposes three human snack foods daily varied in addition to ad libitum control diet [79]. However, Cafeteria diet composition has been modified depending on the experiment. For instance, some researchers use this strategy of varied daily food [38,43,53], while others test the strategy of using a home-made standardized diet which contained a mix of cookies, foie gras, sausage, croissants, sweets, bacon, biscuits, chocolate, peanuts, cheese, and sugary milk [71]. The latter formula is based on the initial work by Sclafani and Springer in 1976 [84]. Surwit et al. developed a high-fat-sucrose diet (HFS) with a calorie density of 5.56 kcal/g with 16.4% of energy from protein, 25.5% from carbohydrates, and 58% from fats, which mimics the Cafeteria diet and causes severe obesity, hyperglycemia, and hyperinsulinemia in mice [90]. This diet is used as a standard of Cafeteria diet in recent research [5,65,73] and might have adverse effects on mothers and fetuses [103]. In summary, fat or fat-sugar selective diets exposure in animal models during the perinatal period negatively regulate homeostatic settings leading to offspring susceptibility to metabolic compromise in adulthood.

Maternal obesity: effects on offspring

Developmental programming hypothesis proposes that during embryonic development there are critical periods of vulnerability to suboptimal conditions, which present as permanent effects in the offspring and alter metabolic and physiologic responses later in life [63]. These periods are related to embryonic states where cells are dividing rapidly, showing a high risk to nutrient over supply or deficiency [63]. In this context, one of the most common models of developmental programming is the exposure to diets during critical periods before pregnancy in order to produce stress in germinal cells disrupting normal physiology. Also, these models can use the maintenance or exposure to hypercaloric diets during other critical stages like gestation and lactation, where excess of nutrients pass from mother to offspring [63] (Fig. 6.1).

Developmental programming in obese mothers promotes a lipotoxic environment, which causes changes in mtDNA content, disturbances in the blood-brain barrier, decrement of fetal size, and abnormalities in offspring [39,56]. Also maternal obesity caused by HFD alters utero-placental hemodynamics and increases risk of stillbirth [28]. It has been reported that maternal energy imbalance can induce epigenetic changes in key organs of metabolism in the offspring, thus leading to a susceptibility to develop insulin resistance [47,51,78]. Likewise, it has been described that HFD administered to mice during pregnancy produces an increase in body

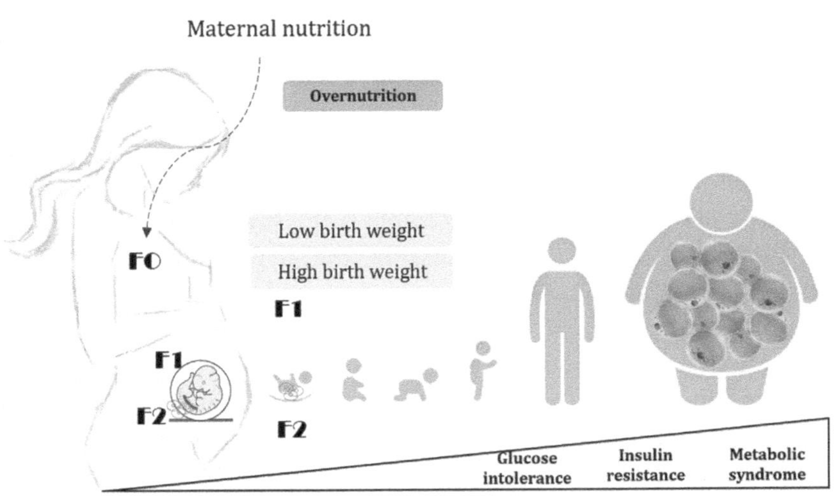

Figure 6.1 Impact of maternal overnutrition and programming of metabolic syndrome in offspring.

length in offspring, as well as a decrease in insulin sensitivity. On the other hand, when the "window" of exposure to a hyperlipidic diet in mice is extended to gestation and lactation, the offsprings increase their predisposition to develop metabolic syndrome [64].

Thus, environmental factors during perinatal period increase the susceptibility to develop obesity in adulthood [49].

In the next section, we will address the effects of toxic insult by lipids oversupply on the central nervous system (CNS) during developmental programming.

Maternal obesity and CNS lipotoxicity during developmental programming alters body energy homeostasis in offspring

CNS is an important region in the regulation of energy intake and expenditure; one of the most prominent brain structures linked to energy homeostasis is the hypothalamus. The hypothalamus is located just dorsal to the median eminence and communicates to the peripheral circulation by the third ventricle [24]. The hypothalamus integrates hormonal and metabolic signals from peripheral organs such as leptin released by adipose tissue and insulin released by pancreas [11,70]. Selective hormonal integration occurs into hypothalamic nucleus, including the arcuate nucleus (ARC), divided into ventromedial part in which orexigenic neuropeptides (appetite promoters) such as the Agouti Related Protein (AgRP) and the Neuropeptide Y (NPY) are expressed. On the other hand, in the ventrolateral part of the arcuate other neurons express the anorexigenic products as pro-opiomelanocortin (POMC), which together favor long-term regulation of body weight and body energy homeostasis [11,70]. Specifically, insulin is known to produce anorexic responses by reducing food intake mainly by activating a neuronal population expressing IRS-1 insulin receptor in ARC which inhibits mRNA expression of orexigenic neuropeptide Y [11,70]. Also, leptin receptors (LepRs) are located throughout the CNS and highly concentrated in the hypothalamus, which are responsible for suppression of food intake and stimulation of energy expenditure [70].

Lipids oversupply could overcome the storage capacity and expandability of adipose tissue leading to accumulation in nonadipose tissues and trigger lipotoxicity and apoptosis in the central nervous system [25]. In particular, maternal obesity might disrupt hormonal or metabolic central integration at the level of hypothalamus leading to changes in the expression of selective neuronal markers, which control food intake in offspring.

For instance, HFD exposure increases density of orexigenic neurons which promote overreaction to fasting signaling due to hypothalamic NPY and AgRP over expression in the offspring [15,69].

One of the most studied lipid species associated to lipotoxicity during maternal obesity is the palmitic acid, which is an ester chemical group located in triglycerides and is the most common lipid specie found in Western diet products [25]. Palmitic acid causes activation of hypothalamic inflammatory response in cells, ER stress, mitochondrial dysfunction, and insulin resistance in individuals with obesity [13,25,52]. Also, exposure to SFAs such as palmitic acid during pregnancy increases plasma inflammatory markers and cytokines including IL-6, sICAM-1, CRP, TNFα [66]. Thus, maternal obesity might impact on ER and mitochondrial homeostasis and activate the inflammatory program disrupting body energy homeostatic settings.

Metabolic and stress dysfunction in offspring programmed by maternal overnutrition

Mitochondria failure: During obesity, mitochondria change dynamically to modulate nutrient oversupply by activating fusion and fission machinery including mitofusins (Mfn1 and Mfn2) and Opa1, Drp1 and MTP18, respectively [97]. Obesity promotes neuronal changes in the expression of Drp1 and mitofusins regulating glucose and leptin sensitivity [80]. Also, obesity induced by HFD in mice decreases expression of Mfn2 in hypothalamus [20]. Maternal programming by high fat/high sucrose diet exposure leads to impaired peripheral insulin signaling in female offspring that is associated with mitochondrial dysfunction and altered fusion-fission dynamic in skeletal muscle, even found at the third generation [78].

Finally, maternal obesity shows impaired homeostasis in ovaries, in part by cellular lipids accumulation [56]. In particular, plasma increase of SFA during obesity promotes changes in energy homeostasis in females creating a fertile soil for epigenetic and mitochondria changes in offspring [32]. For instance, palmitic acid induces cytosolic and mitochondrial reactive oxygen species (ROS) production, promotes oxidative stress by coupling Ca^{2+} over flux from ER to mitochondria [13]. Also, depletion of Ca^{2+} stores in ER leads to ER stress and mitochondria Ca^{2+} accumulation promotes defects in oxidative phosphorylation and ATP depletion [13]. Thus, maternal obesity seems to be a pathway to promote mitochondrial dysfunction in offspring and this effect is transgenerational in animal models.

Systemic and central inflammation: It has been reported that maternal obesity activates the uterine inflammatory response by the upregulation of NF-κB and c-Jun-N-terminal kinase and increases mRNA chemokines (CCL2, CCL5, CCL7, and CxCL10) and regulators (TLR2, CD14, and Ccr1) [86]. This increase of markers of inflammation is associated with lipid accumulation and expression of lipid metabolic genes [86]. In maternal adipose tissue, there is increased secretion and expression of TNFα in HFD and enhanced expression of CD68, a marker of macrophage infiltration [74]. It is known that hypercaloric developmental programming sets to adipose tissue to secrete more inflammatory cytokines, adiponectin, and leptin favoring increase in placental mRNA transcripts of inflammatory markers, such as IL-1B, IL-8, and MCP-1 [66]. In addition, placental infiltration by maternal macrophages exacerbates immune response activation and developmental and metabolic compromise in offspring [66]. Positive inflammatory profile in offspring correlates with liver dysfunction including steatosis and elevated aspartate transaminase (AST) [67,72]. Also, maternal programming by positive energy balance leads to adipose tissue inflammatory response and macrophage infiltration [21].

Proinflammatory markers linked to maternal obesity have also been identified in the CNS of offspring. Maternal obesity induced by HFD causes proinflammatory cytokine expression and increases microglial activation markers in the hippocampus of pups at birth (Bilbo and Tsang, 2010). Also HFD exposure in mothers promotes increased levels of inflammation markers in hypothalamus, including IL-1β mRNA and NFKB in offspring [57].

ER stress activation: Parallel to inflammation and mitochondrial dysfunction, maternal obesity leads to ER stress activation [100]. Endoplasmic reticulum (ER) is an organelle focused in the synthesis and folding of proteins. Thus, an ER stress occurs due to physiological and pathological effects such as inflammatory cytokines [88]. In addition to inflammatory activation programs in offspring linked to HFD during gestation and lactation, hypercaloric surplus also induces hypothalamic ER stress activation by p-PERK, p-eIF2a, XBP1S, GRP78, and GRP94 selective markers [57]. Thus, maternal obesity increases markers of ER stress like GRP78, p-PERK, and p-IRE in adipose tissue and liver of adult offspring [88]. Recently, it was reported that ER stress in hypothalamus of offspring causes mitochondrial dysfunction, which can be diminished by regulating ER stress after birth [64]. Also, mitochondria fusion marker Mfn2 deletion in neurons causes obesity due to ER-stress-induced leptin resistance [83]. These results suggest that ER stress in offspring might be programmed by maternal obesity and postnatal obesogenic diets with severe associated metabolic effects [89].

Metabolic and fetal programming in human models

Obesity during pregnancy has increased considerably, which is of particular concern since maternal obesity is an important risk factor that can affect the pregnancy process and the health of the mother and the newborn, even predisposing the newborn to suffer metabolic diseases in adult stages [55]. Regarding risks to the mother related to obesity during pregnancy are a higher incidence of gestational diabetes and hypertension [54]. On the other hand, maternal obesity during pregnancy has been associated with complications in the neonate.

A study highlights the association of maternal dietary fatty acid composition during pregnancy with normal fetal development and its influence on fetal programming, thus increasing the risk of developing metabolic diseases throughout life [58]. Mothers with higher levels of free fatty acids during early pregnancy are more likely to have children who become obese or overweight by the age of 5–6 years. This effect is also known to influence the progression of metabolic disorders later in life [29]. The maternal omega-3 and omega-6 fatty acid status influences adiposity in the offspring [22,61].

Obesity during pregnancy can result in premature births and higher mortality in early or late fetal stages. Apart from the complications associated with maternal obesity during the fetal stage or at the time of birth, there are other complications related to risk factors for the development of diseases in adulthood. In addition to maternal obesity, the intake of a diet rich in fat during gestation without maternal obesity also contributes to an increase in the incidence of obesity in offspring [101].

An association between the plasma concentration of dihomo-γ-linolenic acid in the mother during pregnancy and an increased body mass index (BMI) and measures of adiposity in children at 7 years of age have been reported [18].

The mechanisms by which maternal obesity during gestation produces these negative effects are not fully understood. But alterations in metabolic pathways related to appetite control and peripheral mechanisms that regulate insulin sensitivity are believed to be responsible. At the molecular level, both processes that increase oxidative stress, inflammation, and certain epigenetic modifications may contribute to the transmission of metabolic diseases from mother to child [75]. Therefore, early exposure to an excess of saturated fat may have late negative effects on the metabolic health of offspring, especially if this exposure occurs during fetal life and childhood, as they are periods of great vulnerability to external factors.

LC-PUFA supplementation during perinatal period

Consumption of LC-PUFAs, especially those found in fatty fish, has a beneficial effect on blood pressure and serum markers of cardiovascular disease risk in adults [7,60]. The consumption of PUFAs during pregnancy and lactation has multiple benefits both to mother and offspring. The increased intake of these fatty acids during pregnancy prevents their decline associated with pregnancy. A previous study reported that pregnant women who had at least two salmon portions per week had higher levels of EPA and DHA in plasma phosphatidylcholine and plasma phosphatidylcholine from umbilical cord blood than control group. The latter indicates enhanced transfer of these functionally important fatty acids to the fetus [59]. High concentrations of SFA and total n-6 PUFA have been reported in higher prepregnancy body mass index and higher gestational weight gain [95].

Lowered serum n-3 PUFA levels have been observed in mothers who developed postpartum depression. The pregnant women who are at risk to develop postpartum depression should be supplemented with n-3 PUFAs. Other studies have had their limitations though [19]. The length of gestation could be influenced by maternal fatty acid consumption. Olsen et al. reported that never consuming fish in pregnancy was a risk factor for preterm delivery [68].

The placental supply of optimal levels of LCPUFA to the fetus during early life is extremely important for the normal growth and development of both placenta and fetus and is considered essential for maturation of the developing brain, retina, and other organs in newborn infants [37]. The omega-3 fatty acids are known to have an effect on fetal programming [96]. However, it is extremely important to consider other fatty acids such as omega-6 fatty acids (AA) in the maternal diet that are transported across the placenta [34]. The omega-6 and omega-3 are known to compete for the same desaturases and elongases and have important opposing physiological effects; therefore a well-balanced omega-6/omega-3 diet is important. There is only one human study that has investigated the effects of maternal supplementation of docosahexaenoic acid (DHA) or DHA + AA during pregnancy and lactation on the brain development of the infant. Supplementation of DHA alone decreased maternal AA status while DHA + AA supplementation restored the DHA/AA balance [94]. LCPUFA are required during all reproductive stages [62]. Fatty acids are transferred during pregnancy through the placenta, and postnatally through breast milk. Breast milk provides both AA and DHA. The level of AA is relatively constant, whereas the level of DHA is variable and depends on maternal dietary habits, culture, and lifestyle [35,41].

During pregnancy, mothers are the sole providers of fatty acids to the growing fetus, since the fetal elongase/desaturase enzyme systems are immature and they are unable to synthesize the required amount [93]. There is rapid accumulation of LCPUFA in the third trimester and the early postnatal period during which the brain growth reaches its peak [98] and is susceptible to any nutritional deficiencies [42].

Maternal PUFAs consumption is important in fetal and new born growth, retinal development, and neurodevelopment [30].There is evidence that people who experience fetal undernutrition or overnutrition have increased adiposity [27]. Metaanalysis of 26 studies showed that maternal omega-3 fatty acids during pregnancy and/or lactation are associated with the offspring's high birth weight and increased waist circumference after birth. However, there was no association with children's birth length, postnatal weight/length, body mass index, fat mass, and the percentage of body fat during postnatal period [46]. A study in Indonesian women showed that inadequate maternal intake of α-linolenic acid, but not omega-3 fatty acids, docosahexaenoic acid, or eicosapentaenoic acid, was associated with lower birth weight [3].

Maternal PUFA status could influence offspring fat mass development. Moon et al. showed results of an observational study where there was a positive association between maternal n-6 PUFA status and offspring fat mass. The statistically significant positive association between maternal n-6 PUFA status and offspring fat mass was observed, but did not find significant effects of maternal n-3 PUFA and body composition [61]. Another study showed that maternal lower n-3 PUFA levels and higher n-6 PUFA levels during pregnancy are associated with a higher body fat percentage and an adverse general and abdominal fat distribution in childhood [95]. The latter studies measured offspring body composition with DXA. In another study, in which an offspring's adiposity was measured with the sum of skinfold thicknesses, showed that higher n-3 PUFA concentrations in the maternal diet and in umbilical cord plasma phospholipids were associated with lower adiposity in children at age 3 [22].

References

[1] Abedi E, Sahari MA. Long-chain polyunsaturated fatty acid sources and evaluation of their nutritional and functional properties. Food Sci Nutr 2014;2(5):443–63. https://doi.org/10.1002/fsn3.121.

[2] Alfaradhi MZ, Ozanne SE. Developmental programming in response to maternal overnutrition. Front Genet 2011;2:27. https://doi.org/10.3389/fgene.2011.00027.

[3] Angkasa D, Tambunan V, Khusun H, Witjaksono F, Agustina R. Inadequate dietary α-linolenic acid intake among Indonesian pregnant women is associated with lower newborn weights in urban Jakarta. Asia Pac J Clin Nutr 2017;26(Suppl. 1):S9–18. https://doi.org/10.6133/apjcn.062017.s1.

[4] Antonow-Schlorke I, Schwab M, Cox LA, Li C, Stuchlik K, Witte OW, et al. Vulnerability of the fetal primate brain to moderate reduction in maternal global nutrient availability. Proc Natl Acad Sci USA 2011;108:3011–6. https://doi.org/10.1073/pnas.1009838108.

[5] Anunciado-Koza RP, Manuel J, Koza RA. Molecular correlates of fat mass expansion in C57BL/6J mice after short-term exposure to dietary fat. Ann N Y Acad Sci 2016;1363(1):50–8.

[6] Armand M. Lipases and lipolysis in the human digestive tract: where do we stand? Curr Opin Clin Nutr Metab Care 2007;10:156–64.

[7] Balk E, Chung M, Lichtenstein A, Chew P, Kupelnick B, Lawrence A, et al. In: Effects of omega-3 fatty acids on cardiovascular risk factors and intermediate markers of cardiovascular disease: evidence Report/Technology Assessment; 2004. No.96.

[8] Bilbo Staci D, Verne Tsang. Enduring consequences of maternal obesity for brain inflammation and behavior of offspring 2010 Jun;24(6):2104–15. https://doi.org/10.1096/fj.09-144014. Epub 2010 Feb 2.

[9] Barker DJ. The fetal and infant origins of adult disease. BMJ Br Med J (Clin Res Ed) 1990;301(6761). 1111-1111.

[10] Barker DJ, Gluckman PD, Godfrey KM, Harding JE, Owens JA, Robinson JS. Fetal nutrition and cardiovascular disease in adult life. Lancet 1993;341(8850):938–41. https://doi.org/10.1016/0140-6736(93)91224-A.

[11] Baskin DG, Figlewicz Lattemann D, Seeley RJ, Woods SC, Porte D, Schwartz MW. Insulin and leptin: dual adiposity signals to the brain for the regulation of food intake and body weight. Brain Res 1999;848(1):114–23. https://doi.org/10.1016/S0006-8993(99)01974-5.

[12] Buettner R, Schölmerich J, Bollheimer LC. High-fat diets: modeling the metabolic disorders of human obesity in rodents. Obesity 2007;15(4):798–808. https://doi.org/10.1038/oby.2007.608.

[13] Cao SS, Luo KL, Shi L. Endoplasmic reticulum stress interacts with inflammation in human diseases. J Cell Physiol 2016;231(2):288–94. https://doi.org/10.1002/jcp.25098.

[14] Cardenas-Perez RE, Fuentes-Mera L, De La Garza AL, Torre-Villalvazo I, Reyes-Castro LA, Rodriguez-Rocha H. Maternal overnutrition by hypercaloric diets programs hypothalamic mitochondrial fusion and metabolic dysfunction in rat male offspring. Nutr Metab 2018;15(1). https://doi.org/10.1186/s12986-018-0279-6.

[15] Chang G-Q, Gaysinskaya V, Karatayev O, Leibowitz SF. Maternal high-fat diet and fetal programming: increased proliferation of hypothalamic peptide-producing neurons that increase risk for overeating and obesity. J Neurosci 2008;28(46):12107–19.
[16] de Souza RJ, Mente A, Maroleanu A, Cozma AI, Ha V, Kishibe T. Intake of saturated and trans unsaturated fatty acids and risk of all cause mortality, cardiovascular disease, and type 2 diabetes: systematic review and meta-analysis of observational studies. Br Med J 2015;351. https://doi.org/10.1136/BMJ.H3978. h3978.
[17] de la Garza AL, Milagro FI, Boque N, Campión J, Martínez JA. Natural inhibitors of pancreatic lipase as new players in obesity treatment. Planta Med 2011;77(8):773–85. https://doi.org/10.1055/s-0030-1270924.
[18] de Vries PS, Gielen M, Rizopoulos D, Rump P, Godschalk R, Hornstra G, et al. Association between polyunsaturated fatty acid concentrations in maternal plasma phospholipids during pregnancy and offspring adiposity at age 7: the MEFAB cohort. Prostaglandins Leukot Essent Fatty Acids 2014;91(3):81–5. https://doi.org/10.1016/j.plefa.2014.04.002.
[19] De Vriese SR, Christophe AB, Maes M. Lowered serum n-3 polyunsaturated fatty acid (PUFA) levels predict the occurrence of postpartum depression: further evidence that lowered n-PUFAs are related to major depression. Life Sci 2003;73(25):3181–7. https://doi.org/10.1016/j.lfs.2003.02.001.
[20] Diaz B, Fuentes-Mera L, Tovar A, Montiel T, Massieu L, Martínez-Rodríguez HG, Camacho A. Saturated lipids decrease mitofusin 2 leading to endoplasmic reticulum stress activation and insulin resistance in hypothalamic cells. Brain Res 2015;1627(Suppl. C):80–9. https://doi.org/10.1016/j.brainres.2015.09.014.
[21] Ding Y, Li J, Liu S, Zhang L, Xiao H, Li J, et al. DNA hypomethylation of inflammation-associated genes in adipose tissue of female mice after multigenerational high fat diet feeding. Int J Obes 2014;38(2):198–204. https://doi.org/10.1038/ijo.2013.98.
[22] Donahue SM, Rifas-Shiman SL, Gold DR, Jouni ZE, Gillman MW, Oken E. Prenatal fatty acid status and child adiposity at age 3 y: results from a US pregnancy cohort. Am J Clin Nutr 2011;93:780–8. https://doi.org/10.3945/ajcn.110.005801.
[23] Dong M, Zheng Q, Ford SP, Nathanielsz PW, Ren J. Maternal obesity, lipotoxicity and cardiovascular diseases in offspring. J Mol Cell Cardiol 2013;55:111–6. https://doi.org/10.1016/j.yjmcc.2012.08.023.
[24] Dudas B. The human hypothalamus: anatomy, functions and disorders. Nova Science Publishers; 2013.
[25] Engin AB. What is lipotoxicity? In: Engin AB, Engin A, editors. Obesity and lipotoxicity. Cham: Springer International Publishing; 2017. p. 197–220.
[26] Fahy E, Subramaniam S, Murphy RC, Nishijima M, Raetz CRH, Shimizu T. Update of the LIPID MAPS comprehensive classification system for lipids 1. JLR (J Lipid Res) 2009;50(Suppl):S9–14. https://doi.org/10.1194/jlr.R800095-JLR200.
[27] Fall CHD. Evidence for the intra-uterine programming of adiposity in later life. Ann Hum Biol 2011;38:410–28. https://doi.org/10.3109/03014460.2011.592513.
[28] Frias AE, Morgan TK, Evans AE, Rasanen J, Oh KY, Thornburg KL, Grove KL. Maternal high-fat diet disturbs uteroplacental hemodynamics and increases the frequency of stillbirth in a nonhuman primate model of excess nutrition. Endocrinology 2011;152(6):2456–64. https://doi.org/10.1210/en.2010-1332.
[29] Gademan MG, Vermeulen M, Oostvogels AJ, Roseboom TJ, Visscher TL, van Eijsden M, et al. Maternal prepregnancy BMI and lipid profile during early pregnancy are independently associated with off- spring's body composition at age 5–6 years: the ABCD study. PloS One 2014;9(4):e94594. https://doi.org/10.1371/journal.pone.0094594.

[30] Greenberg JA, Bell SJ, Ausdal WV. Omega-3 fatty acid supplementation during pregnancy. Rev Obstet Gynecol 2008;1(4):162–9.
[31] Gupta A, Srinivasan M, Thamadilok S, Patel MS. Hypothalamic alterations in fetuses of high fat diet-fed obese female rats. J Endocrinol 2009;200(3):293–300.
[32] Heerwagen MJR, Miller MR, Barbour LA, Friedman JE. Maternal obesity and fetal metabolic programming: a fertile epigenetic soil. Am J Physiol Regul Integr Comp Physiol 2010;299(3):R711.
[33] Hotamisligil GS. Inflammation and endoplasmic reticulum stress in obesity and diabetes. Int J Obes 2008;32(Suppl. 7):S52–4. https://doi.org/10.1038/ijo.2008.238. 2005.
[34] Innis SM. Essential fatty acid transfer and fetal development. Placenta 2005;26:70–5. https://doi.org/10.1016/j.placenta.2005.01.005.
[35] Innis SM. Impact of maternal diet on human milk composition and neurological development of infants. Am J Clin Nutr 2014;99(3):734S–41S. https://doi.org/10.3945/ajcn.113.072595.
[36] Jang H, Serra C. Nutrition, epigenetics, and diseases. Clin Nutr Res 2014;3(1):1–8.
[37] Jasani B, Simmer K, Patole SK, Rao SC. Long chain polyunsaturated fatty acid supplementation in infants born at term. Cochrane Database Syst Rev 2017;3:CD000376. https://doi.org/10.1002/14651858.CD000376.pub4.
[38] Kaur G, Kulkarni S. Antiobesity effect a polyherbal formulation, OB-200G in female rats fed on cafeteria and atherogenic diets. Indian J Pharmacol 2000;32(5):294–9.
[39] Kim DW, Glendining KA, Grattan DR, Jasoni CL. Maternal obesity in the mouse compromises the blood-brain barrier in the arcuate nucleus of offspring. Endocrinology 2016;157(6):2229–42. https://doi.org/10.1210/en.2016-1014.
[40] Kirk SL, Samuelsson A-M, Argenton M, Dhonye H, Kalamatianos T, Poston L, et al. Maternal obesity induced by diet in rats permanently influences central processes regulating food intake in offspring. PloS One 2009;4(6):e5870.
[41] Koletzko B, Lien E, Agostoni C, Böhles H, Campoy C, Cetin I, et al. The roles of long-chain polyunsaturated fatty acids in pregnancy, lactation and infancy: review of current knowledge and consensus recommendations. J Perinat Med 2008;36(1):5–14. https://doi.org/10.1515/JPM.2008.001.
[42] Krabbendam L, Bakker E, Hornstra G, van Os J. Relationship between DHA status at birth and child problem behaviour at 7 years of age. Prostagl Leukot Essent Fat Acids 2007;76(1):29–34. https://doi.org/10.1016/j.plefa.2006.09.004.
[43] La Fleur S, Luijendijk M, Van Der Zwaal E, Brans M, Adan R. The snacking rat as model of human obesity: effects of a free-choice high-fat high-sugar diet on meal patterns. Int J Obes 2014;38(5):643.
[44] Legrand-Poels S, Esser N, L'homme L, Scheen A, Paquot N, Piette J. Free fatty acids as modulators of the NLRP3 inflammasome in obesity/type 2 diabetes. Biochem Pharmacol 2014;92(1):131–41. https://doi.org/10.1016/j.bcp.2014.08.013.
[45] Lewis D, Bertrand H, McMahan C, McGill Jr H, Carey K, Masoro E. Preweaning food intake influences the adiposity of young adult baboons. J Clin Invest 1986;78(4):899.
[46] Li GL, Chen HJ, Zhang WX, Tong Q, Yan YE. Effects of maternal omega-3 fatty acids supplementation during pregnancy/lactation on body composition of the offspring: a systematic review and meta-analysis. Clin Nutr 2017:1–12. https://doi.org/10.1016/j.clnu.2017.08.002.
[47] Li M, Sloboda DM, Vickers MH. Maternal obesity and developmental programming of metabolic disorders in offspring: evidence from animal models. Exp Diabetes Res 2011;9. https://doi.org/10.1155/2011/592408. 2011.

[48] Liang C, Oest ME, Prater MR. Intrauterine exposure to high saturated fat diet elevates risk of adult-onset chronic diseases in C57BL/6 mice. Birth Defects Res B Dev Reprod Toxicol 2009;86(5):377–84. https://doi.org/10.1002/bdrb.20206.

[49] Lillycrop KA, Rodford J, Garratt ES, Slater-Jefferies JL, Godfrey KM, Gluckman PD, et al. Maternal protein restriction with or without folic acid supplementation during pregnancy alters the hepatic transcriptome in adult male rats. Br J Nutr 2010;103(12):1711–9. https://doi.org/10.1017/S0007114509993795.

[50] Llopis M, Sánchez J, Priego T, Palou M, Picó C. Maternal fat supplementation during late pregnancy and lactation influences the development of hepatic steatosis in offspring depending on the fat source. J Agric Food Chem 2014;62(7):1590–601. https://doi.org/10.1021/jf405161e.

[51] Loche E, Ozanne SE. Non-genetic transmission of obesity – it's in your epigenes. Trends Endocrinol Metabol 2016;27(6):349–50. https://doi.org/10.1016/j.tem.2016.04.003.

[52] Ly LD, Xu S, Choi S-K, Ha C-M, Thoudam T, Cha S-K, et al. Oxidative stress and calcium dysregulation by palmitate in type 2 diabetes. Exp Mol Med 2017;49:e291. https://doi.org/10.1038/emm.2016.157.

[53] Martire SI, Holmes N, Westbrook RF, Morris MJ. Altered feeding patterns in rats exposed to a palatable cafeteria diet: increased snacking and its implications for development of obesity. PloS One 2013;8(4):e60407. https://doi.org/10.1371/journal.pone.0060407.

[54] Matusiak K, Barrett HL, Callaway LK, Nitert MD. Periconception weight loss: common sense for mothers, but what about for babies? J Obesity 2014. https://doi.org/10.1155/2014/204295. 204295. 2014.

[55] McCurdy CE, Bishop JM, Williams SM, Grayson BE, Smith MS, Friedman JE, Grove KL. Maternal high-fat diet triggers lipotoxicity in the fetal livers of nonhuman primates. J Clin Invest 2009;119(2):323.

[56] McPherson NO, Bell VG, Zander-Fox DL, Fullston T, Wu LL, Robker RL, Lane M. When two obese parents are worse than one! Impacts on embryo and fetal development. Am J Physiol Endocrinol Metabol 2015;309(6):E568–81. https://doi.org/10.1152/ajpendo.00230.2015.

[57] Melo AM, Benatti RO, Ignacio-Souza LM, Okino C, Torsoni AS, Milanski M, et al. Hypothalamic endoplasmic reticulum stress and insulin resistance in offspring of mice dams fed high-fat diet during pregnancy and lactation. Metabolism 2014;63(5):682–92. https://doi.org/10.1016/j.metabol.2014.02.002.

[58] Mennitti LV, Oliveira JL, Morais CA, Estadella D, Oyama LM, Oller do Nascimiento CM, et al. Type of fatty acids in maternal diets during pregnancy and/or lactation and metabolic consequences of the offspring. J Nutr Biochem 2015;26(2):99–111. https://doi.org/10.1016/j.jnutbio.2014.10.001.

[59] Miles EA, Noakes PS, Kremmyda LS, Vlachava M, Diaper ND, Rosenlund G, et al. The Salmon in Pregnancy Study: study design, subject characteristics, maternal fish and marine n–3 fatty acid intake, and marine n–3 fatty acid status in maternal and umbilical cord blood. Am J Clin Nutr 2011;94(6 Suppl. l):1986S–92S. https://doi.org/10.3945/ajcn.110.001636.

[60] Miller PE, Van Elswyk M, Alexander DD. Long-chain omega-3 fatty acids eicosapentaenoic acid and docosahexaenoic acid and blood pressure: a meta-analysis of randomized controlled trials. Am J Hypertens 2014;27(7):885–96. https://doi.org/10.1093/ajh/hpu024.

[61] Moon RJ, Harvey NC, Robinson SM, Ntani G, Daves JH, Inskip HM, et al. Maternal plasma polyunsaturated fatty acid status in late pregnancy is associated with

offspring body composition in childhood. J Clin Endocrinol Metab 2013;98(1):299–307. https://doi.org/10.1210/jc.2012-2482.
[62] Morse NL. Benefits of docosahexaenoic acid, folic acid, vitamin D and iodine on foetal and infant brain development and function following maternal supplementation during pregnancy and lactation. Nutrients 2012;4(7):799–840. https://doi.org/10.3390/nu4070799.
[63] Nathanielsz PW, Poston L, Taylor PD. In Utero exposure to maternal obesity and diabetes: animal models that identify and characterize implications for future health. Obstet Gynecol Clin N Am 2007;34(2):201–12. https://doi.org/10.1016/j.ogc.2007.03.006.
[64] Nguyen LT, Saad S, Tan Y, Pollock C, Chen H. Maternal high-fat diet induces metabolic stress response disorders in offspring hypothalamus. J Mol Endocrinol 2017:81–92. JME-17-0056.
[65] Nguyen S, Shao D, Tomasi LC, Braun A, de Mattos ABM, Choi YS, et al. The effects of fatty acid composition on cardiac hypertrophy and function in mouse models of diet-induced obesity. J Nutr Biochem 2017:137–42.
[66] O'Reilly JR, Reynolds RM. The risk of maternal obesity to the long-term health of the offspring. Clin Endocrinol 2013;78(1):9–16. https://doi.org/10.1111/cen.12055.
[67] Oben JA, Mouralidarane A, Samuelsson A-M, Matthews PJ, Morgan ML, McKee C, et al. Maternal obesity during pregnancy and lactation programs the development of offspring non-alcoholic fatty liver disease in mice. J Hepatol 2010;52(6):913–20. https://doi.org/10.1016/j.jhep.2009.12.042.
[68] Olsen SF, Osterdal ML, Salving JD, Kesmodel U, Henriksen TB, Hedegaard M, et al. Duration of pregnancy in relation to seafood intake during early and mid pregnancy: prospective cohort. Eur J Epidemiol 2006;21(10):749–58. https://doi.org/10.1007/s10654-006-9053-6.
[69] Page KC, Malik RE, Ripple JA, Anday EK. Maternal and postweaning diet interaction alters hypothalamic gene expression and modulates response to a high-fat diet in male offspring. Am J Physiol Regul Integr Comp Physiol 2009;297(4):R1049–57.
[70] Park H-K, Ahima RS. Physiology of leptin: energy homeostasis, neuroendocrine function and metabolism. Metabolism 2015;64(1):24–34. https://doi.org/10.1016/j.metabol.2014.08.004.
[71] Picó C, Pons A, Gianotti M, Palou A. Sustained changes in blood alpha amino nitrogen compartmentation during recovery from cafeteria feeding in rats. Arch Int Physiol, Biochim Biophys 1991;99(4):345–8.
[72] Pruis MGM, Lendvai Á, Bloks VW, Zwier MV, Baller JFW, de Bruin A, Plösch T. Maternal western diet primes non-alcoholic fatty liver disease in adult mouse offspring. Acta Physiol 2014;210(1):215–27. https://doi.org/10.1111/apha.12197.
[73] Rendina-Ruedy E, Smith BJ. Methodological considerations when studying the skeletal response to glucose intolerance using the diet-induced obesity model. BoneKEy Rep 2016;5.
[74] Reynolds CM, Vickers MH, Harrison CJ, Segovia SA, Gray C. High fat and/or high salt intake during pregnancy alters maternal meta-inflammation and offspring growth and metabolic profiles. Physiol Rep 2014;2(8). https://doi.org/10.14814/phy2.12110.
[75] Rkhzay-Jaf J, O'Dowd JF, Stocker C. Maternal obesity and the fetal origins of the metabolic syndrome. Curr Cardiovasc Risk Rep 2012;6(5):487–95. https://doi.org/10.1007/s12170-012-0257-x.
[76] Romaní-Pérez M, Lépinay AL, Alonso L, Rincel M, Xia L, Fanet H, et al. Impact of perinatal exposure to high-fat diet and stress on responses to nutritional challenges, food-motivated behaviour and mesolimbic dopamine function. Int J Obes 2016;41(4):502–9. https://doi.org/10.1038/ijo.2016.236.

[77] Rustan AC, Drevon CA. Fatty acids: structures and properties. Encyclopedia of life sciences 2005. https://doi.org/10.1038/npg.els.0003894.
[78] Saben JL, Boudoures AL, Asghar Z, Thompson A, Drury A, Zhang W, Moley KH. Maternal metabolic syndrome programs mitochondrial dysfunction via germline changes across three generations. Cell Rep 2016;16(1):1–8. https://doi.org/10.1016/j.celrep.2016.05.065.
[79] Sampey BP, Vanhoose AM, Winfield HM, Freemerman AJ, Muehlbauer MJ, Fueger PT, et al. Cafeteria diet is a robust model of human metabolic syndrome with liver and adipose inflammation: comparison to high-fat diet. Obesity 2011;19(6):1109–17. https://doi.org/10.1038/oby.2011.18.
[80] Santoro A, Campolo M, Liu C, Sesaki H, Meli R, Liu Z-W, et al. DRP1 suppresses leptin and glucose sensing of POMC neurons. Cell Metabol 2017;25(3):647–60. https://doi.org/10.1016/j.cmet.2017.01.003.
[81] Sassa T, Kihara A. Metabolism of very long-chain Fatty acids: genes and pathophysiology. Biomolecules & Therapeutics 2014;22(2):83–92. https://doi.org/10.4062/biomolther.2014.017.
[82] Schaffer JE. Lipotoxicity: when tissues overeat. Curr Opin Lipidol 2003;14(3):281–7.
[83] Schneeberger M, Dietrich MO, Sebastián D, Imbernón M, Castaño C, Garcia A, et al. Mitofusin 2 in POMC neurons connects ER stress with leptin resistance and energy imbalance. Cell 2013;155(1):172–87. https://doi.org/10.1016/j.cell.2013.09.003.
[84] Sclafani A, Springer D. Dietary obesity in adult rats: similarities to hypothalamic and human obesity syndromes. Physiol Behav 1976;17(3):461–71.
[85] Segovia SA, Vickers MH, Gray C, Reynolds CM. Maternal obesity, inflammation, and developmental programming. BioMed Res Int 2014;14. https://doi.org/10.1155/2014/418975.
[86] Shankar K, Zhong Y, Kang P, Lau F, Blackburn ML, Chen J-R, et al. Maternal obesity promotes a proinflammatory signature in rat uterus and blastocyst. Endocrinology 2011;152(11):4158–70. https://doi.org/10.1210/en.2010-1078.
[87] Siri-Tarino PW, Sun Q, Hu FB, Krauss RM. Saturated fat, carbohydrate, and cardiovascular disease. Am J Clin Nutr 2010;91(3):502–9. https://doi.org/10.3945/ajcn.2008.26285.
[88] Soeda J, Cordero P, Li J, Mouralidarane A, Asilmaz E, Ray S. Hepatic rhythmicity of endoplasmic reticulum stress is disrupted in perinatal and adult mice models of high-fat diet-induced obesity. Int J Food Sci Nutr 2017;68(4):455–66. https://doi.org/10.1080/09637486.2016.1261086.
[89] Soeda J, Mouralidarane A, Cordero P, Li J, Nguyen V, Carter R. Maternal obesity alters endoplasmic reticulum homeostasis in offspring pancreas. J Physiol Biochem 2016;72(2):281–91. https://doi.org/10.1007/s13105-016-0476-6.
[90] Surwit R, Feinglos M, Rodin J, Sutherland A, Petro A, Opara E, et al. Differential effects of fat and sucrose on the development of obesity and diabetes in C57BL/6J and AJ mice. Metabolism 1995;44(5):645–51.
[91] Tarrade A, Panchenko P, Junien C, Gabory A. Placental contribution to nutritional programming of health and diseases: epigenetics and sexual dimorphism. J Exp Biol 2015;218(1):50.
[92] Tvrzicka E, Kremmyda L-S, Stankova B, Zak A, Tvrzicka E, Kremmyda L-S. Fatty acids as biocompounds: their role in human metabolism, health and disease – a review. Part 1: classification, dietary sources and biological functions. Biomed Pap Med Fac Univ Palacky Olomouc Czech Repub 2011;(10). https://doi.org/10.5507/bp.2011.038. 1555507.

[93] Uauy R, Mena P, Rojas C. Essential fatty acids in early life: structural and functional role. Proc Nutr Soc 2000;59(1):3–15. https://doi.org/10.1017/S0029665100000021.
[94] van Goor SA, Dijck-Brouwer DA, Doornbos B, Erwich JJ, Schaafsma A, Muskiet FA, et al. Supplementation of DHA but not DHA with arachidonic acid during pregnancy and lactation influences general movement quality in 12-week-old term infants. Br J Nutr 2010;103(2):235–42. https://doi.org/10.1017/S0007114509991528.
[95] Vidakovic A, Jaddoe V, Gishti O, Felix J, Williams M, Hofman A, et al. Body mass index, gestational weight gain and fatty acid concentrations during pregnancy: the Generation R Study. Eur J Epidemiol 2015;30:1175–85. https://doi.org/10.1007/s10654-015-0106-6.
[96] Wadhwani N, Patil V, Joshi S. Maternal long chain polyunsaturated fatty acid status and pregnancy complications. Prostagl Leukot Essent Fat Acids 2017. https://doi.org/10.1016/j.plefa.2017.08.002.
[97] Wai T, Langer T. Mitochondrial dynamics and metabolic regulation. Trends Endocrinol Metabol 2016;27(2):105–17. https://doi.org/10.1016/j.tem.2015.12.001.
[98] Wainwright PE. Dietary essential fatty acids and brain function: a developmental perspective on mechanisms. Proc Nutr Soc 2002;61(1):61–9. https://doi.org/10.1079/PNS2001130.
[99] Warude D, Joshi K, Harsulkar A. Polyunsaturated fatty acids: Biotechnology. Crit Rev Biotechnol 2006;26(2):83–93. https://doi.org/10.1080/07388550600697479.
[100] Westermeier F, Sáez PJ, Villalobos-Labra R, Sobrevia L, Farías-Jofré M. Programming of fetal insulin resistance in pregnancies with maternal obesity by ER stress and inflammation. BioMed Res Int 2014;13. https://doi.org/10.1155/2014/917672. 2014.
[101] White CL, Purpera MN, Morrison CD. Maternal obesity is necessary for programming effect of high-fat diet on offspring. Am J Physiol Regul Integr Comp Physiol 2009;296(5):R1464–72. https://doi.org/10.1152/ajpregu.91015.2008.
[102] Zambrano E, Nathanielsz PW. Mechanisms by which maternal obesity programs offspring for obesity: evidence from animal studies. Nutr Rev 2013;71(Suppl. l_1):S42–54. https://doi.org/10.1111/nure.12068.
[103] Zambrano E, Nathanielsz PW. Relative contributions of maternal western-type high fat high sugar diets and maternal obesity to altered metabolic function in pregnancy. J Physiol 2017;595(14):4573–4. https://doi.org/10.1113/JP274392.

CHAPTER 7

Minerals in pregnancy and newborns

Hamdan Z. Hamdan[1,2] **Ahmed A. Hassan**[3], **Ishag Adam**[3]
[1]Faculty of Medicine, Al-Neelain University, Khartoum, Sudan; [2]Al-Neelain Institute for Medical Research (NIMR), Al-Neelain University, Khartoum, Sudan; [3]Faculty of Medicine, University of Khartoum, Khartoum, Sudan

Contents

Introduction

International Union of Pure and Applied Chemistry (IUPAC) defined trace elements as "any element having an average concentration of less than 100 parts per million (ppm) atoms or less than μg/g" [1]. Many metals are included in this definition, e.g., Zinc (Zn), Selenium (Se), Copper (Cu),

Molecular Nutrition
ISBN 978-0-12-813862-5
https://doi.org/10.1016/B978-0-12-813862-5.00007-4

and Magnesium (Mg). Trace elements like other inorganic elements should be supplied in the diet. Cereals and grains are rich in many trace elements like Zn and Cu. However, grains and legumes may contain phytate which can interfere with the absorption of trace elements in the gastrointestinal tract [2,3].

Pregnancy is accompanied by many physiological changes (including hemodilution) that needed to accommodate the fetus. Hemodilution decreases the levels of trace elements in the blood. Another process is active transport of trace elements which occurs through the placenta to ensure the optimum supply of the trace elements to the growing fetus [4–6]. Increased nutritional requirements are needed to ensure good health status of pregnant woman and her growing fetus. On the other hand, poor maternal nutrition has a deleterious outcome on both mother and the newborn, e.g., Mg, Zn, and Se deficiency is associated with the development of gestational diabetes, which in turn leads to development of type 2 diabetes in both the mother and the newborn in later life [7,8].

The area of molecular trace elements research witnessed much advancement in the last four decades; however, still, there is a gap of knowledge which needs to be removed. In this chapter clinical and molecular aspects of selected trace elements are discussed in regard to obstetrics conditions such as gestational diabetes mellitus and preeclampsia. Molecular mechanisms explaining the mechanism of low birth weight and teratogenicity are discussed too.

Gestational diabetes mellitus

Gestational diabetes mellitus (GDM) is defined as an onset of glucose intolerance during the pregnancy. Its prevalence reached up to 17.8% among pregnant women [9]. GDM can lead to macrosomia, which may result in shoulder dystocia, perinatal injury, and postpartum hemorrhage [10,11]. GDM may lead to development of overt type 2 diabetes in both the mother and the newborn in later life [7,8].

Zinc and its physiological and biological importance

Zn is a divalent cation that is needed in specific concentration to maintain hemostasis in the body [12]. It is involved in many functions that include enhancing immune system, acting as cofactor for over 300 enzymes, improving hormone signaling transduction, and acting as protein antioxidant against free radicals [13–15]. Zn is an important metal component in the cell membrane and it helps in preserving DNA structural integrity [16]. Zn is essential for normal insulin hormone synthesis, storage, and release [17]. Zn is needed for sperm formation, oocyte ovulation, and even zygote formation and reproductive health [16,18]. Zn requirement is increased during pregnancy as a result of increased demands of both mother and the growing fetus [9]. If these requirements are not adequately met, Zn deficiency will occurs.

Zinc and gestational diabetes mellitus

Although the exact cause of GDM is not yet fully understood, trace elements deficiency is suggested as a predisposing factor for GDM. Many studies reported the association between low maternal Zn and GDM [19,20].

Pregnancy is a physiological stress that needs a high amount of antioxidants (vitamins and minerals like Zn, Se, and Cu) [21]. Low Zn level will decrease the antioxidants capacity that is observed in GDM and can further aggravate the oxidative stress condition [22]. Zn supplementation to women with GDM improves the antioxidant capacity, increases serum Zn concentration, decreases inflammatory biomarkers, and improves the glucose homeostasis parameters [23,24].

Zinc transporters in gestational diabetes

There are two families of transporters that govern the movements of Zn in and out of the cell. Firstly, the ZnT family of transporter: this family enhances the secretion of Zn from inside the cell to inside cellular organelle or outside by which cellular Zn content decreases. Secondly, ZIP (Zrt-, Irt-like protein): this transporter enhances the uptake of the Zn by the cell and then increases intracellular Zn content, as illustrated in Fig. 7.1A [25]. ZnT family is composed of 10 members of transporters distributed all over the body including the pancreatic β-cells. The pancreas expresses many ZnT transporters like ZnT3, ZnT5, and ZnT8 [26,27]. These transporters collectively have a synergistic effect that results in unusual intracellular high Zn concentration in pancreatic cells [28]. ZnT8 collects Zn from the cytoplasm and inserts it inside the insulin granules [29]. Autoantibodies directed to the ZnT8 are associated with the development of GDM [30,31], Fig. 7.1B. Gene polymorphism in the coding region of *SLC30A8* gene is associated with the development of type 2 and type 1 diabetes mellitus [32–34]. There is an association between *SLC30A8* polymorphism in the

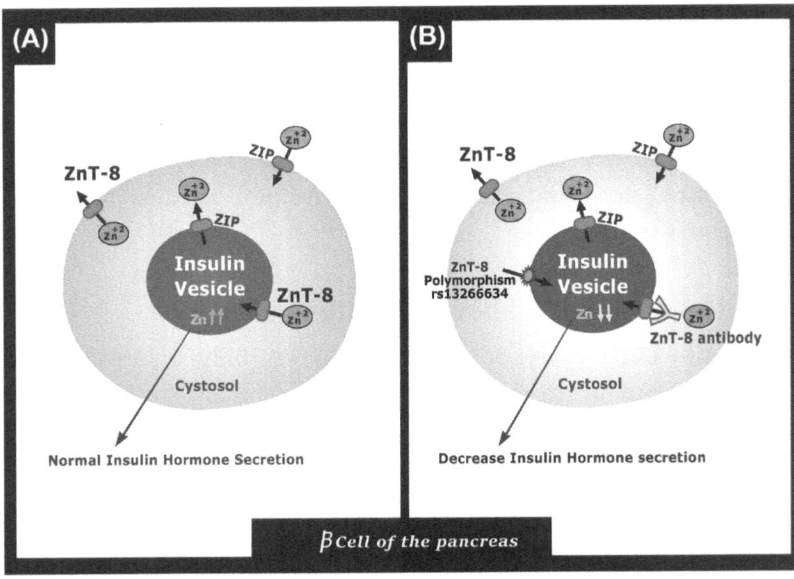

Figure 7.1 Role of zinc transporters ZnT8 and ZIP in transportation of zinc from cytosol of the β-cell to insulin vesicle and outside the β-cell, outside the β-cell to inside the cytosol, respectively. (A): Shows normal movements of zinc inside and outside the cell and its relation to zinc content inside insulin vesicles and its effect on insulin hormone secretion. (B): ZnT 8 binds to its autoantibodies which block the movement of zinc inside the insulin vesicle; it also shows the effect of ZnT 8 gene polymorphism (rs13266634), which results in reduction of zinc movement inside the insulin vesicle.

coding region (rs-13266634) and GDM [35], Fig. 7.1B. In light of the above premises, Zn is an essential metal for the normal insulin hormone synthesis, storage, and secretion. Genetic factors affect the activity of the ZnT transporters, which precipitate development of GDM.

Selenium and gestational diabetes mellitus

Se is an essential trace element with many biological functions in the human body. Dietary source (animal proteins and seafood) is the only source for Se. In addition to animal sources, cereals and grains also contain high amount of Se. However, its content is determined by the content of Se that is found in the soils [36]. Variation in Se concentration internationally may be attributed to geographical distribution of Se in the soils and to the variations in nutritional habits [36]. Se acts as an integral component of many protein enzymes that are known as selenoproteins, which include formate dehydrogenase, glutathione peroxidase, selenoproteins P and W, and the deiodinases [37]. Se is involved in neutralizing free radicals by the action of glutathione peroxidase enzyme and other selenoproteins [38]. It is worth mentioning that more than 60% of the body Se is bound to the glutathione peroxidase enzyme [39]. This indicates the major function of Se in the body cells.

Lower Se levels have been described during normal pregnancy and this is attributed to hemodilution, active transportation of Se to the placenta and fetal circulation, and increased production of antioxidative selenoenzymes to neutralize the gestational oxidative stress which escalates during pregnancy [4–6].

Although Se deficiency is linked with the development of many diseases including type 2 diabetes, there is a controversy on its involvement in GDM [37,40,41]. While some studies linked low Se levels with the GDM, some other studies reported high Se levels in relation to GDM and some others showed no association [41–43]. Se maintains uptake and utilization of the cellular glucose in the peripheral tissues [44]. Se has insulinlike effect, by which it activates sets of regulatory enzymes involved in glycolysis and glycogenesis, resulting in lowering blood glucose levels [45,46]. Se enhances the rate of phosphorylation of the tyrosine residues in the cytoplasmic part of the insulin receptors and IRS-1 [47]. Furthermore, it can enhance the activity of the p42 and p44 of the MAPkinases [47]. Collectively, Se enhances the insulin downstream signaling pathway which ends with activation of glucose transportation and activation of enzymes related to glucose metabolism [47,48].

Se supplementation has a positive effect on GDM, as it decreases the level of fasting blood glucose and inflammatory and oxidative stress markers [49]. Se supplementation can prevent or alleviate the end-organ damage observed in diabetic patients, e.g., diabetic retinopathy, nephropathy, and peripheral neuropathy [43].

Magnesium and gestational diabetes mellitus

Mg is an important metal that assists catalytic activity of over 300 enzymes. It is important for the normal insulin hormone secretion, binding, and receptor function [50,51]. Mg acts as a cofactor for the major glycolytic enzymes that end with reduction of blood glucose [52]. Mg deficiency is implicated in the pathogenicity of type 2 diabetes [51]. There are few studies on Mg and GDM [11,53–55]. Mg supplementation significantly improves insulin sensitivity in type 2 diabetic patients [56,57]. Mg supplementation significantly improves the glucose status in prediabetic patients [58]. These observations consolidate the involvement of Mg in the pathogenicity of the GDM and improving the pregnancy outcome [59].

Preeclampsia

Preeclampsia is a common medical condition that affects about 2%–7% of pregnancies [60]. It is characterized by hypertension (blood pressure >140/90 mmHg) and proteinuria, which is developed after the 20th week of gestation [61]. Preeclampsia is considered the most common obstetrical condition and it is associated with maternal and neonatal adverse outcome [62]. Although preeclampsia has been studied for years, its exact cause still remains uncertain. However, vitamins and minerals deficiency could have a role in the development of preeclampsia [63–65].

Calcium and preeclampsia

Ca is an important divalent cation that is needed for many physiological functions like activation of clotting factors, maintaining of the membrane potential during resting and action potential, muscle contraction and releasing of neurotransmitter [66]. Ca deficiency seems to increase the release of parathyroid hormone and renin angiotensin system, which leads to retention of the calcium in intracellular compartment, especially in smooth muscle and can lead to vasoconstriction which causes rise in blood pressure [67,68], Fig. 7.2. A lower maternal serum Ca has been reported in patients with preeclampsia compared to normal controls [64,65,69]. Ca supplementation could reduce the risk of preeclampsia [70]. It has been suggested that calcium induces the synthesis of vasoactive mediator nitric oxide (NO), which dilates the blood vessels and hence decreases the blood pressure [70].

Magnesium and preeclampsia

Mg is a divalent cation that is ranked as the second major intracellular cation. It is needed for many physiological reactions that include cofactor for more than 300 enzymes, majority of which are related to energy releasing pathways. It is a component of the high energy compound (ATP) [71]. Mg is important for the adaptability, fine-tuning, and contractility of the blood vessels in response to blood pressure [72]. This is the rationale to use magnesium sulfate as a therapy for the prevention of eclampsia attacks [73]. There is wide variation in the maternal serum Mg levels in patients with preeclampsia compared to normal control [74–76]. Interaction between Ca and Mg has been mooted before and authors suggest that to control the blood pressure coordination of both Ca and Mg are highly needed. Ca acts as a vasoconstrictor while Mg acts as a vasodilator. So Mg

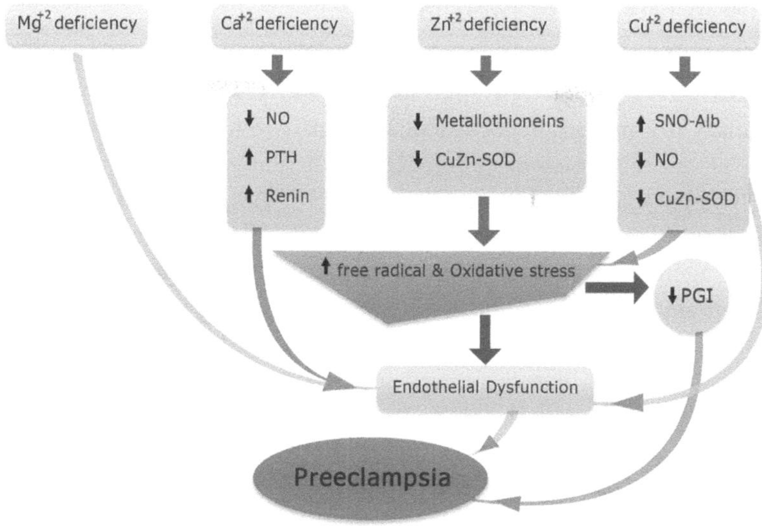

Figure 7.2 Multiple mechanisms of Cu, Zn, Ca, and Mg deficiency in pathogenicity of preeclampsia. Cu deficiency decreases nitric oxide (NO) and copper_zinc superoxide dismutase (CuZn-SOD) and increases S-nitrosoalbumin (SNO-Alb), which contributes to increased oxidative stress and endothelial dysfunction. Zn deficiency decreases the activity of CuZn-SOD and metallothioneins, which contribute directly to increase oxidative stress. Ca deficiency increases both parathyroid hormone and renin levels and decreases NO which contributes to endothelial dysfunction. Mg deficiency is directly involved in endothelial dysfunction. Oxidative stress and increased free radicals decrease levels of prostaglandin-I (PGI). Endothelial dysfunction and reduced PGI both promote preeclampsia.

behaves as if it is a natural calcium channel blocker by which it can reduce the blood pressure [77,78]. Perhaps, decreased Mg levels stimulate epinephrine, norepinephrine, angiotensin-II, serotonin, acetylcholine, and bradykinin, which ultimately raise the blood pressure [79].

Zinc and preeclampsia

Preeclampsia is associated with oxidative stress [80]. Zn is a component in Cu-Zn superoxide dismutase (CuZn-SOD) enzyme structure. It is an inducer element for antioxidant protein metallothioneins, and it is an antioxidant molecule per se that can protect the sulfhydryl group of cysteine containing enzymes [81]. Perhaps, lipid peroxidation as a result of Zn deficiency is the mechanism that can cause endothelial dysfunction in preeclampsia [69], Fig. 7.2. Maternal Zn deficiency can lead to preeclampsia [82,83] and Zn supplementation during pregnancy can decrease the incidence of preeclampsia [82].

Copper in relation to preeclampsia

Cu is an essential cation for the human wellbeing. Cu is cofactor for the antioxidative enzyme activity like catalase and CuZn-SOD. Beside these functions, Cu is important for vascular integrity [84,85]. The bioavailability of NO as vasodilator agent is linked to sufficient availability of blood Cu levels. The circulatory S-nitrosoalbumin (SNO-Alb) act as reservoir for the NO. The NO will be released from SNO-Alb upon binding with a reducing agent like vitamin C or a transitional metal like Cu. Levels of SNO-Alb are high in women with preeclampsia; however, levels of NO are reduced [86], Fig. 7.2. Cu deficiency is associated with oxidative stress as Cu is a component of catalase and superoxide dismutase enzyme which remove cellular free radicals. High levels of superoxide will react with the available NO and generate peroxynitrite ($ONOO^-$), which reduce further the availability of the NO. On the other hand, peroxynitrite is considered as a pathological molecule that can damage the placental vessels and induce vascular resistance, which ultimately increases the blood pressure. Peroxynitrite leads to irreversible nitration of the tyrosine residues in enzymes and proteins, which impair its phosphorylation and activation. By this mechanism peroxynitrite prevents formation of prostaglandin-I2 (PGI2), as tyrosine nitration inhibits the activity of prostaglandin synthase enzyme [87], Fig. 7.2. Lack of PGI2 leads to smooth muscle contraction and increases blood pressure [88], Fig. 7.2. Another potential role of reactive oxygen species is that it can activate and aggregate the platelet inside the blood vessels leading to a generation of intravascular coagulopathy [89]. Genetic knockout of CuZn-SOD or adding a Cu chelating agent resulted in reduced NO vascular response [90,91]. On the contrary adding of CuZn-SOD significantly improves the vessels functions [92].

Low birth weight

Low birth weight (LBW) is defined as a baby weighing less than 2500 g at birth. LBW deliveries are at higher risk for perinatal and infant mortality [93]. Not only this, but LBW babies may develop coronary heart disease, hypertension, diabetes mellitus, chronic obstructive lung disease in their later life [94,95].

Zinc, low birth weight, and fetal growth abnormalities

Zn is the second most abundant trace element after iron [96]. Maternal circulation is the only source of nutrient to the fetus; therefore, maternal nutrition is the main source of Zn to the fetus [97–99].

Zinc and its physiological functions in relation to growth

Maternal and cord Zn deficiency can lead to various fetal growth abnormalities, e.g., LBW, intrauterine growth restriction, preterm birth, congenital malformation (anencephaly), and miscarriage [97–99]. Zn is an important element in the structure of a plethora of metalloenzymes which are important for nucleotide and protein synthesis [98]. Zn is needed for all six enzyme classes named by International Union of Biochemistry and Molecular Biology (IUBMB). It acts as core structure for the enzyme and in such case presence of the Zn is important for stabilizing the quaternary structure of the protein. Therefore, Zn can either enhance or decrease the enzyme efficiency [100]. Zn also is needed for the activity of the DNA binding proteins which regulate the gene expression. Zn is essential for the stability of many hormones' receptors, which include estrogen, glucocorticoids, thyroid hormones, retinoic acid, and vitamin D [101]. The hormone-receptor complex without Zn molecule results in failure of binding to DNA region upon activation, which curtails the gene expression action of these hormones [96].

Zinc effects during embryogenesis

During embryogenesis, Zn is needed for the structure and regulation of chromatin and histone proteins. These proteins are involved directly in the regulation of the gene expression and hence cellular differentiation of the growing embryo [102]. Maternal Zn deficiency can lead to neural tube defects as a failure to cope with the rapid development of the central nervous system during embryonic life [103]. Maternal Zn deficiency can be a result of alcohol consumption, which can lead to fetal alcohol syndrome and growth failure [104]. Fetuses deficient in Zn express low jnsulinlike growth factor binding protein-1(IGF-Binding Protein-1) and low hepatic IGF-1 *mRNA* [105]. Normal expression of IGF-1 and IGFBP is essential for cellular and tissue proliferation, differentiation, survival, and maintaining the maturation process of many embryo systems [105–109].

Zinc effects during fetal period and Zn supplementation trials

Zn is needed during the fetal period to face the expanding and continuous growth requirement. To ensure optimum Zn supply, placenta actively transports Zn from maternal to fetal circulation [110,111]. At 24th week of gestation the fetal liver starts to express metallothioneins (MTs), which are tiny proteins weighing 7 Kd and contain 20 cysteine residues. The unusual high cysteine content allows metallothioneins to store reactive metals like

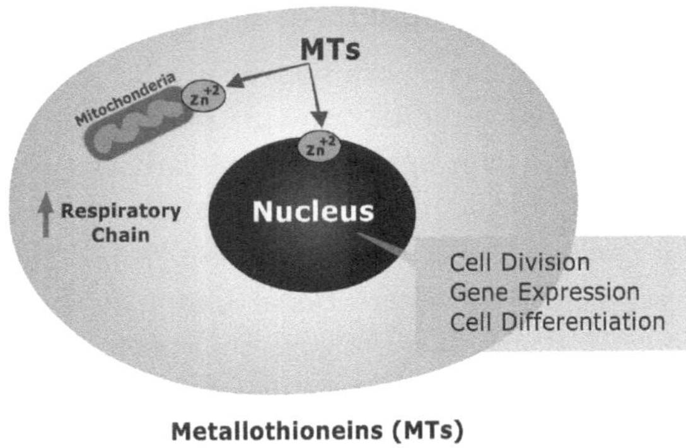

Figure 7.3 Metallothioneins and its role in providing zinc inside the nucleus for gene expression, cell differentiation, and cell division, in addition to respiratory chain reactions in mitochondria.

Zn [112]. In addition, metallothioneins are involved in the transport of Zn from the cytosol to inside the nucleus at the time of cell division and transport of Zn to mitochondrial matrix for respiratory chain reactions. These two functions linked metallothioneins to cell divisions, cell differentiation, gene expression, tissue regenerations, and energy production [113–115] Fig. 7.3. Zn supplementation during pregnancy reduces the rate of preterm delivery and LBW [116,117]. The metallothioneins gene promoter region has seven metal responsive elements (MREs). Upon exposure to high concentration of heavy metals and in case of oxidative stress, MRE-binding transcription factor-1 (MTF-1) will be activated and active MTF-1 binds to MRE region and starts the gene transcription process [118], Fig. 7.4A. There is a promoter region polymorphism in the

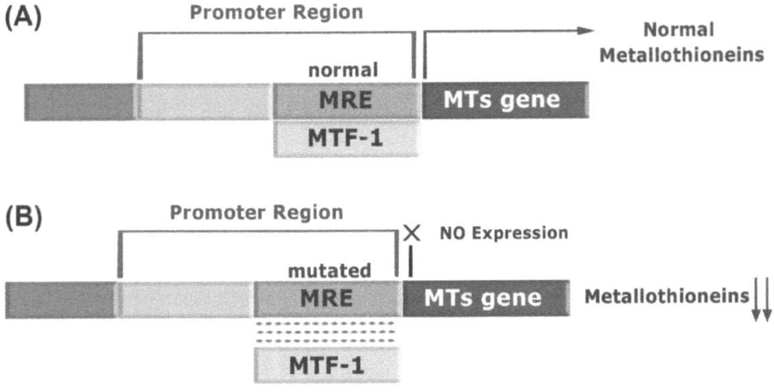

Figure 7.4 (A): Shows normal metallothioneins (MTs) gene expression upon binding of the transcription factor MTF-1 to MRE in the promoter region. (B): Shows failure of expression of metallothioneins as a result of mutation in MRE which decreases the binding affinity of transcription factor MTF-1.

upstream direction of the TATA box. This polymorphism decreases the binding affinity of MTF-1 to MREs, and as a result significant reduction in metallothioneins transcription occurs [119], Fig. 7.4B.

Selenium and low birth weight

There is a positive correlation between the birth weight and cord Se levels [120,121]. It is known that Se is an important component for the structure of thyroid hormone and its involvement in energy metabolism [122]. However, synthesis of thyroid hormone does not decline unless serum Se decreased to more than 80% of the body content [123].

Teratogenesis and mineral involvements

Zinc and its role in teratogenesis

Involvement of Zn deficiency in teratogenicity of human embryo has been postulated early in 1973 by Sever and Emanuel [124]. Pregnant women who have low serum Zn especially in the first and third trimester are subjected to develop a baby with some birth defects [125]. Maternal Zn deficiency decreases the rate of DNA and protein synthesis in the fetus. The reduction in DNA synthesis results in the embryo's chromosomal structure damage. More specifically, the chromosomes show unusual gaps and terminal deletion regions [126,127]. Another mechanism reported indicating that maternal Zn deficiency can induce apoptosis of the embryo's cells, especially in highly sensitive regions [128]. These regions include neural tube, somites, pharyngeal arches, otic placode, optic vesicle, forelimb buds [128,129]. Neural crest cells are the most sensitive cells to Zn deficiency and they will affect either the metabolic profile or migratory movements, and therefore manifested as congenital heart diseases in a rat model [130]. In continuation to apoptotic mechanism, Zn deficiency diminishes ERK signaling pathway, which resulted in reduction of cell proliferation and imposed apoptosis pathway activation. Zn directly can inhibit the apoptotic enzyme caspase-3; this inhibitory action is lost in case of low cellular Zn content [131].

Beside direct apoptosis pathway activation, oxidative stress as a consequence of Zn deficiency was mooted as another mechanism that induces indirectly apoptotic pathways and so leads to teratogenicity. Zn is a core structural component in antioxidative enzymes namely CuZn-SOD. Moreover, Zn per se can protect sulfhydryl group of cysteine containing proteins against the oxidation by free radical [81]. Additionally, Zn deficiency inhibits synthesis of metallothioneins, which acts as a cellular scavenger against free radicals beside its role as storage form and distributor for cellular Zn [132,133] Fig. 7.3. Oxidative stress results in damage of proteins, lipids, and DNA [134,135]. Damaged DNA is usually detected by tumor suppressor protein P53, which arrests the cell cycle and induces either DNA repair mechanism or in case of failure it imposes apoptosis. Interestingly, the DNA binding domain of p53 contains Zn molecule. In case of Zn deficiency, DNA repair will fail and as a consequence apoptosis occurs as an inevitable alternative [136].

Failure of cellular growth observed in Zn deficiency has been considered as a mechanism for teratogenicity. Zn deficiency decreases the velocity of cellular differentiation, especially during the first trimester, which is characterized by organogenesis [137]. This could explain the teratogenicity of Zn deficiency.

Zinc deficiency in newborn

The role of Zn in maintaining cellular growth and tissue differentiation is not limited to intrauterine life period only. Zn deficiency in neonate manifests as growth failure and dermatitis [138,139]. Neonatal skin rash is the most common feature of Zn deficiency and it appears since the first week of life and responds well to Zn supplementation [140]. This skin lesion is most common among preterm babies as they have less Zn store [141]. Skin is the largest organ in the body, with rapid regeneration rate [142]. These two skin's features need high amount of Zn; therefore, signs of Zn deficiency appear first in the skin.

Organs and tissue growth continue after birth and as a result Zn demands continue. Preterm babies are particularly subjected to Zn deficiency as their bodies store less amount of Zn compared to full-term babies. Secondly, their body tissues are eager to grow faster than full-term babies [142]. To gain weight, body tissues have to synthesize enzymes and proteins involved in growth and maturation process and this synthetic process depends on Zn supply. Supplementation of Zn correlates well with weight and tissue growth [143].

Zn has an important role in the integrity of the immune system as it is needed in the synthesis of number of cytokines, differentiation and maturation of immune cells, chemotaxis and squeezing of immune cells between endothelial cells [144]. On the contrary, Zn deficiency is associated with poor immune system and makes the body prone to infections, mainly gastrointestinal and respiratory system infections [145].

Copper and teratogenicity

Cu is involved in many physiological functions that are necessary for normal embryonic life. Cu is found in the structure of many enzymes like cytochrome C, which is involved in the respiratory chain reaction and mitochondrial energy production, metallothioneins, and CuZn-SOD structure, which has antioxidative function. Involvement of Cu deficiency in the teratogenicity has been postulated [146].

Cu is a cofactor for lysyl oxidase enzyme, which is important for the collagen and elastin maturation in the extracellular matrix. In case of Cu deficiency lysyl oxidase enzyme activity is decreased, which leads to formation of abnormal collagen and elastin which resulted in fragile and loose blood vessels [147]. Collagen and elastin are important in the migration and maturation of endothelial cells and hence normal development of cardiovascular system [148,149]. Rats with knockout gene of lysyl oxidase enzyme die at perinatal period as a result of aortic aneurysm and cardiovascular malfunctions [150]. Another point is that the proximal and distal parts of the bronchi are fragmented as they contain abnormal elastin [151]. Additionally, Cu-deficient zebra fish embryo showed abnormally mid- and hind brain region with unusually enlarged ventricles [147]. Lysyl inhibitors result in detachment of the collagen fibers in the notochord region, which resulted in defective notochord, somites, and epidermal blisters [152]. Notochord is the primary structure for the development of the vertebral column, neural tubes, and motor neurons [147].

Cu is a part of the antioxidant enzyme CuZn-SOD SOD. Cu can activate the other non-Cu containing antioxidant enzymes like Se-dependent glutathione peroxidase and catalase enzyme [153]. Cu deficiency results in increased superoxide anion, which reacts with NO to generate peroxynitrite ($ONOO^-$). Peroxynitrite is considered a pathogenic molecule that leads to protein nitration and is involved in many neurodegenerative diseases [154]. Another pathogenic role is that NO acts as important signaling molecule for growing and extending the embryo vasculature. However, overproduction of superoxide consumes this NO and results in fragile embryonic vessels and arrested angiogenesis process [155]. Moreover, NO is crucial for cardiomyocyte growth and differentiation and myocardial angiogenesis [156]. On the contrary, oxidative stress reduction in NO results in excessive apoptosis and teratogenicity [157]. Common defects observed in offspring of Cu-deficient media include septal and valvular defects in addition to contractile dysfunction which ends with early postnatal heart failure [158].

The mechanism for developing teratogenicity in Cu deficiency is multifactorial and both direct Cu deficiency and indirect mechanisms have been documented.

References

[1] McNaught A.D. WA. In: Compendium of chemical terminology: the gold book. 2nd ed. London, UK: Blackwell Science; 1997.

[2] F., I. of Medicine NB. Dietary Reference Intakes for vitamin A, vitamin K, Arsenic, Boron, Chromium, Cu, Iodine, iron, Manganese, Molybdenum, Nickel, Silicon, vanadium, and Zn. Natl. Acad. Press; 2001.

[3] Abdelrahaman SM, Elmaki HB, Idris WH, Hassan AB, Babiker EE, El Tinay AH. Antinutritional factor content and hydrochloric acid extractability of minerals in pearl millet cultivars as affected by germination. Int J Food Sci Nutr 2007;58:6−17.

[4] Mihailović M, Cvetković M, Ljubić A, Kosanović M, Nedeljković S, Jovanović I, Pesut O. Se and malondialdehyde content and glutathione peroxidase activity in maternal and umbilical cord blood and amniotic fluid. Biol Trace Elem Res 2000;73:47−54. https://doi.org/10.1385/BTER:73:1:47.

[5] Kantola M, Purkunen R, Kröger P, Tooming A, Juravskaja J, Pasanen M, Seppänen K, Saarikoski S, Vartiainen T. Se in pregnancy: is Se an active defective ion against environmental chemical stress? Environ Res 2004;96:51−61. https://doi.org/10.1016/j.envres.2004.03.003.

[6] Ferrer E, Alegría A, Barberá R, Farré R, Lagarda MJ, Monleon J. Whole blood Se content in pregnant women. Sci Total Environ 1999;227:139−43.

[7] Weijers RNM, Bekedam DJ. Relationship between gestational diabetes mellitus and type 2 diabetes: evidence of mitochondrial dysfunction. Clin Chem 2007;53:377−83. https://doi.org/10.1373/clinchem.2006.077636.

[8] Kim C, Newton KM, Knopp RH. Gestational diabetes and the incidence of type 2 diabetes: a systematic review. Diabetes Care 2002;25:1862−8.

[9] Swanson CA, King JC. Zn and pregnancy outcome. Am J Clin Nutr 1987;46:763−71.

[10] Ornoy A. Prenatal origin of obesity and their complications: gestational diabetes, maternal overweight and the paradoxical effects of fetal growth restriction and macrosomia. Reprod Toxicol 2011;32:205−12. https://doi.org/10.1016/j.reprotox.2011.05.002.

[11] Wang Y, Tan M, Huang Z, Sheng L, Ge Y, Zhang H, Jiang M, Zhang G. Elemental contents in serum of pregnant women with gestational diabetes mellitus. Biol Trace Elem Res 2002;88:113−8. https://doi.org/10.1385/BTER:88:2:113.

[12] Azhdarzadeh M, Noroozian M, Aghaverdi H, Akbari SM, Baum L, Mahmoudi M. Serum multivalent cationic pattern: speculation on the efficient approach for detection of alzheimer's disease. Sci Rep 2013;3:2782. https://doi.org/10.1038/srep02782.

[13] DiSilvestro RA. Zn in relation to diabetes and oxidative disease. J Nutr 2000;130:1509S−15011S.

[14] Yaman M, Kaya G, Yekeler H. Distribution of trace metal concentrations in paired cancerous and non-cancerous human stomach tissues. World J Gastroenterol 2007;13:612−8. https://doi.org/10.3748/wjg.v13.i4.612.

[15] Tang X, Shay NF. Zn has an insulin-like effect on glucose transport mediated by phosphoinositol-3-kinase and Akt in 3T3-L1 fibroblasts and adipocytes. J Nutr 2001;131:1414−20.

[16] MacDonald RS. The role of Zn in growth and cell proliferation. J Nutr 2000;130:1500S−8S.

[17] Chausmer AB. Zn, insulin and diabetes. J Am Coll Nutr 1998;17:109–15.
[18] Black MM. Zn deficiency and child development. Am J Clin Nutr 1998;68:464S–9S.
[19] Wang Y, Tan M, Huang Z, Sheng L, Ge Y, Zhang H, Jiang M, Zhang G. Elemental contents in serum of pregnant women with gestational diabetes mellitus. Biol Trace Elem Res 2002;88:113–8. https://doi.org/10.1385/BTER:88:2:113.
[20] Bo S, Lezo A, Menato G, Gallo M-L, Bardelli C, Signorile A, Berutti C, Massobrio M, Pagano GF. Gestational hyperglycemia, Zn, Se, and antioxidant vitamins. Nutrition 2005;21:186–91. https://doi.org/10.1016/j.nut.2004.05.022.
[21] Myatt L, Cui X. Oxidative stress in the placenta. Histochem Cell Biol 2004;122:369–82. https://doi.org/10.1007/s00418-004-0677-x.
[22] Suhail M, Patil S, Khan S, Siddiqui S. Antioxidant vitamins and lipoperoxidation in non-pregnant, pregnant, and gestational diabetic women: erythrocytes osmotic fragility profiles. J Clin Med Res 2010;2:266–73. https://doi.org/10.4021/jocmr454w.
[23] Karamali M, Heidarzadeh Z, Seifati SM, Samimi M, Tabassi Z, Hajijafari M, Asemi Z, Esmaillzadeh A. Zn supplementation and the effects on metabolic status in gestational diabetes: a randomized, double-blind, placebo-controlled trial. J Diabet Complicat 2015;29:1314–9. https://doi.org/10.1016/j.jdiacomp.2015.07.001.
[24] Karamali M, Heidarzadeh Z, Seifati S-M, Samimi M, Tabassi Z, Talaee N, Bahardoost H, Asemi Z. Zn supplementation and the effects on pregnancy outcomes in gestational diabetes: a randomized, double-blind, placebo-controlled trial. Exp Clin Endocrinol Diabetes 2015;124:28–33. https://doi.org/10.1055/s-0035-1564146.
[25] Lichten LA, Cousins RJ. Mammalian Zn transporters: nutritional and physiologic regulation. Annu Rev Nutr 2009;29:153–76. https://doi.org/10.1146/annurev-nutr-033009-083312.
[26] Clifford KS, MacDonald MJ. Survey of mRNAs encoding Zn transporters and other metal complexing proteins in pancreatic islets of rats from birth to adulthood: similar patterns in the Sprague-Dawley and Wistar BB strains. Diabetes Res Clin Pract 2000;49:77–85.
[27] Kambe T, Narita H, Yamaguchi-Iwai Y, Hirose J, Amano T, Sugiura N, Sasaki R, Mori K, Iwanaga T, Nagao M. Cloning and characterization of a novel mammalian Zn transporter, Zn transporter 5, abundantly expressed in pancreatic β cells. J Biol Chem 2002;277:19049–55. https://doi.org/10.1074/jbc.M200910200.
[28] Wijesekara N, Chimienti F, Wheeler MB. Zn, a regulator of islet function and glucose homeostasis. Diabetes Obes Metabol 2009;11(Suppl. 4):202–14. https://doi.org/10.1111/j.1463-1326.2009.01110.x.
[29] Seman NA, Mohamud WNW, Östenson C-G, Brismar K, Gu HF. Increased DNA methylation of the SLC30A8 gene promoter is associated with type 2 diabetes in a Malay population. Clin Epigenet 2015;7:30. https://doi.org/10.1186/s13148-015-0049-5.
[30] Rudland VL, Pech C, Harding AJ, Tan K, Lee K, Molyneaux L, Yue DK, Wong J, Ross GP. Zn transporter 8 autoantibodies: what is their clinical relevance in gestational diabetes? Diabet Med 2015;32:359–66. https://doi.org/10.1111/dme.12629.
[31] Arvan P, Pietropaolo M, Ostrov D, Rhodes CJ. Islet autoantigens: structure, function, localization, and regulation. Cold Spring Harb. Perspect. Med. 2012;2. https://doi.org/10.1101/cshperspect.a007658. a007658–a007658.
[32] Xu K, Zha M, Wu X, Yu Z, Yu R, Xu X, Chen H, Yang T. Association between rs13266634 C/T polymorphisms of solute carrier family 30 member 8 (SLC30A8) and type 2 diabetes, impaired glucose tolerance, type 1 diabetes–a meta-analysis. Diabetes Res Clin Pract 2011;91:195–202. https://doi.org/10.1016/j.diabres.2010.11.012.

[33] Jing YL, Sun QM, Bi Y, Shen SM, Zhu DL. SLC30A8 polymorphism and type 2 diabetes risk: evidence from 27 study groups. Nutr Metabol Cardiovasc Dis 2011;21:398–405. https://doi.org/10.1016/j.numecd.2009.11.004.
[34] Wenzlau JM, Liu Y, Yu L, Moua O, Fowler KT, Rangasamy S, Walters J, Eisenbarth GS, Davidson HW, Hutton JC. A common nonsynonymous single nucleotide polymorphism in the SLC30A8 gene determines ZnT8 autoantibody specificity in type 1 diabetes. Diabetes 2008;57:2693–7. https://doi.org/10.2337/db08-0522.
[35] Wang X, Li W, Ma L, Ping F, Liu J, Wu X, Mao J, Wang X, Nie M. Investigation of miRNA-binding site variants and risk of gestational diabetes mellitus in Chinese pregnant women. Acta Diabetol 2017;54:309–16. https://doi.org/10.1007/s00592-017-0969-y.
[36] Kong F-J, Ma L-L, Chen S-P, Li G, Zhou J-Q. Serum Se level and gestational diabetes mellitus: a systematic review and meta-analysis. Nutr J 2016;15:94. https://doi.org/10.1186/s12937-016-0211-8.
[37] Rayman MP. Se and human health. Lancet 2012;379:1256–68. https://doi.org/10.1016/S0140-6736(11)61452-9.
[38] R.F. Burk. Se, an antioxidant nutrient. Nutr Clin Care. (n.d.);5:75–79.
[39] Holben DH, Smith AM. The diverse role of Se within selenoproteins: a review. J Am Diet Assoc 1999;99:836–43. https://doi.org/10.1016/S0002-8223(99)00198-4.
[40] Mueller AS, Mueller K, Wolf NM, Pallauf J. Se and diabetes: an enigma? Free Radic Res 2009;43:1029–59. https://doi.org/10.1080/10715760903196925.
[41] Hamdan HZ, Elbashir LM, Hamdan SZ, Elhassan EM, Adam I. Zn and Se levels in women with gestational diabetes mellitus at Medani Hospital, Sudan. J Obstet Gynaecol 2014;34. https://doi.org/10.3109/01443615.2014.919576.
[42] Molnar J, Garamvolgyi Z, Herold M, Adanyi N, Somogyi A, Rigo J. Serum Se concentrations correlate significantly with inflammatory biomarker high-sensitive CRP levels in Hungarian gestational diabetic and healthy pregnant women at mid-pregnancy. Biol Trace Elem Res 2008;121:16–22. https://doi.org/10.1007/s12011-007-8018-2.
[43] Kilinc M, Guven MA, Ezer M, Ertas IE, Coskun A. Evaluation of serum Se levels in Turkish women with gestational diabetes mellitus, glucose intolerants, and normal controls. Biol Trace Elem Res 2008;123:35–40. https://doi.org/10.1007/s12011-007-8087-2.
[44] Ezaki O. The insulin-like effects of selenate in rat adipocytes. J Biol Chem 1990;265:1124–8.
[45] Douillet C, Tabib A, Bost M, Accominotti M, Borson-Chazot F, Ciavatti M. Se in diabetes: effects of Se on nephropathy in type I streptozotocin-induced diabetic rats. J Trace Elem Exp Med 1999;12:379–92. https://doi.org/10.1002/(SICI)1520-670X. 1999)12:4<379::AID-JTRA12>3.0.CO;2-C.
[46] Antioxidant defense system in differentially hydrogen peroxide sensitive L5178Y sublines. Free Radic Biol Med 1997;22:697–704. https://doi.org/10.1016/S0891-5849(96)00388-7.
[47] Stapleton SR, Garlock GL, Foellmi-Adams L, Kletzien RF. Se: potent stimulator of tyrosyl phosphorylation and activator of MAP kinase. Biochim Biophys Acta 1997;1355:259–69.
[48] Hei YJ, Farahbakhshian S, Chen X, Battell ML, McNeill JH. Stimulation of MAP kinase and S6 kinase by vanadium and Se in rat adipocytes. Mol Cell Biochem 1998;178:367–75.
[49] Asemi Z, Jamilian M, Mesdaghinia E, Esmaillzadeh A. Effects of Se supplementation on glucose homeostasis, inflammation, and oxidative stress in gestational diabetes: randomized, double-blind, placebo-controlled trial. Nutrition 2015;31:1235–42. https://doi.org/10.1016/j.nut.2015.04.014.

[50] Suárez A, Pulido N, Casla A, Casanova B, Arrieta FJ, Rovira A. Impaired tyrosine-kinase activity of muscle insulin receptors from hypomagnesaemic rats. Diabetologia 1995;38:1262–70.
[51] Sales CH, Pedrosa L de FC. Mg and diabetes mellitus: their relation. Clin Nutr 2006;25:554–62. https://doi.org/10.1016/j.clnu.2006.03.003.
[52] MacLeod D, MacLeod J. Mg: physiology and pharmacology. Br J Anaesth 1999;83:972–3.
[53] Akhlaghi F, Bagheri SM, Rajabi O. A comparative study of relationship between micronutrients and gestational diabetes. ISRN Obstet. Gynecol 2012:1–4. https://doi.org/10.5402/2012/470419. 2012.
[54] Goker Tasdemir U, Tasdemir N, Kilic S, Abali R, Celik C, Gulerman HC. Alterations of ionized and total Mg levels in pregnant women with gestational diabetes mellitus. Gynecol Obstet Invest 2015;79:19–24. https://doi.org/10.1159/000365813.
[55] Ertbeg P, Nørgaard P, Bang L, Nyholm H, Rudnicki M. Ionized Mg in gestational diabetes. Magnes Res 2004;17:35–8.
[56] Guerrero-Romero F, Rodríguez-Morán M. Mg improves the beta-cell function to compensate variation of insulin sensitivity: double-blind, randomized clinical trial. Eur J Clin Invest 2011;41:405–10. https://doi.org/10.1111/j.1365-2362.2010.02422.x.
[57] Mooren FC, Krüger K, Völker K, Golf SW, Wadepuhl M, Kraus A. Oral Mg supplementation reduces insulin resistance in non-diabetic subjects - a double-blind, placebo-controlled, randomized trial. Diabetes Obes Metabol 2011;13:281–4. https://doi.org/10.1111/j.1463-1326.2010.01332.x.
[58] Guerrero-Romero F, Simental-Mendía LE, Hernández-Ronquillo G, Rodriguez-Morán M. Oral Mg supplementation improves glycaemic status in subjects with prediabetes and hypomagnesaemia: a double-blind placebo-controlled randomized trial. Diabetes Metab 2015;41:202–7. https://doi.org/10.1016/j.diabet.2015.03.010.
[59] Asemi Z, Karamali M, Jamilian M, Foroozanfard F, Bahmani F, Heidarzadeh Z, Benisi-Kohansal S, Surkan PJ, Esmaillzadeh A. Mg supplementation affects metabolic status and pregnancy outcomes in gestational diabetes: a randomized, double-blind, placebo-controlled trial. Am J Clin Nutr 2015;102:222–9. https://doi.org/10.3945/ajcn.114.098616.
[60] Adam I, Haggaz AED, Mirghani OA, Elhassan EM. Placenta previa and pre-eclampsia: analyses of 1645 cases at medani maternity hospital, Sudan. Front Physiol 2013;4:28–31. https://doi.org/10.3389/fphys.2013.00032. FEB.
[61] Cunningham FG WK, Leveno KJ, Bloom SL, Hauth JC, Gilstrap LC. Hypertensive disorders in pregnancy. In: Cunningham FG, Leveno KJ, Bloom SL, Hauth JC, editors. Gilstrap LC, wenstrom KD williams obstet. 22nd ed. New York: McGraw-Hill; 2005. p. 761–808.
[62] N. Vasiljević, M. Vasiljević, D. Plećas. [The role of nutritional factors in pre-eclampsia and eclampsia]. Srp Arh Celok Lek. (n.d.);124:156–159.
[63] V Raman L S. Nutrition during pregnancy and lactation. Textb. Hum. Nutr. 2002:509.
[64] Elmugabil A, Hamdan HZ, Elsheikh AE, Rayis DA, Adam I, Gasim GI. Serum calcium, Mg, Zn and Cu levels in Sudanese women with preeclampsia. PloS One 2016;11:e0167495. https://doi.org/10.1371/journal.pone.0167495.
[65] Jain S, Sharma P, Kulshreshtha S, Mohan G, Singh S. The role of calcium, Mg, and Zn in pre-eclampsia. Biol Trace Elem Res 2010;133:162–70. https://doi.org/10.1007/s12011-009-8423-9.
[66] PA F. Agents affecting mineral ion homeostasis and bone turnover. In: Brunton LLL, P.K.G., s JS G, editors. Pharmacol. Basis ther. 11th ed. Mc Graw-Hill; 2006.

[67] V Kanagal D, Rajesh A, Rao K, Devi UH, Shetty H, Kumari S, Shetty PK. Levels of serum calcium and Mg in pre-eclamptic and normal pregnancy: a study from coastal India. J Clin Diagn Res 2014;8:OC01–4. https://doi.org/10.7860/JCDR/2014/8872.4537.
[68] Belizán JM, Villar J, Repke J. The relationship between calcium intake and pregnancy-induced hypertension: up-to-date evidence. Am J Obstet Gynecol 1988;158:898–902.
[69] Farzin L, Sajadi F. Comparison of serum trace element levels in patients with or without pre-eclampsia. J Res Med Sci 2012;17:938–41.
[70] Khaing W, Vallibhakara SA-O, Tantrakul V, Vallibhakara O, Rattanasiri S, McEvoy M, Attia J, Thakkinstian A. Calcium and vitamin D supplementation for prevention of preeclampsia: a systematic review and network meta-analysis. Nutrients 2017;9:1141. https://doi.org/10.3390/nu9101141.
[71] Saris NE, Mervaala E, Karppanen H, Khawaja JA, Lewenstam A. Mg. An update on physiological, clinical and analytical aspects. Clin Chim Acta 2000;294:1–26.
[72] Walsh SB, Zdebik AA, Unwin RJ. Mg: the disregarded cation. Mayo Clin Proc 2015;90:993–5. https://doi.org/10.1016/j.mayocp.2015.06.011.
[73] Sibai BM. Mg sulfate is the ideal anticonvulsant in preeclampsia-eclampsia. Am J Obstet Gynecol 1990;162:1141–5.
[74] Kumru S, Aydin S, Simsek M, Sahin K, Yaman M, Ay G. Comparison of serum Cu, Zn, calcium, and Mg levels in preeclamptic and healthy pregnant women. Biol Trace Elem Res 2003;94:105–12. https://doi.org/10.1385/BTER:94:2:105.
[75] Sanders GT, Huijgen HJ, Sanders R. Mg in disease: a review with special emphasis on the serum ionized Mg. Clin Chem Lab Med 1999;37:1011–33. https://doi.org/10.1515/CCLM.1999.151.
[76] Sukonpan K, Phupong V. Serum calcium and serum Mg in normal and preeclamptic pregnancy. Arch Gynecol Obstet 2005;273:12–6. https://doi.org/10.1007/s00404-004-0672-4.
[77] Skjærven R, Wilcox AJ, Lie RT. The interval between pregnancies and the risk of preeclampsia. N Engl J Med 2002;346:33–8. https://doi.org/10.1056/NEJMoa011379.
[78] Power ML, Heaney RP, Kalkwarf HJ, Pitkin RM, Repke JT, Tsang RC, Schulkin J. The role of calcium in health and disease. Am J Obstet Gynecol 1999;181:1560–9.
[79] Altura BM, Altura BT. Mg, electrolyte transport and coronary vascular tone. Drugs 1984;28(Suppl. 1):120–42.
[80] Ilhan N, Ilhan N, Simsek M. The changes of trace elements, malondialdehyde levels and superoxide dismutase activities in pregnancy with or without preeclampsia. Clin Biochem 2002;35:393–7.
[81] Niles BJ, Clegg MS, Hanna LA, Chou SS, Momma TY, Hong H, Keen CL. Zn deficiency-induced iron accumulation, a consequence of alterations in iron regulatory protein-binding activity, iron transporters, and iron storage proteins. J Biol Chem 2008;283:5168–77. https://doi.org/10.1074/jbc.M709043200.
[82] Ma Y, Shen X, Zhang D. The relationship between serum Zn level and preeclampsia: a meta-analysis. Nutrients 2015;7:7806–20. https://doi.org/10.3390/nu7095366.
[83] Zhu Q, Zhang L, Chen X, Zhou J, Liu J, Chen J. Association between Zn level and the risk of preeclampsia: a meta-analysis. Arch Gynecol Obstet 2016;293:377–82. https://doi.org/10.1007/s00404-015-3883-y.
[84] Danks DM. Cu deficiency in humans. Annu Rev Nutr 1988;8:235–57. https://doi.org/10.1146/annurev.nu.08.070188.001315.
[85] Gibson RS. Assessment of trace element status in humans. Prog Food Nutr Sci 1989;13:67–111.

[86] Gandley RE, Tyurin VA, Huang W, Arroyo A, Daftary A, Harger G, Jiang J, Pitt B, Taylor RN, Hubel CA, Kagan VE. S-nitrosoalbumin-mediated relaxation is enhanced by ascorbate and Cu: effects in pregnancy and preeclampsia plasma. Hypertension (Dallas) 2005;45:21–7. https://doi.org/10.1161/01.HYP.0000150158.42620.3e. Dallas, Tex. 1979.
[87] Ullrich V, Bachschmid M. Superoxide as a messenger of endothelial function. Biochem Biophys Res Commun 2000;278:1–8. https://doi.org/10.1006/bbrc.2000.3733.
[88] Kirk EA, Dinauer MC, Rosen H, Chait A, Heinecke JW, LeBoeuf RC. Impaired superoxide production due to a deficiency in phagocyte NADPH oxidase fails to inhibit atherosclerosis in mice. Arterioscler Thromb Vasc Biol 2000;20:1529–35.
[89] Matsubara K, Higaki T, Matsubara Y, Nawa A. Nitric oxide and reactive oxygen species in the pathogenesis of preeclampsia. Int J Mol Sci 2015;16:4600–14. https://doi.org/10.3390/ijms16034600.
[90] Didion SP, Ryan MJ, Didion LA, Fegan PE, Sigmund CD, Faraci FM. Increased superoxide and vascular dysfunction in CuZnSOD-deficient mice. Circ Res 2002;91:938–44.
[91] Falcone JC, Lominadze D, Johnson WT, Schuschke DA. Endothelial cell-derived nitric oxide mobilization is attenuated in Cu-deficient rats. Appl Physiol Nutr Metabol 2008;33:1073–8. https://doi.org/10.1139/H08-091.
[92] Gibson E, A., Lilley. Superoxide anions, free-radical scavengers, and nitrergic neurotransmission. Gen Pharmacol 1997:489–93.
[93] Wilcox AJ. On the importance–and the unimportance–of birthweight. Int J Epidemiol 2001;30:1233–41.
[94] Stein CE, Fall CH, Kumaran K, Osmond C, Cox V, Barker DJ. Fetal growth and coronary heart disease in south India. Lancet (London, England) 1996;348:1269–73.
[95] Curhan GC, Willett WC, Rimm EB, Spiegelman D, Ascherio AL, Stampfer MJ. Birth weight and adult hypertension, diabetes mellitus, and obesity in US men. Circulation 1996;94:3246–50.
[96] King JC. Zn: an essential but elusive nutrient. Am J Clin Nutr 2011;94:679S–84S. https://doi.org/10.3945/ajcn.110.005744.
[97] Abass RM, Hamdan HZ, Elhassan EM, Hamdan SZ, Ali NI, Adam I. Zn and Cu levels in low birth weight deliveries in Medani Hospital, Sudan. BMC Res Notes 2014;7:386. https://doi.org/10.1186/1756-0500-7-386.
[98] Costello AM de L, Osrin D. Micronutrient status during pregnancy and outcomes for newborn infants in developing countries. J Nutr 2003;133:1757S–64S.
[99] Siddiqui MKJ, Srivastava S, Mehrotra PK, Srivastava SP. Some essential elements in maternal and cord blood in relation to birth weight and gestational age of the baby Biol Trace Elem Res 2002;86:097–106. https://doi.org/10.1385/BTER:86:2:097.
[100] Vallee BL, Auld DS. Active Zn binding sites of Zn metalloenzymes. Matrix Suppl 1992;1:5–19.
[101] Evans RM. The steroid and thyroid hormone receptor superfamily. Science 1988;240:889–95. 80-.
[102] Falchuk KH. The molecular basis for the role of Zn in developmental biology. Mol Cell Biochem 1998;188:41–8.
[103] Hambidge M, Hackshaw A, Wald N. Neural tube defects and serum Zn. Br J Obstet Gynaecol 1993;100:746–9.
[104] McClain CJ, Kasarskis EJ, Allen JJ. Functional consequences of Zn deficiency. Prog Food Nutr Sci 1985;9:185–226.

[105] Hanna LA, Clegg MS, Ellis-Hutchings RG, Niles BJ, Keen CL. The influence of gestational Zn deficiency on the fetal insulin-like growth factor axis in the rat. Exp Biol Med (Maywood) 2010;235:206–14. https://doi.org/10.1258/ebm.2009.009018.
[106] Thornburg KL, Louey S, Giraud GD. The role of growth in heart development. In: Wind. Oppor. Pre-pregnancy to 24 Mon. Age. Basel: KARGER; 2008. p. 39–51. https://doi.org/10.1159/000113169.
[107] Cannarella R, Condorelli RA, La Vignera S, Calogero AE. Effects of the insulin-like growth factor system on testicular differentiation and function: a review of the literature. Andrology 2018;6:3–9. https://doi.org/10.1111/andr.12444.
[108] Joseph D'Ercole A, Ye P. Expanding the mind: insulin-like growth factor I and brain development. Endocrinology 2008;149:5958–62. https://doi.org/10.1210/en.2008-0920.
[109] Wang Y, Nishida S, Sakata T, Elalieh HZ, Chang W, Halloran BP, Doty SB, Bikle DD. Insulin-like growth factor-I is essential for embryonic bone development. Endocrinology 2006;147:4753–61. https://doi.org/10.1210/en.2006-0196.
[110] Bax CMR, Bloxam DL. Two major pathways of Zn(II) acquisition by human placental syncytiotrophoblast. J Cell Physiol 1995;164:546–54. https://doi.org/10.1002/jcp.1041640312.
[111] Donangelo CM, King JC. Maternal Zn intakes and homeostatic adjustments during pregnancy and lactation. Nutrients 2012;4:782–98. https://doi.org/10.3390/nu4070782.
[112] Vašák M. Advances in metallothionein structure and functions. J Trace Elem Med Biol 2005;19:13–7. https://doi.org/10.1016/j.jtemb.2005.03.003.
[113] Cherian MG, Kang YJ. Metallothionein and liver cell regeneration. Exp Biol Med (Maywood) 2006;231:138–44.
[114] Ye B, Maret W, Vallee BL. Zn metallothionein imported into liver mitochondria modulates respiration. Proc. Natl. Acad. Sci. U.S.A 2001;98:2317–22. https://doi.org/10.1073/pnas.041619198.
[115] Tsujikawa K, Imai T, Kakutani M, Kayamori Y, Mimura T, Otaki N, Kimura M, Fukuyama R, Shimizu N. Localization of metallothionein in nuclei of growing primary cultured adult rat hepatocytes. FEBS Lett 1991;283:239–42.
[116] Soltani H, Duxbury AMS, Rundle R, Chan L-N. A systematic review of the effects of dietary interventions on neonatal outcomes in adolescent pregnancy. Evid. Based Midwifery. 2015;13:29–34 6p.
[117] Ota E, Mori R, Middleton P, Tobe-Gai R, Mahomed K, Miyazaki C, Bhutta ZA. Zn supplementation for improving pregnancy and infant outcome. In: Mori R, editor. Cochrane database syst. Rev. Chichester, UK: John Wiley & Sons, Ltd; 2015. CD000230. 10.1002/14651858.CD000230.pub5.
[118] Suzuki K, Koizumi S. Individual metal responsive elements of the human metallothionein-IIA gene independently mediate responses to various heavy metal signals. Ind Health 2000;38:87–90.
[119] Koizumi S, Suzuki K, Ogra Y, Yamada H, Otsuka F. Transcriptional activity and regulatory protein binding of metal-responsive elements of the human metallothionein-IIA gene. Eur J Biochem 1999;259:635–42.
[120] Makhoul IR, Sammour RN, Diamond E, Shohat I, Tamir A, Shamir R. Se concentrations in maternal and umbilical cord blood at 24-42 weeks of gestation: basis for optimization of Se supplementation to premature infants. Clin Nutr 2004;23:373–81. https://doi.org/10.1016/j.clnu.2003.08.004.
[121] Scholl JDBWK-GPO. Low-normal serum Se early in human pregnancy predicts lower birth weight. Nutr Res 2006;26:497–502. https://doi.org/10.1016/J.NUTRES.2006.08.008.

[122] Hawkes WC, Keim NL. Dietary Se intake modulates thyroid hormone and energy metabolism in men. J Nutr 2003;133:3443–8.
[123] Bates JM, Spate VL, Morris JS, Germain DLS, Galton VA. Effects of Se deficiency on tissue Se content, deiodinase activity, and thyroid hormone economy in the rat during development [1]. Endocrinology 2000;141:2490–500. https://doi.org/10.1210/endo.141.7.7571.
[124] Sever LE, Emanuel I. Is there a connection between maternal Zn deficiency and congenital malformations of the central nervous system in man? Teratology 1973;7:117–8. https://doi.org/10.1002/tera.1420070116.
[125] Keen CL, Uriu-Adams JY, Skalny A, Grabeklis A, Grabeklis S, Green K, Yevtushok L, Wertelecki WW, Chambers CD. The plausibility of maternal nutritional status being a contributing factor to the risk for fetal alcohol spectrum disorders: the potential influence of Zn status as an example. Biofactors 2010;36:125–35. https://doi.org/10.1002/biof.89.
[126] Eckhert CD, Hurley LS. Reduced DNA synthesis in Zn deficiency: regional differences in embryonic rats. J Nutr 1977;107:855–61.
[127] Bell LT, Branstrator M, Roux C, Hurley LS. Chromosomal abnormalities in maternal and fetal tissues of Mg- or Zn-deficient rats. Teratology 1975;12:221–6. https://doi.org/10.1002/tera.1420120302.
[128] Rogers JM, Taubeneck MW, Daston GP, Sulik KK, Zucker RM, Elstein KH, Jankowski MA, Keen CL. Zn deficiency causes apoptosis but not cell cycle alterations in organogenesis-stage rat embryos: effect of varying duration of deficiency. Teratology 1995;52:149–59. https://doi.org/10.1002/tera.1420520307.
[129] Jankowski MA, Uriu-Hare JY, Rucker RB, Rogers JM, Keen CL. Maternal Zn deficiency, but not Cu deficiency or diabetes, results in increased embryonic cell death in the rat: implications for mechanisms underlying abnormal development. Teratology 1995;51:85–93. https://doi.org/10.1002/tera.1420510207.
[130] Lopez V, Keen CL, Lanoue L. Prenatal Zn deficiency: influence on heart morphology and distribution of key heart proteins in a rat model. Biol Trace Elem Res 2008;122:238–55. https://doi.org/10.1007/s12011-007-8079-2.
[131] Hashemi M, Ghavami S, Eshraghi M, Booy EP, Los M. Cytotoxic effects of intra and extracellular Zn chelation on human breast cancer cells. Eur J Pharmacol 2007;557:9–19. https://doi.org/10.1016/j.ejphar.2006.11.010.
[132] Szczurek EI, Bjornsson CS, Taylor CG. Dietary Zn deficiency and repletion modulate metallothionein immunolocalization and concentration in small intestine and liver of rats. J Nutr 2001;131:2132–8.
[133] Maret W. Metallothionein redox biology in the cytoprotective and cytotoxic functions of Zn. Exp Gerontol 2008;43:363–9. https://doi.org/10.1016/j.exger.2007.11.005.
[134] Carter JE, Truong-Tran AQ, Grosser D, Ho L, Ruffin RE, Zalewski PD. Involvement of redox events in caspase activation in Zn-depleted airway epithelial cells. Biochem Biophys Res Commun 2002;297:1062–70. https://doi.org/10.1016/S0006-291X(02)02292-1.
[135] Oteiza PI, Olin KL, Fraga CG, Keen CL. Zn deficiency causes oxidative damage to proteins, lipids and DNA in rat testes. J Nutr 1995;125:823–9.
[136] Corniola RS, Tassabehji NM, Hare J, Sharma G, Levenson CW. Zn deficiency impairs neuronal precursor cell proliferation and induces apoptosis via p53-mediated mechanisms. Brain Res 2008;1237:52–61. https://doi.org/10.1016/j.brainres.2008.08.040.
[137] O'Dell BL, Browning JD. Impaired calcium entry into cells is associated with pathological signs of Zn deficiency. Adv. Nutr. 2013;4:287–93. https://doi.org/10.3945/an.112.003624.

[138] Islam MN, Chowdhury AK, Siddika M, Hossain MA, Hossain MK. Effect of Zn on growth of preterm babies. Mymensingh Med J 2009;18:125–30.
[139] Arlette JP, Johnston MM. Zn deficiency dermatosis in premature infants receiving prolonged parenteral alimentation. J Am Acad Dermatol 1981;5:37–42.
[140] Zattra E, Belloni Fortina A. Transient symptomatic Zn deficiency resembling acrodermatitis enteropathica in a breast-fed premature infant: case report and brief review of the literature. G Ital Dermatol Venereol 2013;148:699–702.
[141] Wulf K, Wilhelm A, Spielmann M, Wirth S, Jenke AC. Frequency of symptomatic Zn deficiency in very low birth weight infants. Klin Padiatr 2013;225:13–7. https://doi.org/10.1055/s-0032-1312610.
[142] Wang T, Zhu L, Pei M. Insight into skin cell-based osteogenesis: a review. F1000Research. 2017;6:291. https://doi.org/10.12688/f1000research.10280.1.
[143] Ram Kumar TV, Ramji S. Effect of Zn supplementation on growth in very low birth weight infants. J Trop Pediatr 2012;58:50–4. https://doi.org/10.1093/tropej/fmr036.
[144] Bonaventura P, Benedetti G, Albarède F, Miossec P. Zn and its role in immunity and inflammation. Autoimmun Rev 2015;14:277–85. https://doi.org/10.1016/j.autrev.2014.11.008.
[145] McDonald CM, Manji KP, Kisenge R, Aboud S, Spiegelman D, Fawzi WW, Duggan CP. Daily Zn but not multivitamin supplementation reduces diarrhea and upper respiratory infections in Tanzanian infants: a randomized, double-blind, placebo-controlled clinical trial. J Nutr 2015;145:2153–60. https://doi.org/10.3945/jn.115.212308.
[146] Bennetts FE, H.W., Chapman. Cu deficiency in sheep in Western Australia: a preliminary account of the aetiology of enzootic ataxia of lambs and anemia of the Ewe. Aust Vet J 1937:138–49.
[147] Mendelsohn BA, Yin C, Johnson SL, Wilm TP, Solnica-Krezel L, Gitlin JD. Atp7a determines a hierarchy of Cu metabolism essential for notochord development. Cell Metabol 2006;4:155–62. https://doi.org/10.1016/j.cmet.2006.05.001.
[148] George EL, Baldwin HS, Hynes RO. Fibronectins are essential for heart and blood vessel morphogenesis but are dispensable for initial specification of precursor cells. Blood 1997;90:3073–81.
[149] Reeves PG, DeMars LCS. Cu deficiency reduces iron absorption and biological half-life in male rats. J Nutr 2004;134:1953–7.
[150] Hornstra IK, Birge S, Starcher B, Bailey AJ, Mecham RP, Shapiro SD. Lysyl oxidase is required for vascular and diaphragmatic development in mice. J Biol Chem 2003;278:14387–93. https://doi.org/10.1074/jbc.M210144200.
[151] Mäki JM, Sormunen R, Lippo S, Kaarteenaho-Wiik R, Soininen R, Myllyharju J. Lysyl oxidase is essential for normal development and function of the respiratory system and for the integrity of elastic and collagen fibers in various tissues. Am J Pathol 2005;167:927–36. https://doi.org/10.1016/S0002-9440(10)61183-2.
[152] Geach TJ, Dale L. Members of the lysyl oxidase family are expressed during the development of the frog *Xenopus laevis*. Differentiation 2005;73:414–24. https://doi.org/10.1111/j.1432-0436.2005.00041.x.
[153] Uriu-Adams JY, Keen CL. Cu, oxidative stress, and human health. Mol Aspect Med 2005;26:268–98. https://doi.org/10.1016/j.mam.2005.07.015.
[154] Freixes M, Rodríguez A, Dalfó E, Ferrer I. Oxidation, glycoxidation, lipoxidation, nitration, and responses to oxidative stress in the cerebral cortex in Creutzfeldt-Jakob disease. Neurobiol Aging 2006;27:1807–15. https://doi.org/10.1016/j.neurobiolaging.2005.10.006.

[155] Yang SJ, Keen CL, Lanoue L, Rucker RB, Uriu-Adams JY. Low nitric oxide: a key factor underlying Cu-deficiency teratogenicity. Free Radic Biol Med 2007;43:1639–48. https://doi.org/10.1016/j.freeradbiomed.2007.08.031.
[156] Schulz R, Rassaf T, Massion PB, Kelm M, Balligand J-L. Recent advances in the understanding of the role of nitric oxide in cardiovascular homeostasis. Pharmacol Ther 2005;108:225–56. https://doi.org/10.1016/j.pharmthera.2005.04.005.
[157] Haremaki T, Fraser ST, Kuo Y-M, Baron MH, Weinstein DC. Vertebrate Ctr1 coordinates morphogenesis and progenitor cell fate and regulates embryonic stem cell differentiation. Proc. Natl. Acad. Sci. U.S.A 2007;104:12029–34. https://doi.org/10.1073/pnas.0701413104.
[158] Feng Q, Song W, Lu X, Hamilton JA, Lei M, Peng T, Yee S-P. Development of heart failure and congenital septal defects in mice lacking endothelial nitric oxide synthase. Circulation 2002;106:873–9.

CHAPTER 8

Perinatal nutritional intervention: current and future perspectives

Cristina Campoy[1,2] Mireia Escudero-Marín[1,2] Estefanía Diéguez[1,2], Tomás Cerdó[1,2]
[1]Department of Pediatrics, School of Medicine, University of Granada, Granada, Spain; [2]EURISTIKOS Excellence Centre for Pediatric Research, University of Granada, Granada, Spain

Contents

Introduction

During the past decades, developmental biology has spotlighted the fundamental nature of epigenetic control of cell fate. From the study carried out by John Gordon in the 1960s about the amphibian somatic cell nuclear transfer to Azim Surani's groundbreaking studies on the nonequivalence of the maternal and paternal genomes, recent findings of Shinya Yamanaka about the creation of induced pluripotent stem cells should be highlighted [1–3].

Perinatal development is a critical window for the fetus that can cause alterations in gene expression related to later diseases [4]. At the end of World War II, during the winter of 1944–45, Germans cut down the food supplies to the Netherlands, causing widespread famine, known as the Dutch Famine. The Dutch Hunger Winter provided knowledge about the importance of maternal nutrition to influence offspring health in later life. Several studies suggested that the timing of the nutritional constraint is important, as the first trimester famine exposure increased the risk of obesity and cardiovascular disease (CVD), whereas exposure in later stages of

Molecular Nutrition
ISBN 978-0-12-813862-5
https://doi.org/10.1016/B978-0-12-813862-5.00008-6

gestation increased the risk of later insulin resistance and hypertension [5,6]. Accordingly, it is important to ensure a good nutrition status during pregnancy, especially the maintenance of a healthy glucose homeostasis, to avoid the increased risk for developing type 2 diabetes (T2D), obesity, and CVD [7,8] in mothers and their offspring.

It should be noted that the perinatal period is a window of opportunity to carry out nutritional interventions that may avoid the development of diseases in later stages of life. However, despite the aforementioned studies, few interventional studies have been conducted in humans on this regard.

Given the above, in the present chapter, we review recent evidence on the potential role of maternal diet during pregnancy and breastfeeding to counteract epigenetic alterations and phenotypic outcomes in offspring. Furthermore, we will propose and present knowledge about potential mechanisms of action and ways to intervene for disease prevention and treatments with possible medical and industrial applications in the future.

Molecular bases of early nutrition programming

Epigenetic processes, such as DNA methylation, histone modifications, or microRNAs (miRNAs) (Fig. 8.1), induce heritable changes in gene expression without a change in DNA sequence [9]. As a consequence, the fetus develops adaptive responses that allow it to predict and be prepared for later environmental experiences, but excessive alterations can degenerate in future diseases [10].

On one hand, DNA methylation consists of the addition of a methyl group along the DNA strand where a cytosine base is located beside a guanine base (CpG site), which might confer stable silencing of transcription [11]. On the other hand, aminoacidic histone tails can be post-transcriptionally modified, including their acetylation, methylation, phosphorylation, ubiquitinylation, and SUMOylation, and these modifications *(among other epigenetic marks)* might determine whether the chromatin is active or inactive. As a result, the gene expression within that chromatin region is affected [12]. Moreover, miRNAs are short RNAs composed of 20–22 nucleotides, which are evolutionarily conserved and located within the introns and exons of protein-coding genes (70%) or in intergenic regions (30%). Although the role of miRNAs in fetal programming remains largely understudied, dietary factors have been shown to modify their expression profiling, notably in maternal nutrition-induced epigenetic modifications in offspring with lipid metabolism, insulin resistance, and inflammation [13,14].

In addition to all these epigenetic alterations, recent evidences implicate the role of gut microbiota in mother's and offspring's metabolism [15,16].

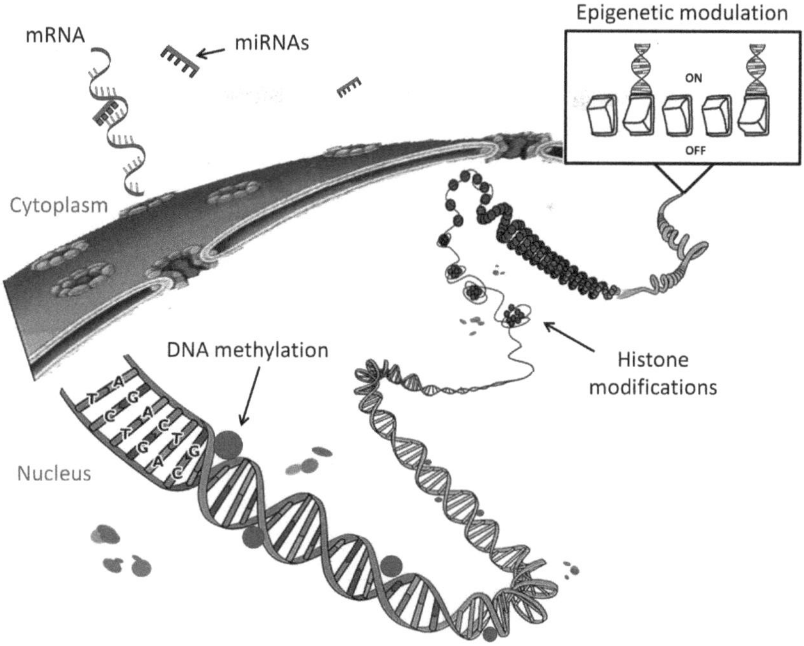

Figure 8.1 Epigenetic mechanisms. Methylation, histone modification, and miRNA are examples of mechanisms determining changes on DNA and gene expression. These changes do not alter the underlying DNA sequence.

Probiotics may modulate glucose tolerance through balancing gut microbiota, normalizing increased intestinal permeability, and lowering systemic and local low-grade inflammation, reducing the risk of developing gestational diabetes mellitus (GDM) [17].

It should be noted that DNA methylation as well as histone modifications require methyl donors from dietary folate and need the presence of choline, vitamins B6 and B12, methionine, and methyltransferases *(nutrients involved in one-carbon metabolism)* [18]. Therefore, new intervention studies supplementing women before pregnancy with probiotics and prebiotics could provide new advances to improve maternal vitamin B6, vitamin B12, vitamin D, and zinc status, optimizing maternal glycemia and glucose supply to the fetus-placental unit to promote healthy offspring growth and body composition.

Nutrigenomics is the future of personalized nutrition. It deals with the effect of nutrients and bioactive compounds of foods on gene expression using "omics" technologies to understand the interplay of diets with the genome of individuals and population groups. On this matter, nutrients can be considered as *"signaling molecules"* transmitting dietary signals that cause changes in gene, protein, and metabolite expression. Thus, on a genomic level, nutrients make an imprint in cells linked to the phenotype. Therefore, nutrigenomics could make a difference on the prevention of chronic diseases, such as diabetes, obesity, and CVD, among others [19].

Nutritional intervention during pregnancy

Intrauterine environment and maternal habits during pregnancy (Fig. 8.2) determine offspring short- and long-term outcomes by affecting cell differentiation and organ growth, as well as reprograming plasticity of the embryo [20] with transgenerational effects, affecting the germ cells of the fetus, which could perpetuate the cycle [21]. Long-term effects depend on the stability of epigenetic marks, which are reversible and affected by endogenous and environmental stimuli [20].

On one hand, the addition of a methyl group along the DNA strand, where a cytosine base is located beside a guanine base (CpG site), might confer stable silencing of transcription [11,22]. As an example, a prospective study has shown that significant seasonal variations in methyl-donor nutrient intake of mothers around the time of conception is influenced 13 relevant plasma biomarkers. Moreover, they found that the level of several of these maternal biomarkers predicted increased/decreased

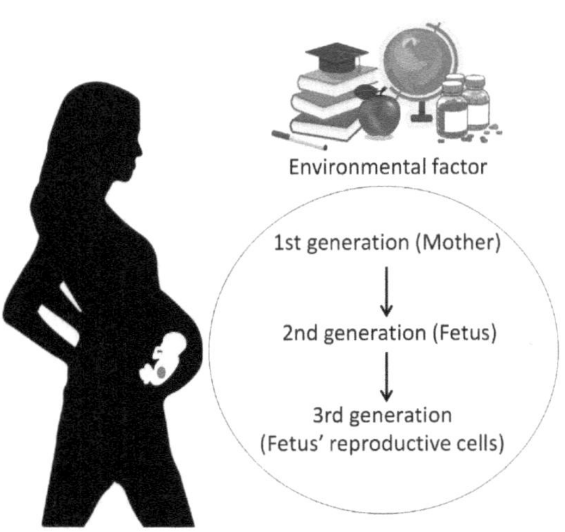

Figure 8.2 Different environmental factors during pregnancy could influence DNA methylation which may affect children's epigenome, even in their germ cells.

methylation at metastable epialleles in DNA extracted from lymphocytes and hair follicles in infants postnatally [23].

An inadequate intake of methyl donors (methionine, betaine, serine, and glycine) and cofactors (vitamins B6, B12, and B2) affects the DNA methylation pattern and mechanisms of transcriptional regulation developing *"nutritional imprinting"* [24], with particular relevance during pregnancy The timing of maternal insult, the offspring gender, and the severity of nutritional changes determine the outcome [25].

Recent nutritional interventions during pregnancy are based on nutrients supplementation or dietary counseling. Despite the reducing comparability of results due to the differences in the methodology employed, such as the follow-up period and dietary monitoring and intervention methods, dietary counseling studies have shown improvements in the quality of the dietary intake [26]; healthier birth outcomes were observed when the intervention was focused on dietary patterns (DPs) before and during pregnancy rather than on isolated nutrients [27]. Nutritional intervention during pregnancy is of particular relevance in poverty situation, and in the presence of eating disorders and high adiposity levels [25], observed in both developed populations and those undergoing rapid socioeconomic transitions [21].

- ***Epigenetic effects of maternal undernutrition during pregnancy***

Undernutrition during pregnancy programs the fetus for increased energy retention and weight gain [27] facing a life of scarcity ("thrifty phenotype" hypothesis) [20] possibly as a consequence of impaired insulin secretion (Fig. 8.3). However, the effect depends on the timing of the nutritional insult [25]. Early gestation famine is related to normal birth weight and higher risk of offspring obesity [25,27] with epigenetic effects on hypothalamic programming and reduced DNA methylation rate at the insulinlike growth factor II (IGF2) gene [20], observed up to six decades later in severe periconceptional undernutrition [24]. Regarding this matter, women exposed to the 1959–61 famine in China, during pregnancy or early childhood, were reported to have a greater risk of metabolic syndrome [28]. Similarly, in Spain during the Civil War (1936–39), there were two main health issues derived from the famine, pellagra and lathyrism, among other health issues [29].

Later in pregnancy, famine is associated with lower birth weight [25]. Early postnatal affluence produces later accelerated growth or *"catch-up,"* resulting in fat deposition and obesity [20] and increased risk of developing hypertension, T2D, and CVD later in life [25].

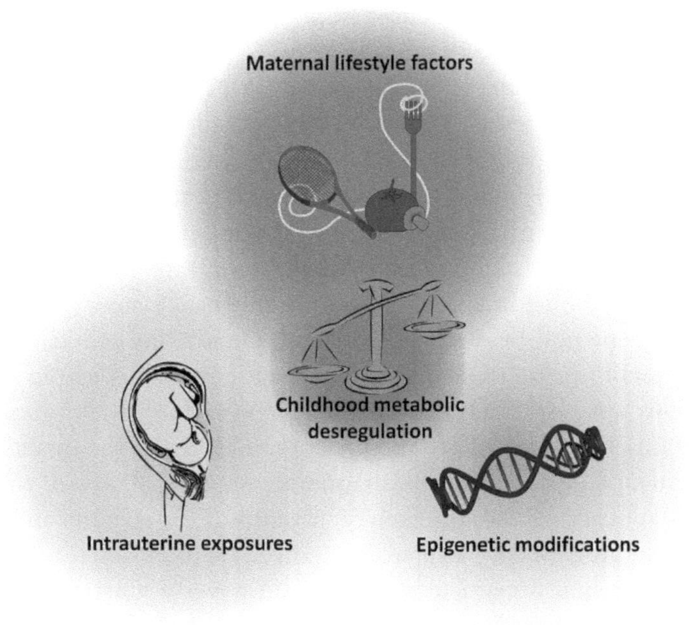

Figure 8.3 Interactions among maternal lifestyle factors *(stress, diet, physical activity)*, intrauterine exposures *(hyperglycaemia, weight gain, obesity)*, and epigenetic modifications *(methylation, histones modifications, miRNA)* will cause childhood metabolic deregulation and future adult diseases *(obesity, type 2 diabetes, cardiovascular disease, ...)*.

Routinely, during pregnancy and lactation the micronutrient supplementation strategy is 60 mg of iron and 400 μg of folic acid, and for severe malnutrition, lipid-based nutrient supplements with varying amounts of protein and energy [22]. Nevertheless, prenatal iron and folic acid supplementation may reduce zinc absorption [30].

Pregnancy fasting state produces hypoaminoacidemia, specifically in glucogenic amino acids, becoming an indicator of maternal protein intake and metabolism. Milk supplementation with vitamin B12 (500 mL/d+10 mg) in South Indian pregnant women from the first trimester of pregnancy increased remethylation rates of methionine cycle during the third trimester, with no effects on placental vascular endothelial growth factor (VEGF) promoter region or long interspersed nuclear element 1 (LINE-1). [24]

Animal models and human studies have shown increased placental gene expression of micronutrient receptors as a consequence of maternal nutritional deficiencies, such as zinc uptake proteins.Additionally, Jobarteh et al.

found lower cord ferritin status in spite of placental expression of transferrin receptor 1 (TfR1) increased after iron deficiency [22].

Accordingly, the PREGGIO study [31] cohort showed that the micronutrient intake was largely predicted by changes in carbohydrate quality. Particularly, low dietary glycemic index and glycemic load were the best predictors of a favorable micronutrient profile [32]. Therefore, several studies focus the intervention on reducing the glycemic index of the diet [27].

Hypothalamic structural variations and changes in neuropeptides gene expression from the arcuate nucleus (ARC) have been observed in rodent models. These changes affect the regulation of food intake and energy expenditure. Moreover, it has been shown that moderate early gestation undernutrition increases glucocorticoid receptor (GR) hypothalamic expression levels, sustaining this effect up to adult life, as well as increases neuropeptide Y (NPY) expression and decreases propiomelanocortin (POMC) expression in animal models. Folic acid supplementation and protein restriction in maternal diet seem to prevent epigenetic changes in GR gene in the offspring's liver [25].

- ***Gestational diabetes mellitus and risk of glucose impairment in the offspring.*** During pregnancy exists a relative maternal insulin resistance that allows the transport of glucose from mother to fetus. In contrast to other nutrients, there is no limit of placental transport of glucose [21]. GDM is characterized by insulin resistance as well as impaired pancreatic β-cells function with its first detection during pregnancy [26,33], increasing risk of embryonic mortality, premature delivery, dystocia, macrosomia, neonatal hypoglycemia, hyperbilirubinemia, and hypocalcemia [30], as well as obesity, diabetes, and metabolic disease in the offspring later in life [21]. Impaired glucose tolerance (IGT) is more critical especially at the beginning of the second trimester of pregnancy [30]. The most relevant GDM risk factors are lower mother's birth weight, family history of T2D, prepregnancy overweight or obesity, excessive gestational weight gain, advanced maternal age, previous pregnancy with GDM and ethnicity, with lower risk in non-Hispanic white women. GDM is related to an increased prevalence of obesity and diabetes in their offspring, perpetuating the vicious cycle [21,26,33,34].

According to a recent metaanalysis, low glycemic index (LGI) diets reduce the risk of having a child large for gestational age (LGA). It has been shown that dietary advice, leading to dietary changes, reduces the energy intake and weight gain during pregnancy but the studies are heterogeneous regarding nutritional interventions, glucose monitoring methods, exercise measurement, mixed interventions with physical activity counseling, weight gain, and probiotic use [33].

Impaired insulin secretion and insulin resistance have been frequently associated with impaired levels of micronutrients, mainly chromium, magnesium, selenium, vanadium, zinc, and copper [30,35], while vitamin D and B12 deficiencies provide a possible causal pathway to offspring's adiposity [21,24]. Other nonessential nutrients, such as myoinositol could reduce insulin resistance during pregnancy [21].

Vitamin D or zinc supplementation could produce beneficial effects on glycemia, by reducing the risk of insulin resistance. Nevertheless, different studies found inconclusive results regarding zinc serum and blood glucose levels, because of the variation in zinc supplementation doses, duration, chemical form and the participants' characteristics. A recent study found increased zinc serum levels and decreased fasting glucose on Iranian pregnant women with impaired glucose tolerance after supplementation of 30 mg/day of zinc gluconate tablet during eight consecutive weeks [30].

Recent interventional studies are focused on reducing GDM incidence in high risk women, primarily obese pregnant women or with family history of diabetes, by dietary counseling or supplementation before and during pregnancy. In this regard, dietary and healthy life habits counseling during pregnancy included weight control in RADIEL [26] reduced in 39% the incidence of GDM, increasing physical activity and improving the quality of the diet in Finnish pregnant women [33]. Furthermore, NiPPeRaims to observe epigenetic changes in offspring after nutritional intervention, but the results have not been published yet [21].

- ***Maternal obesity and oxidative stress***

Firstly, prepregnancy overweight, especially obesity, is linked to higher risk of miscarriage, induced preterm delivery, preterm premature membrane rupture, and cesarean delivery, as well as infants born LGA. Moreover, fetal growth restriction, together with maternal overnutrition during pregnancy, increases fetal fat deposition and fetal number of adipocytes [24,25,27] and hence, the risk of developing obesity and CVD later in life according to the *"Developmental origins of adult disease"* (DoHAD) hypothesis [20]. Maternal obesity has been related to the reduction of energy expenditure on the offspring throughout epigenetic programming of anorexigenic neurons. Similar permanent changes have been described in animal studies [25]. In this sense, breastfeeding is shorter and less prevalent in obese mothers due to physiological difficulties in milk production [27].

On the other hand, in rodents it has been observed that a high fat diet increases maternal obesity and hyperglycemia together with the risk of developing metabolic disease in their offspring, such as obesity or overweight, associated with epigenetic changes, such as DNA methylation of genetic loci, which is involved in metabolic functions [21]. Inflammatory cytokines are involved in development of pregnancy complications including insulin resistance and GDM. The adipose tissue and placenta of GDM women produce higher levels of tumor necrosis factor-α (TNF-α) after the placental exposure to high glucose levels. Nonetheless, antiinflammatory cytokines, such as adiponectin, and VEGF placental expression and VEGF umbilical cord blood levels are lower in GDM mothers in comparison to their healthy siblings. Different studies [35] have shown changes in the expression of proinflammatory genes after selenium supplementation throughout inhibition of MAP kinase pathways and NF-κB, increasing the production of glutathione peroxidase (GPx). Selenium supplementation in animal models has shown inconsistent results depending on the chemical form of the supplements and the addition of other antioxidants. In the first epigenetic study performed in humans with selenium supplementation, 200 μg/day, during 6 weeks in GDM women, the authors found downregulated TNF-α and transforming growth factor beta (TGF-β) gene expression, and upregulated VEGF gene expression in lymphocytes, with no effect on interleukin (IL) 1β and IL-8 [35].

Therefore, the supplementation with chemical chaperones and antioxidant vitamins could be an alternative therapy that reduces the oxidative stress, caused by high blood glucose levels induced by placental endoplasmic reticulum stress in GDM [36].

Finally, Chase et al. carried out a pilot trial to determine the effect of DHA supplementation to mothers in the last trimester of pregnancy and during breastfeeding and to formula-fed and breastfed infants, on levels of red blood cells (RBC) membrane DHA and on whole-blood stimulated inflammatory cytokine production in infants with a high genetic risk for developing type 1 diabetes. As a consequence of the supplementation of infant diets with DHA, an increase of at least 20% in RBC DHA levels was shown at 12 months and 61%–100% at 6–36 months. However, it was not seen a substantial reduction in the production of inflammatory cytokines at 12 months [37].

- ***Prenatal programming and the role of gut microbiota***

In the past years, several studies have demonstrated that the pregnancy period is of high importance on the acquisition of an initial microbiome for infants, where microbial DNA has been detected in the placenta, umbilical cord, amnion fluids, and the meconium [38–41]. These findings have led to the drafting of several hypotheses about the invasion of the placenta breaking the *"sterile womb paradigm"* and proposing that microbiome acquisition begins in utero [42]. A study carried out by Rescigno et al. suggested the existence of a route for bacterial invasion, where dendritic cells could actively penetrate the epithelium, sample microbes from the gut lumen, and possibly transport the bacteria to the placenta during pregnancy [43]. Nevertheless, several studies with axenic animals and germ-free humans, via cesarean sections, strongly support sterility of the fetal environment in mammals [44].

Type 1 T helper (Th1) and type 2 T helper (Th2) cells represent two polarized forms of the CD4+ Th cell, mediating specific immune responses against different pathogens [45]. During pregnancy, the maternal environment promotes Th2 polarity in the fetal immune system, giving rise to a nonallergic Th1 phenotype occurring after birth. If this transition is altered during early postnatal life, there is an increased risk of suffering atopic disease including asthma [46]. Therefore, bacterial enterotypes could influence the immune system of the mother during pregnancy, affecting infant's health and immunity [47]. Kumar et al. investigated the association of gut microbiota with epigenetic changes during pregnancy and their postpartum methylation profile. Intriguingly, they found that the microbiota profiles correlated with differential methylation status of gene promoters functionally associated with CVDs [48]. Furthermore, recent research indicate that microbial exposure during pregnancy may be even more important for the allergy preventive effect in the offspring [49,50]. Immunoglobulin A (sIgA) plays a critical role in infant gut mucosal immunity because a delay in its production is associated with greater risk of allergic disease [51]. Kang et al. investigated differences in infant fecal sIgA concentrations according to the presence of maternal depressive symptoms during and after pregnancy. They found that infants born to mothers with depressive symptoms appeared to have lower fecal sIgA concentrations, predisposing them to higher risk for allergic disease [52].

Long chain polyunsaturated fatty acids (LCPUFAs) have been shown to influence the DNA methylation patterns, affecting the expression of relevant genes, which can lead to clinical effects [53]. Different nutritional intervention studies with DHA and EPA have been carried out during pregnancy. Nonetheless, no long-term effects have been found regarding infants' growth [54,55]. But, NUHEALstudy found differences in offspring neurodevelopment [56,57]. However, there are no human studies where supplementation with LCPUFAs given during pregnancy reported both the epigenetic mechanisms of action and later effects in infants' neurodevelopment and growth.

The epigenetic mechanisms elicited for environmental factors during pregnancy are hypothesized to be the key to understand how they mediate their numerous health promoting effects from the gut to overall health status in the offspring throughout the gut microbiota community.

Influences of breastfeeding versus infant formula on postnatal epigenetic modulation

- ***Influences of breastfeeding on postnatal epigenetic***

Infant feeding plays a key role in determining lifelong health and disease via epigenetic mechanisms. Human breast milk is universally considered the normative standard for infant feeding, as it confers unique nutritional and nonnutritional benefits that could be partly explained by epigenetics [58]. The WHO recommends exclusive breastfeeding during the first 6 months of life. When breastfeeding is not possible, it is necessary to use a suitable nutritional substitute. Currently, the optionis infant formulas, which intend to mimic the composition of breast milk [59]. Breastfeeding has been associated with lower risk of overweight and obesity during the first years of life, as well as lower levels of blood pressure, lower total- and LDL-cholesterol levels, and lower risk of diabetes in adulthood [60].

The "hygiene hypothesis" was introduced by David Strachan in 1989, where it is postulated that infections during childhood can cause an incorrect response of the immune system to innocuous antigens later in life [61]. Drawing on this hypothesis, the number of investigations around early life environmental exposures that modify infant contact with microbes were increased, to better understand what predisposes some children to develop food allergy while others do not [62]. These discoveries have allowed to find risk factors during the perinatal period, such as caesarean section, early cessation of breastfeeding, and antibiotic treatment, which may alter the gut microbiota composition, interfering with the mechanisms involved in the development of immunological tolerance [63—65].

Breast milk is composed of carbohydrates, proteins, fats, vitamins, minerals, digestive enzymes, and hormones. It is rich in immune cells, such as macrophages, stem cells, and other bioactive molecules. It is worth noting that the antimicrobial properties of human milk oligosaccharides

(HMOs) in the infant gastrointestinal tract, and their role in the development of a diverse and balanced microbiota, are vital for appropriate immune responses. Additionally, human breast milk is a good source of linoleic acid and α-linolenic acid, which are respectively converted to arachidonic acid (AA) and eicosapentaenoic acid (EPA), which in turn is converted to docosahexaenoic acid (DHA). All these three fatty acids are essential and important for regulating growth, inflammatory responses, immune function, vision, and cognitive and motor development in newborns [59]. Colostrum contains high concentration of lactoferrin, which regulates gene expression by binding to proinflammatory bacterial DNA sequences in Peyer's patches and intestinal mucosa. This binding inhibits the transcriptional activation of nuclear factor-κB (NF-κB) in human intestinal B-lymphocytes and downregulates IL-8 synthesis, which is involved in the amplification of the local inflammatory response [66]. Moreover, colostrum presents high concentration of IgA. Collado et al. found that an aberrant IgA responsiveness to the gut microbiota during infancy precedes asthma and allergy development, possibly indicating an impaired mucosal barrier function in allergic children [67].

From 5 days to 2 weeks postpartum, there is a production of transitional milk, which shares some characteristics with colostrum [53]. The omega-3 LCPUFA DHA, an antiinflammatory fatty acid, has been assigned as a beneficial factor that alters microbiota composition by increasing butyrate-producing bacteria [68,69]. Scopesi et al. showed a positive correlation between total saturated fatty acids (SFAs) and monounsaturated fatty acids (MUFAs) in transitional breast milk (collected 4–7 days postpartum) and maternal dietary intake ($r = 0.60$, $P < .01$) in an observational study [70].

Finally, 2 weeks after the delivery the milk can be considered as mature and its composition tends to be stable over the time [71].

- ***Formula feeding and epigenetic influences***

The period of the highest vulnerability for epigenetic dysregulation phenomena that extends from preconception to early infancy and during which epigenetic DNA activity is the most active has also been called the *"1000 days period"* [72]. So, during pregnancy and the first 2 years of life, perdurable patterns of gene expression are being established. Nevertheless, there are opportunities to improve health outcomes apart from critical developmental periods during development. Daily dietary patterns, as well as the lifestyle, are very important to disease prevention, even more in those subjects who are genetically susceptible. It is important to highlight that the effect of nutrition on health status is not a result only from individual biology and behavior, but it is a consequence of a complex interaction between the subject and the environment [73].

Although AA and DHA are the most important essential LCPUFAs recommended for infant formula supplementation, there is no enough evidence about the minimal concentration linked to long-term effects on growth and neurodevelopment. In this way, Uhl et al. conducted a randomized, double-blind, controlled intervention study in 4-month-old healthy term infants to receive either a formula supplemented with AA and DHA or a control one; they recruited also exclusively breastfeeding infants as a reference group. They investigated the effect of the supplemented formula on the different plasma phospholipid species during the first month of life; they concluded that the intake of the supplemented formula increased related phospholipid species, improving infants' LCPUFA status [74].

Additionally, a recent metaanalysis of randomized controlled trials (RCTs) was carried out by Wang et al. to evaluate the effects of nucleotides supplementation of infant formulas on erythrocyte and plasma fatty acid composition. As a result, infants who were fed the formula supplemented with nucleotides showed increased plasma levels of linoleic and AA (n-6 PUFAs), as well as decreased plasma levels of α-linolenic acid (n-3 PUFA) [75]. Perinatal PUFAs are essential for infant growth, neurodevelopment, and health. In fact, PUFAs have been observed to better visual acuity, as well as better scores in Bayley test [76]. Nevertheless, the nucleotides supplementation did not affect the concentration of PUFAs, neither n-3 or n-6, in erythrocyte membranes [75].

Cheatham et al. performed a study in mothers and their 16-month-old infants to investigate the relationship between maternal genetic and epigenetic fatty acid desaturase 2 (FADS2) profiles and toddlers' n-6 and n-3 PUFAs metabolism. The authors concluded that maternal FADS2 methylation was a predictor for α-linolenic acid plasma concentration in all toddlers and AA concentrations in boys [77].

According to a longitudinal observational study performed by Yeates et al. in two mother-child cohorts with high fish intake, maternal FADS genotype rs3834458 was significantly associated with maternal LCPUFA status, particularly with AA and linoleic acid:AA ratio. Nevertheless, no association was found with either serum EPA or DHA composition. Additionally, there was not significant association of the FADS genotype with the offspring's neurodevelopment; the authors found: (a) a trend for improved psychomotor development among infants born to mothers with the variant allele for rs3834458 in both cohorts; and (b) significant adverse associations between higher maternal n-6/n-3 ratios and both infant psychomotor development and communicative skills at 20 months of age. Therefore, the balance between AA and DHA might be important for a child's neurodevelopment [78].

It is vital to identify the new biomarkers associated with obesity/metabolic alterations in order to carry out early interventions. On this matter, Priego et al. performed a study in 237 children, aged 2–9 years old, as part of the IDEFICS project. They found that breastfed children presented higher levels of *SLC27A2, FASN, PPARα,* and *INSR*, previously described as biomarkers of metabolic health, in peripheral blood cells in comparison to formula-fed infants. This suggests a protective effect of breastfeeding, since breastfed infants have higher expression levels of these biomarkers, which could serve to discriminate formula-fed children to a higher risk of developing metabolic alterations later in life, such as insulin resistance and dyslipidemia [79].

On the other hand, it should be noted that preterm infants are particularly at risk of developing eating behavior disorders, which can potentially affect their growth, compared to full-term infants. The mechanisms are still unclear, but it is possible that involves developmental alterations and altered epigenetic control of genes responsible for the neuroendocrine regulation of energy homeostasis and food intake. There is growing evidence that eating behavior is established very early in life under the influence of complex interactions between biological mechanisms and environmental factors [80]. In this context, Amarger et al. performed a study in a cohort of preterm infants (born before 33 weeks of gestational age) to assess the eating behavior at 2 years of age. The authors identified a common single nucleotide polymorphism (SNP) in the *INSR* gene potentially associated with eating difficulties in preterm infants at 2 years of age [80].

Regarding infants' visual acuity, neurodevelopment, and growth, according to a systematic review the results of whether the LCPUFA supplementation in term infants has long-term beneficial or harmful effects on visual function or neurodevelopment are inconclusive. Similarly, no effect was found on physical growth. The inconsistency of the results could be attributed to the heterogeneity of methodologies employed [81].

So far, nutrigenomics research often has excluded the role of microbiota to host responses to nutritive molecules, in spite of its role in host metabolism and immune maturation [82].

- ***Probiotic and prebiotic supplementation during breastfeeding***

Feeding type, among others factors (Fig. 8.4), has been demonstrated to influence microbiota composition, as it provides the necessary substrates for

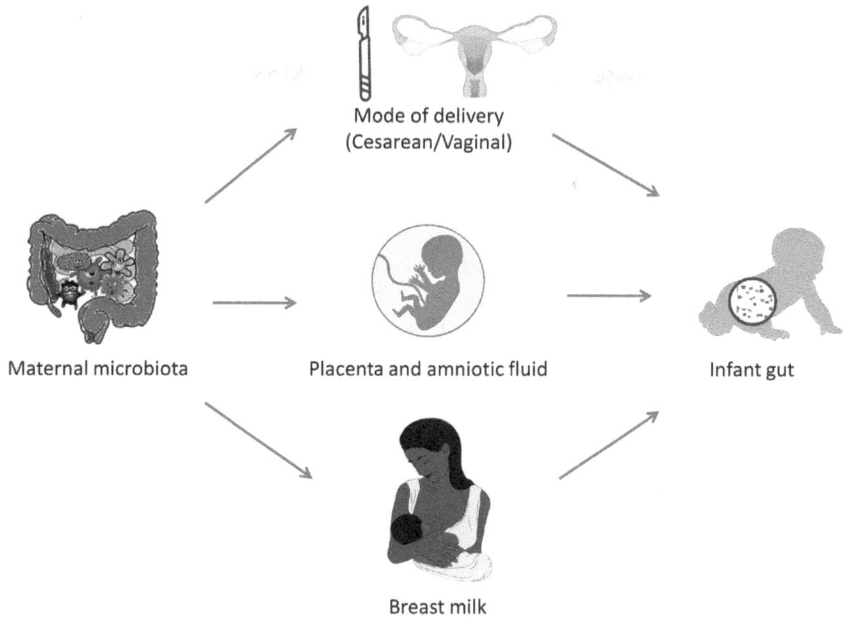

Figure 8.4 Mother-to-newborn bacteria transmission. Mother's gut microbiota influences the colonization and maturation of the infant gut microbiota through placenta and amniotic fluid, mode of delivery, and breast milk.

bacterial colonization and maturation and this has an indirect effect over the morphology and physiology of the intestinal mucosa [83]. Probiotics and prebiotics play a role in a variety of human diseases, such as prevention of allergic disease and asthma or protection against atopic disease in the offspring during pregnancy and breastfeeding [84–86].

It has been proved that probiotics use reduces the duration of antibiotic therapy and improves the immune-related disease, such as inflammatory bowel diseases (IBDs), celiac disease, metabolic syndrome, and diabetes [87,88]. *Faecalibacterium prausnitzii,* a natural probiotic of human milk, has been classified as one of the most important butyrate producer, which is a short chain fatty acid (SCFA) that inhibits histone deacetylases (HDACs) [89,90]. It showed that this SCFA has the ability to activate epigenetically silenced genes in cancer cells, to repress angiogenesis and reduce the expression of proangiogenic factors [91,92].

Within the group of substances recognized for their ability to influence gastrointestinal health are certain soluble fermentable fibers, some nondigestible oligosaccharides, and the oligosaccharides present in human milk called prebiotics [93]. HMOs, an important component of human milk, act as prebiotics, favoring the growth of certain beneficial bacteria, such as *Bifidobacterium infantis*, which protect the infant from colonization by pathogenic bacteria and prevent neonatal diarrheal and respiratory tract infections [94,95]. Although infant milk formulations have evolved greatly during the past years, it is necessary to continue studying the complex composition and the positive effects of breast milk versus infant formulas to improve the outcomes.

Recently, different studies have analyzed the impact of infant formula supplemented with probiotics on infants' health. Bazanella et al. in a double-blind, randomized, and placebo controlled trial, found that the metabolite profile in infants fed with formula supplemented with bifidobacteria was significantly different in comparison to those who fed the placebo formula and the breastfed group. Additionally, the authors observed that the experimental formula modulated the infant microbiome during early life with no detectable long-term effects on gut microbiota function [96]. In this regard, infants who fed a formula supplemented with *Bifidobacterium longum* BB536 showed an improved Th1 immune response and a tendency to establish a healthy intestinal microbiota early in life compared to those who fed a nonsupplemented formula. The authors suggest that this type of probiotic supplementation could be potentially useful for the prevention and treatment of immune-mediated diseases. Furthermore, they concluded that in order to establish efficient interventions with better effects, the supplementation should start before 4 months of age; after this period, the introduction of solid food and the composition of the host-microbiota might weaken the effects of probiotics [97].

On the other hand, in preterm infants fed with formula supplemented with *Saccharomyces boulardii*, improved feeding tolerance and weight gain have been observed [98]. Meanwhile, children with cow's milk allergy have shown better tolerance with the consumption of an extensively hydrolyzed casein formula supplemented with *Lactobacillus rhamnosus* GG. Thus, the first years of life could constitute a window of opportunity for the prevention of food allergies based on the modulation of gut microbiota [99].

In other blinded RCT the consumption of an oral probiotic, *Lactobacillus reuteri* DSM 17938, together with vitamin D3 during the first 3 months of life in full-term exclusively breastfed infants was associated with a reduction of pediatric consultations for infantile colic and the use of medication, as well as the necessity of infant formula. Therefore, this orally administered probiotic might be useful for the reduction of the intensity and frequency of infantile colic episodes [100].

When it comes to formula supplementation with prebiotics, infant formula with galacto-oligosaccharides has been associated with increased abundance of bifidobacteria and reduced α-diversity of the microbiota in healthy term infants, closer to the microbiota composition of exclusively breastfed infants [101]. A major public health issue is the rising prevalence of allergy in general and food allergies in pediatric population. Nevertheless, in a recent RCT carried out by Bozensky et al. in full-term infants with a history of allergy in their families, the consumption of an experimental hypoallergenic formula supplemented with galacto-oligosaccharides did not influence the severity of atopic dermatitis [102]. Finally, preterm neonates who were fed prebiotics enriched formula presented increased motilin levels, resulting in reduced gastric residue, good feeding tolerance, increased frequency of stools, lower mean cholesterol without any increase in LDL-cholesterol, and lower weight gain, compared with a standard preterm formula; this could imply a hypolipidemic protective effect of prebiotics [103].

Therefore, it is vital to perform more intervention studies during early stages of life in order to clarify the role of pro- and prebiotics in the treatment and prevention of noncommunicable diseases.

Future directions and problems

The increase in metabolic diseases, such as diabetes, obesity, and CVD, has led to significant consequences in terms of clinical burden and economic costs derivate from their complications. More recently, research has demonstrated the vital importance of epigenomic programming disorders, especially during pregnancy and the first days of life, and their possible preventive actions [104].

So-called personalized nutrition has given rise to nutrigenetics studies about the effects of genetic variations on the interaction between diet and health, reaching a variety of direct-to-consumer tests widely customized in different countries, although they present some ethical and legal issues, as well as doubts about the processing and interpretation of the genetic information [105].

At the present, genome characterization can be checked both in utero and at birth, although this pathway has not been fully explored yet. This method may be used to find genes involved in energy expenditure, genes involved in appetite control and food intake, as well as in adipogenesis and lipid metabolism or other polymorphisms of interest involved in specific diseases [106]. However, this knowledge is still of very limited value due to the scarce evidence available and its high cost. Thus, it is difficult to translate the research results to clinical practice. Despite this fact study results obtained so far indicate that an individual genome characterization will increase in importance over the coming years.

As a consequence of lifestyle changes derived from a globalized world and rural-urban migration, it is necessary to develop new public health interventions based on the current evidence [107,108]. Furthermore, recent reviews clearly underline that many groups of environmental pollutants, such as endocrine disrupting chemicals (i.e., phthalate esters, dioxins, hydrocarbons) and various groups of pesticides may influence upon epigenomic programming throughout life, particularly during pregnancy and childhood [109,110]. Accordingly, dietary and environmental databases could be the key in the observed increase in noncommunicable diseases and the application of medicine systems in the era of precision medicine.

Regarding microbiome characterization, numerous studies in vivo and in vitro have been carried out in order to know the influence of gut microbiota on the host's metabolism. Although, there is growing evidence of in vivo experiments in animals, it is necessary to perform more RCTs in humans in order to clarify the molecular mechanisms involved in the metabolism [111,112]. As replacement to traditional techniques to confront the metabolic or psychiatric diseases, an option could be the manipulation of the gut ecosystem by recombinant probiotics expressing therapeutic biomolecules [110,113] or fecal microbiota transplant [114]. Other alternative for the future could be phage cocktails customized, which would target directly to preidentified bacterial pathogens. However, the main inconvenience would be the high interindividual variation of the gut microbiome and the legislative approval [115,116]. Several evidences have suggested that prebiotics might represent novel strategies to prevent the progression of some diseases [117]. Future prebiotics research should strive to confirm causality between an observed health benefit and microbiota-mediated mechanisms.

In summary, further studies are still needed to confirm and clarify the possible mechanisms involved. Understanding those mechanisms associating early nutrition and later health outcomes could have a tremendous preventive potential. Thus, the first years of life constitute a window of opportunity in the effective primary prevention of adult chronic diseases. The areas of knowledge listed above will allow us to investigate epigenomic programming, even reprograming, to move toward more personalized therapy.

References

[1] Gurdon JB. The developmental capacity of nuclei taken from intestinal epithelium cells of feeding tadpoles. Development 1962;10(4):622–40.

[2] Takahashi K, Tanabe K, Ohnuki M, Narita M, Ichisaka T, Tomoda K, et al. Induction of pluripotent stem cells from adult human fibroblasts by defined factors. Cell 2007;131(5):861–72.

[3] Surani M, Barton S, Norris M. Nuclear transplantation in the mouse: heritable differences between parental genomes after activation of the embryonic genome. Cell 1986;45(1):127–36.

[4] Cantone I, Fisher AG. Epigenetic programming and reprogramming during development. Nat Struct Mol Biol 2013;20(3):282.

[5] Roseboom T, de Rooij S, Painter R. The Dutch famine and its long-term consequences for adult health. Early Human Development 2006;82(8):485–91.

[6] Painter RC, Roseboom TJ, Bleker OP. Prenatal exposure to the Dutch famine and disease in later life: an overview. Reprod Toxicol 2005;20(3):345–52.

[7] Hammoud NM, de Valk HW, Biesma DH, Visser GH. Intrauterine adiposity and BMI in 4-to 5-year-old offspring from diabetic pregnancies. Neonatology 2017;111(2):177–81.

[8] Godfrey KM, Reynolds RM, Prescott SL, Nyirenda M, Jaddoe VW, Eriksson JG, et al. Influence of maternal obesity on the long-term health of offspring. Lancet Diabetes Endocrinol 2017;5(1):53–64.

[9] Bird A, Macleod D, editors. Reading the DNA methylation signal. Cold Spring Harbor symposia on quantitative biology. Cold Spring Harbor Laboratory Press; 2004.

[10] Gluckman PD, Hanson MA, Spencer HG. Predictive adaptive responses and human evolution. Trends Ecol Evol 2005;20(10):527–33.

[11] Bird A. DNA methylation patterns and epigenetic memory. Genes Dev 2002;16(1):6–21.

[12] Cheng X, Blumenthal RM. Coordinated chromatin control: structural and functional linkage of DNA and histone methylation. Biochemistry 2010;49(14):2999–3008.

[13] Alejandro EU, Gregg B, Wallen T, Kumusoglu D, Meister D, Chen A, et al. Maternal diet–induced microRNAs and mTOR underlie β cell dysfunction in offspring. J Clin Invest 2014;124(10):4395–410.

[14] Zhang J, Zhang F, Didelot X, Bruce KD, Cagampang FR, Vatish M, et al. Maternal high fat diet during pregnancy and lactation alters hepatic expression of insulin like growth factor-2 and key microRNAs in the adult offspring. BMC Genomics 2009;10(1):478.

[15] Luoto R, Laitinen K, Nermes M, Isolauri E. Impact of maternal probiotic-supplemented dietary counselling on pregnancy outcome and prenatal and post-natal growth: a double-blind, placebo-controlled study. Br J Nutr 2010;103(12):1792–9.

[16] Cerdó T, Ruiz A, Jáuregui R, Azaryah H, Torres-Espínola FJ, García-Valdés L, et al. Maternal obesity is associated with gut microbial metabolic potential in offspring during infancy. J Physiol Biochem 2017:1–11.

[17] Isolauri E, Rautava S, Collado M, Salminen S. Role of probiotics in reducing the risk of gestational diabetes. Diabetes Obes Metabol 2015;17(8):713–9.
[18] Anderson OS, Sant KE, Dolinoy DC. Nutrition and epigenetics: an interplay of dietary methyl donors, one-carbon metabolism and DNA methylation. J Nutr Biochem 2012;23(8):853–9.
[19] Vyas P, Singh D, Singh N, Kumar V, Dhaliwal HS. Nutrigenomics: advances, opportunities and challenges in understanding the nutrient-gene interactions. Curr Nutr Food Sci 2017;13:1–12.
[20] Navarro E, Funtikova AN, Fíto M, Schröder H. Prenatal nutrition and the risk of adult obesity: long-term effects of nutrition on epigenetic mechanisms regulating gene expression. J Nutr Biochem 2017;39:1–14.
[21] Godfrey KM, Cutfield W, Chan S-Y, Baker PN, Chong Y-S. Nutritional intervention preconception and during pregnancy to maintain healthy glucose metabolism and offspring health ("NiPPeR"): study protocol for a randomised controlled trial. Trials 2017;18(1):131.
[22] Jobarteh ML, McArdle HJ, Holtrop G, Sise EA, Prentice AM, Moore SE. mRNA levels of placental iron and zinc transporter genes are upregulated in Gambian women with low iron and zinc status. J Nutr 2017;147(7):1401–9.
[23] Dominguez-Salas P, Moore SE, Baker MS, Bergen AW, Cox SE, Dyer RA, et al. Maternal nutrition at conception modulates DNA methylation of human metastable epialleles. Nat Commun 2014;5:3746.
[24] Devi S, Mukhopadhyay A, Dwarkanath P, Thomas T, Crasta J, Thomas A, et al. Combined vitamin B-12 and balanced protein-energy supplementation affect homocysteine remethylation in the methionine cycle in pregnant South Indian women of low vitamin B-12 status–4. J Nutr 2017;147(6):1094–103.
[25] Gali Ramamoorthy T, Begum G, Harno E, White A. Developmental programming of hypothalamic neuronal circuits: impact on energy balance control. Front Neurosci 2015;9:126.
[26] Valkama A, Koivusalo S, Lindström J, Meinilä J, Kautiainen H, Stach-Lempinen B, et al. The effect of dietary counselling on food intakes in pregnant women at risk for gestational diabetes: a secondary analysis of a randomised controlled trial RADIEL. Eur J Clin Nutr 2016;70(8):912.
[27] Paliy O, Piyathilake CJ, Kozyrskyj A, Celep G, Marotta F, Rastmanesh R. Excess body weight during pregnancy and offspring obesity: potential mechanisms. Nutrition 2014;30(3):245–51.
[28] Vineis P, Stringhini S, Porta M. The environmental roots of non-communicable diseases (NCDs) and the epigenetic impacts of globalization. Environ Res 2014;133:424–30.
[29] Culebras JM. Neurological changes related to malnutrition during the Spanish civil war (1936-1939). Nutr Hosp 2014;29(4):712–8.
[30] Roshanravan N, Alizadeh M, Hedayati M, Asghari-Jafarabadi M, Alamdari NM, Anari F, et al. Effect of zinc supplementation on insulin resistance, energy and macronutrients intakes in pregnant women with impaired glucose tolerance. Iran J Public Health 2015;44(2):211.
[31] Cleary J, Casey S, Hofsteede C, Moses RG, Milosavljevic M, Brand-Miller J. Does a low glycaemic index (GI) diet cost more during pregnancy? Nutrients 2012;4(11):1759–66.
[32] Goletzke J, Buyken AE, Louie JC, Moses RG, Brand-Miller JC. Dietary micronutrient intake during pregnancy is a function of carbohydrate quality, 2. Am J Clin Nutr 2015;102(3):626–32.

[33] Koivusalo SB, Rönö K, Klemetti MM, Roine RP, Lindström J, Erkkola M, et al. Gestational diabetes mellitus can be prevented by lifestyle intervention: the Finnish Gestational Diabetes Prevention Study (RADIEL): a randomized controlled trial. Diabetes Care 2016;39(1):24–30.
[34] Schwartz N, Nachum Z, Green MS. The prevalence of gestational diabetes mellitus recurrence—effect of ethnicity and parity: a metaanalysis. Am J Obstet Gynecol 2015;213(3):310–7.
[35] Jamilian M, Samimi M, Ebrahimi FA, Aghadavod E, Mohammadbeigi R, Rahimi M, et al. Effects of selenium supplementation on gene expression levels of inflammatory cytokines and vascular endothelial growth factor in patients with gestational diabetes. Biol Trace Elem Res 2018;181(2):199–206.
[36] Yung H-w, Alnæs-Katjavivi P, Jones CJ, El-Bacha T, Golic M, Staff A-C, et al. Placental endoplasmic reticulum stress in gestational diabetes: the potential for therapeutic intervention with chemical chaperones and antioxidants. Diabetologia 2016;59(10):2240–50.
[37] Chase HP, Boulware D, Rodriguez H, Donaldson D, Chritton S, Rafkin-Mervis L, et al. Effect of docosahexaenoic acid supplementation on inflammatory cytokine levels in infants at high genetic risk for type 1 diabetes. Pediatr Diabetes 2015;16(4):271–9.
[38] Jiménez E, Marín ML, Martín R, Odriozola JM, Olivares M, Xaus J, et al. Is meconium from healthy newborns actually sterile? Res Microbiol 2008;159(3):187–93.
[39] Rautava S, Collado MC, Salminen S, Isolauri E. Probiotics modulate host-microbe interaction in the placenta and fetal gut: a randomized, double-blind, placebo-controlled trial. Neonatology 2012;102(3):178–84.
[40] Satokari R, Grönroos T, Laitinen K, Salminen S, Isolauri E. Bifidobacterium and Lactobacillus DNA in the human placenta. Lett Appl Microbiol 2009;48(1):8–12.
[41] Jiménez E, Fernández L, Marín ML, Martín R, Odriozola JM, Nueno-Palop C, et al. Isolation of commensal bacteria from umbilical cord blood of healthy neonates born by cesarean section. Curr Microbiol 2005;51(4):270–4.
[42] Walker R, Clemente J, Peter I, Loos R. The prenatal gut microbiome: are we colonized with bacteria in utero? Pediatric obesity 2017;12(Suppl. 1):3–17.
[43] Rescigno M, Urbano M, Valzasina B, Francolini M, Rotta G, Bonasio R, et al. Dendritic cells express tight junction proteins and penetrate gut epithelial monolayers to sample bacteria. Nat Immunol 2001;2(4):361.
[44] Perez-Muñoz ME, Arrieta M-C, Ramer-Tait AE, Walter J. A critical assessment of the "sterile womb" and "in utero colonization" hypotheses: implications for research on the pioneer infant microbiome. Microbiome 2017;5(1):48.
[45] Romagnani S. T-cell subsets (Th1 versus Th2). Ann Allergy Asthma Immunol 2000;85(1):9–21.
[46] Holt PG, Upham JW, Sly PD. Contemporaneous maturation of immunologic and respiratory functions during early childhood: implications for development of asthma prevention strategies. J Allergy Clin Immunol 2005;116(1):16–24.
[47] Azad MB, Kozyrskyj AL. Perinatal programming of asthma: the role of gut microbiota. Clin Dev Immunol 2011;2012.
[48] Kumar H, Lund R, Laiho A, Lundelin K, Ley RE, Isolauri E, et al. Gut microbiota as an epigenetic regulator: pilot study based on whole-genome methylation analysis. MBio 2014;5(6):e02113–4.
[49] Jenmalm MC. The mother–offspring dyad: microbial transmission, immune interactions and allergy development. J Intern Med 2017;282(6):484–95.

[50] Garcia-Larsen V, Ierodiakonou D, Jarrold K, Cunha S, Chivinge J, Robinson Z, et al. Diet during pregnancy and infancy, and risk of allergic or autoimmune disease: a systematic review and meta-analysis. PLoS Med 2018;15(2). e1002507.
[51] Brandtzaeg P. Secretory IgA: designed for anti-microbial defense. Front Immunol 2013;4:222.
[52] Kang LJ, Koleva PT, Field CJ, Giesbrecht GF, Wine E, Becker AB, et al. Maternal depressive symptoms linked to reduced fecal Immunoglobulin A concentrations in infants. Brain Behav Immun 2018;68:123–31.
[53] Khot V, Chavan-Gautam P, Joshi S. Proposing interactions between maternal phospholipids and the one carbon cycle: a novel mechanism influencing the risk for cardiovascular diseases in the offspring in later life. Life Sciences 2015;129:16–21.
[54] van Dijk SJ, Zhou J, Peters TJ, Buckley M, Sutcliffe B, Oytam Y, et al. Effect of prenatal DHA supplementation on the infant epigenome: results from a randomized controlled trial. Clin Epigenet 2016;8(1):114.
[55] Wood K, Mantzioris E, Lingwood B, Couper J, Makrides M, Gibson R, et al. The effect of maternal DHA supplementation on body fat mass in children at 7 years: follow-up of the DOMInO randomized controlled trial. Prostagl Leukot Essent Fat Acids 2018;139:49–54.
[56] Campoy C, Escolano-Margarit MV, Ramos R, Parrilla-Roure M, Csábi G, Beyer J, et al. Effects of prenatal fish-oil and 5-methyltetrahydrofolate supplementation on cognitive development of children at 6.5 y of age–. Am J Clin Nutr 2011;94(Suppl. l_6). 1880S-8S.
[57] Catena A, Muñoz-Machicao JA, Torres-Espínola FJ, Martínez-Zaldívar C, Diaz-Piedra C, Gil A, et al. Folate and long-chain polyunsaturated fatty acid supplementation during pregnancy has long-term effects on the attention system of 8.5-y-old offspring: a randomized controlled trial–3. Am J Clin Nutr 2015;103(1):115–27.
[58] Witkowska-Zimny M, Kaminska-El-Hassan E. Cells of human breast milk. Cell Mol Biol Lett 2017;22(1):11.
[59] Martin CR, Ling P-R, Blackburn GL. Review of infant feeding: key features of breast milk and infant formula. Nutrients 2016;8(5):279.
[60] Agostoni C, Baselli L, Mazzoni MB. Early nutrition patterns and diseases of adulthood: a plausible link? Eur J Intern Med 2013;24(1):5–10.
[61] Strachan DP. Hay fever, hygiene, and household size. BMJ Br Med J (Clin Res Ed) 1989;299(6710):1259.
[62] Dunlop JH, Keet CA. Epidemiology of food allergy. ImmunolAllergy Clin 2018;38(1):13–25.
[63] Gensollen T, Blumberg RS. Correlation between early-life regulation of the immune system by microbiota and allergy development. J Allergy Clin Immunol 2017;139(4):1084–91.
[64] Cerdó T, Ruiz A, Campoy C. Human gut microbiota and obesity during development. Adiposity-Omics and Molecular Understanding: InTech. 2017.
[65] Candy DC, Van Ampting MT, Nijhuis MMO, Wopereis H, Butt AM, Peroni DG, et al. A synbiotic-containing amino-acid-based formula improves gut microbiota in non-IgE-mediated allergic infants. Pediatr Res 2018;83(3):677–86.
[66] Minekawa R, Takeda T, Sakata M, Hayashi M, Isobe A, Yamamoto T, et al. Human breast milk suppresses the transcriptional regulation of IL-1β-induced NF-κB signaling in human intestinal cells. Am J Physiol Cell Physiol 2004;287(5):C1404–11.
[67] Dzidic M, Abrahamsson TR, Artacho A, Björkstén B, Collado MC, Mira A, et al. Aberrant IgA responses to the gut microbiota during infancy precede asthma and allergy development. J Allergy Clin Immunol 2017;139(3):1017–25. e14.

[68] Balfegó M, Canivell S, Hanzu FA, Sala-Vila A, Martínez-Medina M, Murillo S, et al. Effects of sardine-enriched diet on metabolic control, inflammation and gut microbiota in drug-naïve patients with type 2 diabetes: a pilot randomized trial. Lipids Health Dis 2016;15(1):78.
[69] Noriega BS, Sanchez-Gonzalez MA, Salyakina D, Coffman J. Understanding the impact of omega-3 rich diet on the gut microbiota. Case reports in medicine 2016;2016.
[70] Scopesi F, Ciangherotti S, Lantieri P, Risso D, Bertini I, Campone F, et al. Maternal dietary PUFAs intake and human milk content relationships during the first month of lactation. Clin Nutr 2001;20(5):393–7.
[71] Ballard O, Morrow AL. Human milk composition: nutrients and bioactive factors. Pediat Clin 2013;60(1):49–74.
[72] Simeoni U, Yzydorczyk C, Siddeek B, Benahmed M. Epigenetics and neonatal nutrition. Early Human Develop 2014;90:S23–4.
[73] Herman DR, Baer MT, Adams E, Cunningham-Sabo L, Duran N, Johnson DB, et al. Life Course Perspective: evidence for the role of nutrition. Matern Child Health J 2014;18(2):450–61.
[74] Uhl O, Fleddermann M, Hellmuth C, Demmelmair H, Koletzko B. Phospholipid species in newborn and 4 month old infants after consumption of different formulas or breast milk. PloS One 2016;11(8). e0162040.
[75] Wang L, Liu J, Lv H, Zhang X, Shen L. Effects of nucleotides supplementation of infant formulas on plasma and erythrocyte fatty acid composition: a meta-analysis. PloS One 2015;10(6). e0127758.
[76] Jasani B, Simmer K, Patole SK, Rao SC. Long chain polyunsaturated fatty acid supplementation in infants born at term. Cochrane Database Syst Rev 2017;(3).
[77] Cheatham CL, Lupu DS, Niculescu MD. Genetic and epigenetic transgenerational implications related to omega-3 fatty acids. Part II: maternal FADS2 rs174575 genotype and DNA methylation predict toddler cognitive performance. Nutr Res (NY) 2015;35(11):948–55.
[78] Yeates AJ, Love TM, Engström K, Mulhern MS, McSorley EM, Grzesik K, et al. Genetic variation in FADS genes is associated with maternal long-chain PUFA status but not with cognitive development of infants in a high fish-eating observational study. Prostagl Leukot Essent Fat Acids 2015;102:13–20.
[79] Priego T, Sánchez J, Picó C, Ahrens W, Bammann K, De Henauw S, et al. Influence of breastfeeding on blood-cell transcript-based biomarkers of health in children. Pediatric obesity 2014;9(6):463–70.
[80] Amarger V, Bouvagnet A, Moyon T, Vaiman D, Darmaun D, de Lauzon-Guillain B, et al. A common genetic variant in the insulin receptor gene is associated with eating difficulties at 2 Years of age in a cohort of preterm infants. J Nutrigenetics Nutrigenomics 2015;8(4–6):153–63.
[81] Campoy C, Escolano-Margarit MV, Anjos T, Szajewska H, Uauy R. Omega 3 fatty acids on child growth, visual acuity and neurodevelopment. Br J Nutr 2012;107(S2):S85–106.
[82] Sela DA, Mills DA. The marriage of nutrigenomics with the microbiome: the case of infant-associated bifidobacteria and milk–. Am J Clin Nutr 2014;99(3):697S–703S.
[83] Guaraldi F, Salvatori G. Effect of breast and formula feeding on gut microbiota shaping in newborns. Front CellulInfect Microbiol 2012;2:94.
[84] Al-muzafar HM, Amin KA. Probiotic mixture improves fatty liver disease by virtue of its action on lipid profiles, leptin, and inflammatory biomarkers. BMC ComplementAlternat Med 2017;17(1):43.

[85] Zhang G-Q, Hu H-J, Liu C-Y, Zhang Q, Shakya S, Li Z-Y. Probiotics for prevention of atopy and food hypersensitivity in early childhood: a PRISMA-compliant systematic review and meta-analysis of randomized controlled trials. Medicine 2016;95(8).
[86] West CE, Jenmalm MC, Kozyrskyj AL, Prescott SL. Probiotics for treatment and primary prevention of allergic diseases and asthma: looking back and moving forward. Expet Rev Clin Immunol 2016;12(6):625–39.
[87] Rayes N, Seehofer D, Hansen S, Boucsein K, Müller AR, Serke S, et al. Early enteral supply of lactobacillus and fiber versus selective bowel decontamination: a controlled trial in liver transplant recipients. Transplantation 2002;74(1):123–8.
[88] Ivanov II, Honda K. Intestinal commensal microbes as immune modulators. Cell Host & Microbe 2012;12(4):496–508.
[89] Davie JR. Inhibition of histone deacetylase activity by butyrate. J Nutr 2003;133(7). 2485S-93S.
[90] Louis P, Flint HJ. Diversity, metabolism and microbial ecology of butyrate-producing bacteria from the human large intestine. FEMS Microbiol Lett 2009;294(1):1–8.
[91] Canani RB, Di Costanzo M, Leone L. The epigenetic effects of butyrate: potential therapeutic implications for clinical practice. Clin Epigenet 2012;4(1):4.
[92] Zgouras D, Wächtershäuser A, Frings D, Stein J. Butyrate impairs intestinal tumor cell-induced angiogenesis by inhibiting HIF-1α nuclear translocation. Biochem Biophys Res Commun 2003;300(4):832–8.
[93] Cerdó T, Ruíz A, Suárez A, Campoy C. Probiotic, prebiotic, and brain development. Nutrients 2017;9(11):1247.
[94] Ward RE, Ninonuevo M, Mills DA, Lebrilla CB, German JB. In vitro fermentation of breast milk oligosaccharides by Bifidobacterium infantis and Lactobacillus gasseri. Appl Environ Microbiol 2006;72(6):4497–9.
[95] Newburg DS, Walker WA. Protection of the neonate by the innate immune system of developing gut and of human milk. Pediatr Res 2007;61(1):2.
[96] Bazanella M, Maier TV, Clavel T, Lagkouvardos I, Lucio M, Maldonado-Gòmez MX, et al. Randomized controlled trial on the impact of early-life intervention with bifidobacteria on the healthy infant fecal microbiota and metabolome. Am J Clin Nutr 2017;106(5):1274–86.
[97] Wu B-B, Yang Y, Xu X, Wang W-P. Effects of Bifidobacterium supplementation on intestinal microbiota composition and the immune response in healthy infants. World J Pediatr 2016;12(2):177–82.
[98] Xu L, Wang Y, Wang Y, Fu J, Sun M, Mao Z, et al. A double-blinded randomized trial on growth and feeding tolerance with Saccharomyces boulardii CNCM I-745 in formula-fed preterm infants. J Pediatr 2016;92(3):296–301.
[99] Canani RB, Sangwan N, Stefka AT, Nocerino R, Paparo L, Aitoro R, et al. Lactobacillus rhamnosus GG-supplemented formula expands butyrate-producing bacterial strains in food allergic infants. ISME J 2016;10(3):742.
[100] Savino F, Ceratto S, Poggi E, Cartosio M, Cordero di Montezemolo L, Giannattasio A. Preventive effects of oral probiotic on infantile colic: a prospective, randomised, blinded, controlled trial using Lactobacillus reuteri DSM 17938. Benef Microbes 2014;6(3):245–51.
[101] Matsuki T, Tajima S, Hara T, Yahagi K, Ogawa E, Kodama H. Infant formula with galacto-oligosaccharides (OM55N) stimulates the growth of indigenous bifidobacteria in healthy term infants. Benef Microbes 2016;7(4):453–61.
[102] Boženský J, Hill M, Zelenka R, Skýba T. Prebiotics do not influence the severity of atopic dermatitis in infants: a randomised controlled trial. PloS One 2015;10(11). e0142897.

[103] Dasopoulou M, Briana DD, Boutsikou T, Karakasidou E, Roma E, Costalos C, et al. Motilin and gastrin secretion and lipid profile in preterm neonates following prebiotics supplementation. J Parenter Enteral Nutr 2015;39(3):359–68.
[104] Shenderov BA, Midtvedt T. Epigenomic programing: a future way to health? Microb Ecol Health Dis 2014;25(1):24145.
[105] Allyse MA, Robinson DH, Ferber MJ, Sharp RR, editors. Direct-to-consumer testing 2.0: emerging models of direct-to-consumer genetic testing. Mayo clinic proceedings. Elsevier; 2018.
[106] Goni L, Cuervo M, Milagro FI, Martínez JA. Future perspectives of personalized weight loss interventions based on nutrigenetic, epigenetic, and metagenomic data–3. J Nutr 2015;146(4). 905S-12S.
[107] da Costa Louzada ML, Baraldi LG, Steele EM, Martins APB, Canella DS, Moubarac J-C, et al. Consumption of ultra-processed foods and obesity in Brazilian adolescents and adults. Prev Med 2015;81:9–15.
[108] Carrillo-Larco RM, Bernabé-Ortiz A, Pillay TD, Gilman RH, Sanchez JF, Poterico JA, et al. Obesity risk in rural, urban and rural-to-urban migrants: prospective results of the Peru MIGRANT study. Int J Obes 2016;40(1):181.
[109] Solecki R, Kortenkamp A, Bergman Å, Chahoud I, Degen GH, Dietrich D, et al. Scientific principles for the identification of endocrine-disrupting chemicals: a consensus statement. Arch Toxicol 2017;91(2):1001–6.
[110] LaRocca J, Johnson KJ, LeBaron MJ, Rasoulpour RJ. The interface of epigenetics and toxicology in product safety assessment. Curr Opin Toxicol 2017;6:87–92.
[111] Ooi L-G, Liong M-T. Cholesterol-lowering effects of probiotics and prebiotics: a review of in vivo and in vitro findings. Int J Mol Sci 2010;11(6):2499–522.
[112] Burton JP, Drummond BK, Chilcott CN, Tagg JR, Thomson WM, Hale JD, et al. Influence of the probiotic Streptococcus salivarius strain M18 on indices of dental health in children: a randomized double-blind, placebo-controlled trial. J Med Microbiol 2013;62(6):875–84.
[113] Paton AW, Jennings MP, Morona R, Wang H, Focareta A, Roddam LF, et al. Recombinant probiotics for treatment and prevention of enterotoxigenic *Escherichia coli* diarrhea. Gastroenterology 2005;128(5):1219–28.
[114] Kang D-W, Adams JB, Gregory AC, Borody T, Chittick L, Fasano A, et al. Microbiota Transfer Therapy alters gut ecosystem and improves gastrointestinal and autism symptoms: an open-label study. Microbiome 2017;5(1):10.
[115] Mirzaei MK, Maurice CF. Menage a trois in the human gut: interactions between host, bacteria and phages. Nat Rev Microbiol 2017;15(7):397–408.
[116] Cooper CJ, Mirzaei MK, Nilsson AS. Adapting drug approval pathways for bacteriophage-based therapeutics. Front Microbiol 2016;7.
[117] Verma A, Shukla G. Administration of prebiotic inulin suppresses 1, 2 dimethylhydrazine dihydrochloride induced procarcinogenic biomarkers fecal enzymes and preneoplastic lesions in early colon carcinogenesis in Sprague Dawley rats. J Func Foods 2013;5(2):991–6.

CHAPTER 9

Perinatal nutrition and metabolic disease

Gonzalo Cruz[1], Daniela Fernandois[2], Gonzalo Jorquera[1], Paola Llanos[3], Manuel Maliqueo[4], Ximena Palma[5]
[1]Centro de Neurobiología y Fisiopatología Integrativa (CENFI), Instituto de Fisiología, Facultad de Ciencias, Universidad de Valparaíso, Valparaíso, Chile; [2]Development and Plasticity of the Neuroendocrine Brain, INSERM, Lille, France; [3]Instituto de Investigación en Ciencias Odontológicas, Facultad de Odontología, Universidad de Chile, Santiago, Chile; [4]Laboratory of Endocrinology and Metabolism, West Division, Faculty of Medicine, Universidad de Chile, Santiago, Chile; [5]Escuela de Nutrición y Dietética, Facultad de Farmacia, Universidad de Valparaíso, Valparaíso, Chile

Contents

Effects of maternal obesity during pregnancy on fetal development and body weight

Several studies demonstrate that maternal overweight or obesity increases the birth weight of the newborns [1–6]. Different techniques which analyze body composition such as air plethysmography, skinfold measurements, bioimpedance, dual-energy X-ray absorptiometry, and magnetic resonance imaging, have demostrated a positive association between pre--pregnancy obesity and gestational body weight (BW) gain with increased

Molecular Nutrition
ISBN 978-0-12-813862-5
https://doi.org/10.1016/B978-0-12-813862-5.00009-8

fat accumulations, suggesting a higher risk to develop metabolic abnormalities from early infancy.

Several metabolic adaptations occur during pregnancy to ensure a proper transfer of nutrients to the fetus. In humans, food intake increases 10%–15% during pregnancy [7], and maternal stores of subcutaneous body fat increase from the 6th to the 35th week of pregnancy [8]. In the third trimester, an increase of diabetogenic hormones produces a marked reduction of insulin sensitivity, concomitantly with fat accumulation and BW gain of the fetus. According to Pedersen hypothesis, in women with gestational diabetes mellitus (GDM), maternal hyperinsulinemia induces fetal overgrowth. This occurs due to placenta transports glucose by a gradient concentration mechanism. Moreover, maternal insulin resistance and elevated body mass index (BMI) are also associated with higher maternal circulating free fatty acids (FAA) and triglycerides, both of them, contributing to neonatal adiposity storage [9–11].

In women without GDM, maternal adiposity and the amount of adipokines and cytokines secreted, such as leptin, are the strongest determinants of having large gestational development rather than glucose tolerance and lipid levels [12]. Indeed, inflammatory markers, such as C-reactive protein, interleukin 6 (IL-6), and monocyte chemoattractant protein-1 (MCP-1), are increased in obese pregnant women compared with normo-weight pregnant women [13–16]. Interestingly, cord blood of overweight and obese women presents increased levels of IL-6, tumor necrosis factor alpha (TNF-α), leptin, and adiponectin [17–20]. An effect of adiponectin is inhibiting the insulin-stimulated amino acid transport, which is important for reducing fetal growth under elevated insulin levels, as occurs in obesity and GDM [21,22].

Different studies in women with high BMI showed that placental adaptations, including placental biometry or histopathology, depend on fetal sex [23,24]. For example, one study showed that the uptake of oleic acid, and gene expression of fatty acid binding proteins 5 (FABP5) and fatty acid transport proteins (FAT) CD36 were decreased in the placentas of male fetuses from obese women in contrast to the enhanced uptake of oleic acid observed in the placentas of female fetuses, suggesting a gender-dependent mechanism in the control of fatty acid uptake [25]. In the same way, a high maternal weight gain in the first trimester was associated with a reduction in placental thickness and low levels of n-3 long chain polyunsaturated fatty acids (LCPUFAs) in cord blood of male offspring but not in females [26]. Recently, one study showed that maternal obesity was associated with higher fat mass, insulin resistance, and higher leptin levels in girls, but not in boys [4]. Other authors have shown that total cholesterol, high-density lipoprotein cholesterol (HDL-C), low-density lipoprotein cholesterol (LDL-C), and triglycerides are higher in cord blood of females compared to males born to obese mothers. Then, sex dimorphism could be an important factor regulating fetal adaptations to maternal environment, influencing the susceptibility to develop metabolic disorders (Fig. 9.1).

Fetal environment is key for skeletal muscle development and function because there is no increase in the number of muscle skeletal fibers after birth [27]. The skeletal muscle is the main site for glucose and fatty acids utilization, with both nutrients being the principal sources of energy of muscle tissue [28]. Thus, a limited fetal skeletal muscle development impairs glucose and fatty acid metabolism, predisposing the offspring to suffer obesity and diabetes later in life [29]. Bayol et al. reported that maternal overnutrition reduces muscle force production in offspring, which affects the ability to exercise in adult life [30]. In this same context, Bucci et al. studying a subgroup from the Helsinki Birth Cohort Study, explored the metabolic effects of resistance exercise in frail elderly women born to either obese or normo-weight mothers [31]. Interestingly, women born to obese/overweight mothers tended to be insulin resistant and to have impaired skeletal muscle glucose uptake compared to women born to normo-weight mothers. Beauchamp et al. reported that maternal undernutrition promotes low birth weight but is associated with higher adiposity, impaired skeletal muscle energetics, and weight loss resistance as long-term effects [32]. This study reports a reduced mitochondrial content and an altered mitochondrial bioenergetics in skeletal muscle [32]. These findings mean over- and undernutrition during pregnancy can have deleterious effects in skeletal muscle physiology associated to obesity and insulin resistance.

During fetal muscle development, the mesenchymal stem cells commit to myogenesis; however, muscle-derived stem cells are also capable of differentiating to adipocytes and fibroblasts cells [33]. Maternal obesity alters fetal muscle development by shifting mesenchymal stem cells differentiation from myogenesis toward adipogenesis or fibrogenesis promoting impaired muscle function [29]. Zhu et al. observed that maternal obesity enhanced the expression of adipogenic markers in fetal muscle, which was associated with a systemic inflammatory response [34]. In this report, the authors showed that both TNF-α and peroxisome proliferator-activated receptor gamma (PPAR-γ) were increased in skeletal muscle indicating increased inflammatory state and enhanced adipogenesis in fetuses from an obese pregnant sheep model [34] (Fig. 9.1).

Several studies show that offspring born to obese mothers have more intrahepatic fat content than those born to normo-weight mothers, having also a higher risk for developing nonalcoholic fatty liver disease (NAFLD). For example, a study using magnetic resonance spectroscopy in 25 human infants born to mothers with obesity (pre-pregnancy BMI >30 kg/m^2) and GDM or normo-weight nondiabetic mothers (pre-pregnancy BMI <25 kg/m^2), found a 68% increase in intrahepatic fat content in neonates exposed to maternal obesity during prenatal life [35]. Another study with a cohort of 1170 adolescents aged 17 years old, analyzed fatty liver composition by hepatic ultrasound. This study showed that 15% of adolescents presented NAFLD correlated with lower time of breastfeeding (less than 6 months), early use of supplementary milk formula, maternal pre-pregnancy obesity, and adolescent obesity [36].

In animal models, the offspring of female baboons fed with high fat diet (HFD) and free access to sugar-containing drinks at least 9 months before and throughout pregnancy develop bigger waist-hip circumferences, higher LDL blood levels, hypercholesterolemia, and hypertriglyceridemia, and a higher percentage of body fat compared with matched females who received a control diet. Primate's fetuses of 165 days of gestation from mothers fed with an HFD presented hyperinsulinemia and three times more lipid accumulation in the liver when compared with control ones [37].

Influence of maternal obesity during pregnancy on breast milk composition: macronutrients, micronutrients, and hormones

Human milk composition is complex with an energy content ranging between individuals, going from 50 to 86 kcal/dL [38]. Evidence has been inconclusive in demonstrating an association between maternal BMI and macronutrients content of breast milk (BM). However, some findings are indicative of a link between these two factors.

Proteins

Overall, BM contains over 400 different proteins providing not only nutritional functions but also antimicrobial and immunomodulatory activities [39]. Since lactocytes produce approximately 80%–90% of BM proteins and only around 10%–20% are taken up from the maternal circulation via transcytosis, protein concentration is remarkably conserved in term BM (0.9–1.2 g protein/dL) [40]. When considering maternal nutritional status, some studies have reported a positive association between total BM protein content and maternal adiposity, while others have not shown differences [41–43]. Interestingly, the concentration of nonprotein nitrogen-containing compounds, particularly free branched-chain amino acids (BCAAs), has been shown to be higher in BM from obese mothers compared with normo-weight mothers [44]. In addition, milk formulas also have higher BCAA concentration than milk of normo-weight mothers. This is important because BCAAs stimulate insulin secretion and could be associated with increased BW in infants [45]. In this sense, a higher BCAA concentration has been observed in formula-fed infants compared with BM-fed infants from normo-weight mothers [46].

Lipids

Lipids represent around 40%–50% of the BM energy content, being the most variable macronutrient of milk [39]. Particularly important are LCPUFA because their concentration in milk varies in relation to maternal diet, mobilization of endogenous stores, and de novo synthesis of fatty acids. Therefore, when analyzing fatty acid composition, several studies have observed that BM from overweight/obese women have significantly lower content of total n-3 polyunsaturated fatty acid (PUFA), alpha linolenic acid, eicosapentaenoic acid (EPA), and docosahexaenoic acid (DHA) and higher n-6:n-3 PUFA ratio when compared with normo-weight women [47–49]. This is relevant considering the participation of EPA and DHA on infant neuroprotection and their contribution to neural and visual development [50]. In addition, proinflammatory effects have been related to high n-6:n-3 PUFA ratio, which could contribute to metabolic dysregulations in offspring. Despite this, fatty acid composition reflects dietary habits of mothers; therefore, PUFA and specially EPA and DHA supplementation could reduce this gap [51,52].

Carbohydrates

The principal sugar of human BM is the disaccharide lactose. Given the fact that lactose is important for maintaining a constant osmotic pressure in BM, it is the least variable nutrient and evidence shows that maternal nutritional status should not have a significant impact on its concentration [53].

Micronutrients

Vitamins and minerals are transported from the maternal peripheral blood, across the mammary epithelium, into BM. For instance, concentration of vitamins A, B_1, B_2, B_6, B_{12}, C, D, E, and iodine can vary depending on maternal diet and body stores [54,55]. In addition, vitamin D was found to be 38% lower in BM from obese mothers, with or without adjustment for maternal race [48].

Other bioactive factor concentrations such as lutein, zeaxanthin (involved in infant neuronal development), cryptoxanthin, α-carotene, and β-carotene were also significantly lower in BM from obese mothers (50%, 37%, 76%, 67%, and 74%, respectively) [48]. In addition, polyamines, essential compounds in the regulation of intestinal and immune function in newborns and infants, were also significantly lower in obese compared with normo-weight mothers [56].

Hormones and cytokines

Several studies conducted in humans and animal models show that besides nutrients, BM transports growth factors, cytokines, and hormones such as leptin, insulin, ghrelin, glucagon-like peptide 1 (GLP-1), adiponectin, resistin, and obestatin [57−59]. Regrettably, the lack of standardized collection methods and techniques to quantify hormones in BM has not allowed to establish standardized reference ranges for hormones in BM [60]. The mammary gland of lactating women, mice, ewes, cows, and goats synthetizes and secretes hormones, but mammary epithelial cells can also transfer hormones from maternal blood into the milk, making difficult determining the origin of hormones in BM.

Rodents fed with an HFD during pregnancy and lactation have elevated BM levels of leptin [61], ghrelin, and obestatin [62]. Moreover, a positive correlation between hormonal BM content and plasmatic offspring hormone concentration has been described for leptin, ghrelin, obestatin, and insulin [62−65]. Interestingly, leptin supplied orally to neonatal rats results in increased leptin levels in serum [66], meaning that leptin from milk could have physiological effects on lactating offspring. Indeed, leptin is essential in the development of hypothalamic neural circuitry controlling food intake and energy balance [67]. On the other hand, BM from overweight women, 1 month after delivery, has decreased levels of cytokines as TGF-β2, IL-6, and soluble CD14 when compared with normo-weight mothers. Along with this, BM microbiota composition is also different in overweight mothers compared with normo-weight mothers. Both cytokines and microbiota are crucial factors in the acquisition of oral tolerance to antigens, and a failure in this process has been linked to several diseases, including food allergies, celiac disease, and inflammatory bowel diseases. Therefore, changes in BM hormones, cytokines, and soluble receptors could be affecting the newborns immune system, metabolism, and the development of their organs [68]. Therefore, the impact of altered levels of BM hormones/cytokines or the lack of them (i.e., in milk formulas or pasteurized BM) could have a long-term impact in the descendants.

Long-term effects of maternal obesity during pregnancy on metabolic features in adult offspring

Maternal pre-pregnancy obesity and excessive BW gain during pregnancy increase nutrient supply to the fetus, which lead to adaptive responses by the fetus resulting in altered development of its organs and tissues, which usually are evidenced as long-term functional changes [69,70]. In fact, maternal obesity is associated with increased risk to develop childhood obesity, diabetes, insulin resistance, hypertension, hyperlipidemia, and cardiovascular complications including coronary heart disease and stroke [18,71–73].

In humans, macrosomia and excessive gestational weight gain are the strongest predictors of higher BMI at 1 year of age (being 1 year old BMI a predictive parameter for weight status between 5 to 8 years of age) [74]. Boney et al. in an early study revealed an association between metabolic syndrome in childhood obesity at 11 years old and maternal obesity during pregnancy, concluding that metabolic syndrome in childhood is associated with birth weight, maternal obesity, and GDM [72].

The impact of maternal obesity during gestation was elegantly investigated in a cross-sectional study where the records of 2054 obese women who underwent bariatric surgery were analyzed [75]. Among them, 42 had children before and after surgery. Children born after bariatric surgery presented reduced macrosomia at birth, and during preadolescence they have less BMI, body fat percentage, and waist circumference compared with their adolescent siblings born before maternal surgery. Besides, children born before bariatric surgery showed more severe cases of obesity, dyslipidemia, insulin resistance, and chronic inflammation [75]. These data suggest that development of obesity and derived metabolic alterations is not only purely associated to genetic background and specific familial environments but also highly associated with gestational epigenetic modifications.

A longitudinal study performed in aboriginal Pima people in Arizona is very valuable in this respect. Pima people have one of the highest prevalence for type 2 diabetes in the world. Researchers wanted to isolate gestational hyperglycemia as a risk factor. They selected 19 families in which at least one sibling was born before and at least one after the mother was diagnosed with type 2 diabetes. Siblings had the same parents, so the main difference between these pregnancies was the exposure to intrauterine hyperglycemia. Glucose tolerance test, height, weight, and blood pressure were measured periodically from 1965 to 1969 and family relations were registered. Analysis showed that siblings exposed to high glucose levels had higher risks to develop obesity and type 2 diabetes at earlier age than their siblings exposed to gestational euglycemia [76].

Another study analyzed data from 1400 people born between 1974 and 1976 and their mothers. Data showed and found that pre-pregnancy and gestational obesity is positively associated with higher BMI and adiposity, and bigger waist circumference in offspring at age 32 [77]. Authors showed that adults with mothers with higher BMI before pregnancy had higher blood pressure, elevated fasting insulin, cholesterol, and triglycerides plasma levels. Researchers conclude that maternal weight excess and weight gain in pregnancy increase cardiometabolic risk in offspring during adulthood, and diseases such as myocardial infarction and stroke are more frequent in these people [77]. Moreover, a study performed in 37,709 people found that maternal obesity is a risk factor for premature death due to cardiovascular events in adulthood [78].

Similarly, several animal models explore the effects of maternal nutrition and obesity on the progeny. Guo et al. suggested an increase in BW and adiposity in weaned offspring of rats fed with HFD during pregnancy and lactation [79]. Likewise maternal overnutrition in rats induce not only lipogenesis but also lipolysis through a compensation oxidation pathway, leading to an increased BW, impaired glucose tolerance, elevated serum cholesterol, and hepatic steatosis at weaning [80]. A systematic review on animal models of maternal HFD feeding showed a real risk to develop type 2 diabetes and obesity in male offspring exposed to an HFD during maternal gestation period and during gestation plus lactation period [81]. Even more, offspring of HFD-fed mothers had elevated concentrations of circulating leptin and corticosterone, high BW gain and food intake, modest preference for fat-containing food types, and early onset of hypothalamic leptin resistance. The authors suggest that maternal HFD exposure during the perinatal period modifies caloric input in the offspring, and as a consequence, secretion of metabolic signals that affect synaptic plasticity in the brain [82].

Samuelsson et al. fed female C57BL/6J mice for 6 weeks previous mating, during pregnancy and lactation with an obesogenic/cafeteria diet.

Authors found that adult offspring born to obese mothers had an increase in BW and fat mass and a reduction in skeletal muscle mass at 3- and 6-month-old. At 3-month-old, young adult mice born to obese mothers had dyslipidemia, hyperinsulinemia, hyperleptinemia, intolerance to glucose, and hypertension. Mice at 6-month-old continue with all previous described metabolic alterations, plus a declining in beta pancreatic cells function [83]. These studies provided strong evidences that diet-induced maternal obesity during pregnancy is associated with increased risk of metabolic and cardiovascular disease in the offspring.

Interestingly, gestational obesity has effects on puberty onset. A study performed in 15,267 girls ranging from 6 to 11 years old established that a higher maternal BMI during pregnancy correlates with early signs of puberty such as breast growth and pubic hair development. Authors proposed that intrauterine exposure to hyperglycemia leads to higher adiposity, tissue that could contribute to estrogen production triggering precocious puberty [84]. In rodents, female offspring born to rats fed with HFD 1 month before mating and until weaning showed increased estrogen levels during early development compared with offspring of control dams. Females born to obese mothers also had increased BW since day 1 to 120 after birth and an early vaginal opening, manifesting a precocious puberty [85].

Early puberty is also linked to metabolic alterations. A study in a big cohort of Caucasians (250,037 women and 197,714 men) showed an association between early menarche and higher risk for developing type 2 diabetes and cardiovascular disease [86]. They also reported for the first time a positive association between early puberty and cardiometabolic alterations in men [86].

Overall, these data shed light on how crucial is regulating nutritional environment in intrauterine and early postnatal life and is a warning sign for medical professionals to advise women to lose weight before pregnancy (Fig. 9.2).

Epigenetics in offspring of obese mothers

Epigenetics is a term first referred as "the branch of biology which studies the causal interactions between genes and their products which bring the phenotype into being" [87]. Currently, epigenetics is defined as the study of long-lived but reversible modifications in DNA which lead changes in gene expression without affecting DNA sequence [88]. Three main epigenetic mechanisms modulate gene expression: (1) DNA methylation, (2) post-translational histone modifications, and (3) noncoding RNAs [89–91].

Epigenetics is fundamental because its participation in key physiological processes, including cell growth and differentiation, organisms' development, and adaptation of living beings to the environment.

Gestational and neonatal stages are sensitive periods of life. During these periods, the development of new tissues and organs is characterized by massive cell differentiation and the establishment of strong epigenetic marks determining the lineage commitment of each cell [92]. Importantly, epigenetic machinery is susceptible to be controlled or influenced by nutrients and hormones. Therefore, affecting the epigenetic machinery and/or its function through environmental challenges in these vulnerable periods of life could result in long term or even permanent alterations in gene expression without affecting DNA sequence, thus leading to altered morphology and function of the organs.

The power of modulating epigenetic marks during development altering diet is observed in the agouti mice. The murine Agouti gene (a or A) encodes a paracrine signaling molecule that regulates either the production of black eumelanin (a) or yellow pheomelanin (A). Between them, some mutations in the regulatory region of the agouti locus result in the dominant allele A^{vy} (viable yellow agouti). The isogenic A^{vy}/a mice exhibit stochastic and systemic interindividual variation in DNA methylation at A^{vy}, which in turn regulates variable degrees of ectopic agouti expression [93]. Because of the structural similitude with agouti-related protein (Agrp), agouti protein is a high affinity antagonist of MCR3 and MCR4 melanocortin receptors, which is related to orexigenic behavior and obesity [94]. The variability of ectopic agouti expression leads a different degree of pheomelanin synthesis resulting in ranging phenotypes between the brown furred lean mice and the yellow furred obese mice [93,95]. Descendants of A^{vy} (yellow furred mice) obese females inherit obesity; however, when A^{vy} mice are fed with a diet enriched in methyl donors during pregnancy (e.g., betaine, folic acid, vitamin B12, and choline), the offspring present a global hypermethylation of DNA, including the agouti gene, therefore resulting in a brown furred descendant and lean phenotype [96]. Similarly, Tamashiro et al. [97] showed that two genetically identical mice, being one of them produced by cloning, had different phenotypes. Intriguingly, the cloned mice were heavier and presented metabolic alterations consistent with obesity [97]. Because cloning was performed by a microinjection of a somatic cell into an enucleated oocyte, the authors conclude that obesity phenotype could be a result of an epigenetic shift [93].

In humans, a good example of the influence of epigenetics is the Prader–Willi syndrome (PWS), which is a neurodevelopmental and neuroendocrine disorder that among several impairments produces a development of central obesity between 1 and 4 years of age, due to a concurrent hyperphagia. The most common cause of PWS is a genomic deletion of a large portion of chromosome 15, caused by paternal gene deletion (about 70% of the cases), maternal uniparental disomy (20%–30%), and a subset of sporadic cases (1%–3%), which are caused by an abnormal DNA methylation pattern leading to silencing that genomic region [93,98,99].

Maternal obesity induced by high fat or high fat/high sucrose diet in rodents leads to changes in methylation patterns of regulatory regions of proopiomelanocortin (*POMC*) gene. Specifically, both the promoter region and two enhancer regions are hypermethylated in offspring of obese mothers. These modifications decrease the leptin-mediated stimulation of POMC expression, thus affecting energy homeostasis. As POMC is the precursor of the anorexigenic α-melanocyte-stimulating hormone (α-MSH), a main neuropeptide involved in the homeostatic control of food intake, the decrease of POMC expression in offspring born to obese mothers could alter their food intake behavior [100]. Maternal obesity also produces a DNA hypomethylation in promoter regions of pre-pro enkephalin and μ-opioid receptor in nucleus accumbens, prefrontal cortex, and hypothalamus, key centers in the hedonic control of food intake [101]. In fact, the reprogramed prefrontal cortex is associated with BW gain, decreased motivation, and increased sucrose preference in offspring of obese mothers. Yet, a pre- and postnatal diet rich in methyl donors groups is able to normalize some of the prefrontal cortex impairments in offspring [102,103].

Beyond the brain, several epigenetic modifications have found to increase the vulnerability of offspring to suffer metabolic diseases. Masuyama et al. showed that maternal obesity decreases offspring adiponectin expression in fat by lowering acetylation in H3K9 histone (related to activation) and increases its dimethylations (related to repression) in the adiponectin promoter. Likewise, increased expression of leptin in offspring of obese mothers was associated to increased methylation of H4K20 (related to activation) in the leptin promoter region [104].

Offspring of obese mothers has an increase in zinc finger protein 423 (*zfp423*) expression, which correlates with a decreased DNA methylation in its promoter region. This leads to adipogenic lineage committing and differentiation during fetal development in mice, limiting the adipose tissue expansion and plasticity and favoring adipocyte hypertrophy associated to inflammation in the adult offspring [105,106]. In addition, Ding et al. demonstrated that macrophage infiltration in fat could be increased due to an overexpression of toll-like receptor (TLR) 1/4 and linker for activation of T cells (LAT), whose DNA promoter regions are hypomethylated in offspring of obese mothers [107]. Interestingly, DNA hypomethylation and increased expression of TLR1, TLR4, and LAT are maintained until F2 generation, showing a high stability of the transgenerational effect of maternal obesity in epigenetic-related impairments [107].

As mentioned above, offspring of HFD-fed mothers exhibit inflammation and steatosis. This is accompanied by higher profibrogenic gene expression on 82 differentially methylated regions of hepatic genes [108]. In addition, offspring of HFD-fed primate mothers have an increase in hepatic H3K14 acetylation and related key components of the epigenetic machinery [109]. Similarly, offspring of HFD-fed mice mothers show increased acetylation of H3K14 and trimethylation of H3K9 in the promoter regions of genes associated to lipid metabolism, such as Ppar-α, Ppar-γ, Rora, and Roxra during the fetal development [110]. In the same line, hypermethylation of Ppar-γ, LXRa, and CD36 could be responsible for lipid accumulation and altered glucose metabolism observed in offspring of obese mothers. Furthermore, phosphoenolpyruvate carboxykinase (PEPCK) enzyme, which participates in glycerol synthesis, was increased in adult rats born to obese mothers as a result of increased H3 acethylation and H3K4 dimethylation and decreased H3K9 trimethylation levels in its promoter [111]. Similarly, histone modification in the upstream, promoter, and coding regions of the gluconeogenic gene pck1 produces an increase in PEPCK expression and potentially programs an overproduction of glucose in the livers of HFD-fed mothers offspring [112].

In addition, offspring of obese mothers have a decreased expression of miR-122 in the liver [113,114]. miR-122 is involved in multiple metabolic processes including cholesterol and fatty acid biosynthesis and oxidation. In fact, miR-122 knockout mice develop steatohepatitis, fibrosis, and cellular carcinoma [115], and decreased miR-122 leads to protein-tyrosine phosphatase 1B induction, which is associated with liver insulin resistance [113].

Pharmacological and nonpharmacological treatment of maternal obesity during pregnancy: Docosahexaenoic acid (DHA) and metformin

In the last years, the consumption of dietary supplements, such as folic acid, vitamins, minerals, and DHA, has increased in pregnant women. However, their benefits on preventing long-term consequences of maternal obesity are under debate. LCPUFAs, mainly DHA and arachidonic acid (AA), are essential for neural development and cellular functions in fetal organs. Although the liver and adipose fetal tissues synthesize them from glucose, the bulk of DHA and AA is supplied by a selective transplacental transport from maternal circulation resulting in its biomagnification in fetal circulation near the onset of the period of maximum fetal growth.

In general, pre-pregnancy obesity more than gestational weight gain (GWG) is associated with an adverse fatty acid profile in erythrocytes from maternal circulation characterized by an increase of saturated fatty acid and higher n-6:n-3 PUFA ratio [116–118]. Moreover, in women with GDM, fatty acids in the umbilical artery had lower proportions of AA, DHA, and total n-6 and n-3 PUFAs, indicating an enhanced utilization by fetal tissues [119]. Interestingly, high ratio of n-6:n-3 PUFAs in cord plasma is associated with a higher adiposity measured by skinfold thicknesses and the development of obesity at age 3 years [120]. Similarly, elevated maternal n-6 PUFA at second trimester of gestation predicts higher body fat and abdominal fat evaluated by DEXA in children at 6 years old [121]. However, others have shown that higher maternal concentrations of n-3 PUFA, mainly DHA, are related with higher total cholesterol, HDL-C, and insulin levels at 6 years old in the offspring. A study in Danish population did not show any relationship between dietary intake of n-3 PUFA during second trimester of pregnancy with cardiometabolic risk, including cholesterol, triglycerides, and lipoproteins in blood at 19–20 years old in the offspring [122,123].

Supplementation with n-3 PUFA from second trimester of gestation to term reduces placental expression of IL-6, IL-8, and TNF-α in overweight and obese pregnant women [124]. In turn, 800 mg DHA from 26th week to term decreased placental amino acid transport and the expression of fatty acid transporting protein 4 [125]. Similar studies have shown that maternal PUFA status during pregnancy affects fetal lipid and insulin metabolism and cytokine profile in cord blood. In healthy pregnant women, the dietary intervention with fish oil supplement providing 1020 mg DHA and 180 mg EPA throughout pregnancy reduced the n-6:n-3 LCPUFA ratio in maternal and cord blood plasma [126]. Supplementation with 500 mg of DHA plus 150 mg EPA and 400 μg of methyl-tetra-hydrofolic acid in healthy pregnant patients from the second trimester, decreased the mRNA expression of proinflammatory cytokines, such as IL-4, IL-13, and CCR4, in cord blood of newborns [127]. In contrast, in obese pregnant women, EPA-rich fish oil (1060 mg EPA plus 274 mg DHA) reduced levels of several inflammatory cytokines in maternal plasma, while the supplementation of DHA-rich fish oil (900 mg DHA plus 180 mg EPA) had no significant effect on cytokine concentrations. In both cases, no significant effect on umbilical cord blood cytokine concentration was observed [128]. Interestingly, maternal concentration of DHA in erythrocytes at the 32 week of gestation was positively related to birth weight [126]. However, other study using functional food enriched in DHA (214 mg DHA/d) consumed from second trimester of gestation reported a lower infant ponderal index at birth and also decreased umbilical cord insulin concentrations compared with infants of mothers consuming a placebo [129]. Nevertheless, a study in Norwegian pregnant women supplemented with cod liver oil (approximately 1000 mg DHA/day and 800 mg EPA/day) showed no effect of n-3 PUFA supplementation on infant birth weight or length [130].

The multicenter randomized control trial, DHA to Optimize Mother Infant Outcome (DOMInO), has analyzed the effect of DHA-enriched fish oil (800 mg/d) supplementation in women during the second half of pregnancy (from 20 weeks of gestation until birth) on maternal and neonatal outcomes and also the long-term effects on infant adiposity. Interestingly, this trial show that DHA supplementation did not reduce the risk of GDM or preeclampsia [131] and was not associated with BMI z-score and percentage of body fat at 3, 5, and 7 years of age [132,133]. Similar results were observed by Foster et al. who did not find difference in the BMI z-score between the offspring of mothers supplemented with DHA versus a placebo; however, they found a significant association when breastfeeding and measured DHA levels were considered [134]. On the other hand, offspring born to women who received 600 mg of DHA from second trimester of gestation until term, showed that maternal DHA status during pregnancy is related to higher fat-free mass at 5 years old [135]. It is striking to note that DHA intake during pregnancy results in sex-specific changes in DNA methylation at birth with 127 diferentially methylated regions (DMRs) in males and 72 DMRs in females. However, only some of them were maintained until 5 years old, indicating that DHA supplementation can induce epigenetics modifications [136]. In summary, the evidence regarding the long-term effects of DHA on offspring adiposity seems to be not conclusive and dependent of the kind and source of n-3 PUFA supplementation.

Maternal obesity during pregnancy is a risk factor for developing GDM [137]. One of the proposed treatments for GDM is metformin because its properties in reducing hepatic glucose output and increasing insulin sensitivity. These effects reduce glycemia without a high risk of hypoglycemia or weight gain. However, metformin can cross placental barrier and can have unknown effects in the fetus, which have limited a wide use of the drug [138]. In a randomized trial, 751 women with GDM at 20–33 weeks of gestation received metformin (plus insulin if required) or insulin only until delivery [139]. Metformin treatment (2500 mg as maximum daily dose) was effective in regulating maternal glycemia, with no statistical difference compared with insulin treatment. Women receiving metformin had lower weight gain during pregnancy and lost weight more easily postpartum. This study did not find significant increase in neonatal complications in infants born to women with GDM who received metformin compared with those receiving insulin as treatment. Neonatal hypoglycemia, one of the possible complications, was similar in both groups, and even severe hypoglycemia was significantly less present in neonates from mothers who were treated with metformin. More women in the metformin group stated they will repeat treatment again compared with those in the insulin group. Authors concluded metformin alone or supplemented with insulin is a safe treatment for pregnant women with GDM and their infants [139]. In another study, 150 women with GDM were treated with metformin or insulin, macrosomia at birth was significantly reduced in offspring of metformin-treated mothers compared to those born to women receiving insulin injections. Metformin (3000 mg as maximum daily dose) helped in reducing gestational weight gain, controlled maternal glycemia as good as insulin treatment, and even neonatal complications were reduced in metformin group [140].

In addition, metformin has been used in nondiabetic pregnant obese women. In a double-blind, placebo-controlled trial, two groups of 225 obese pregnant women each with BMI >35 kg/m^2 were treated with metformin (up to 3000 mg) or placebo from 12 to 18 weeks of pregnancy to delivery. This study wanted to analyze macrosomia at birth, maternal gestational weight gain, GDM, and preeclampsia. Metformin treatment failed reducing neonatal weight but diminished maternal gestational weight and the incidence of preeclampsia [141]. Metformin treatment was not associated to pregnancy complications or adverse fetal or neonatal outcomes [141].

We have reviewed that metformin has positive effects in obese and diabetic pregnant women and their babies at birth. However, controversial data are available about long-term effects of in utero exposure to metformin on the offspring metabolic health during early infancy and adulthood. In animal models, pregnant mice have been fed with control chow and treated with metformin dissolved in the water (5 mg/mL). Researchers then analyzed metabolic parameters in adult progeny. They found metformin group had no difference in BW, fasting blood glucose, and fasting and after fed blood insulin compared with mice from control dams. They also showed that young males from metformin group had improved glucose tolerance after intraperitoneal glucose injections, and they released more insulin in response to glucose. Female offspring from metformin group did not show any difference in the above-mentioned tests compared with controls, but older females at 1–2 years old presented improved glucose tolerance [142]. Another study administered metformin orally (300 mg/kg per day) to dams on control diet. Female offspring from metformin group presented higher BW at 4.5–7 weeks old than control ones. When mice were fed with an HFD, metformin intrauterine–exposed group gained more weight than mice that did not receive metformin during fetal life. In addition, metformin prenatally exposed male offspring presented impaired glucose tolerance and elevated fasting blood glucose when they were fed with HFD [143]. In a third study in animals, female progeny of obese pregnant rats treated with metformin (200 mg/kg per day) showed higher BW, hyperleptinemia, and increased retroperitoneal fat depot than female offspring born to obese dams who were not treated with metformin [144].

In humans, few studies have analyzed long-term effect of intrauterine metformin treatment. Two-year-old children from mothers with GDM (treated with metformin or insulin) participated in a study where body composition was assessed. Authors did not find any difference in central fat measures, total fat mass, percentage body fat, or central-to-peripheral fat between metformin group and insulin group [145]. They found larger upper arm circumferences and bigger biceps and subscapular skinfolds, in children who received metformin in utero, which may suggest more subcutaneous fat deposit and less visceral fat. According to authors, these

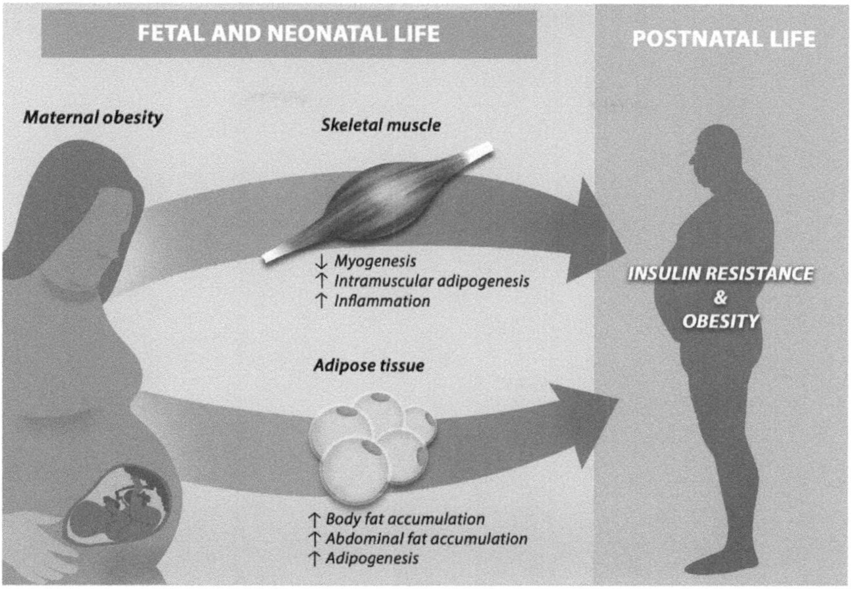

Figure 9.1 Key organs with a high metabolic function, as skeletal muscle and adiposse tissue, show functional alterations in offspring born to obese mothers.

findings could represent a more favorable pattern of fat distribution for in utero metformin-exposed children [145]. A recent study analyzed height, weight, and BMI in 4-year-old children whose mothers were treated with metformin (2000 mg maximum daily dose) or placebo during pregnancy. This research analyzed data from 292 children [146]. Authors found a higher BW and higher BMI in metformin group than placebo and more overweight and obese children in the metformin group. Researchers concluded that metformin exposure during intrauterine life increased the prevalence of overweight and obesity in children [146].

In summary, it is urgent to have more data about long-term effects of metformin gestational treatment with new studies in animals and humans. Metformin appears to be effective for preventing maternal complications associated to GDM, but long-term effects on offspring metabolism are much less clear.

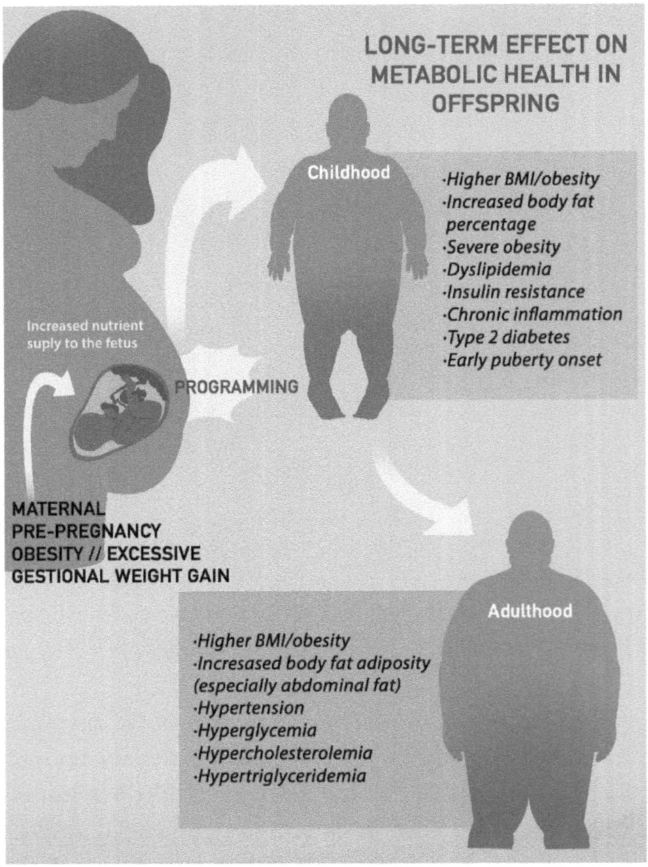

Figure 9.2 Offspring born to obese mothers have a higher risk to develop cardiometabolic disturbances during childhood and adulthood.

References

[1] Cedergren MI. Maternal morbid obesity and the risk of adverse pregnancy outcome. Obstet Gynecol 2004;103(2):219–24.

[2] Gaudet L, et al. Maternal obesity and occurrence of fetal macrosomia: a systematic review and meta-analysis. BioMed Res Int 2014;2014:640291.

[3] Martin KE, et al. The influence of maternal BMI and gestational diabetes on pregnancy outcome. Diabetes Res Clin Pract 2015;108(3):508–13.

[4] Mitanchez D, et al. Effect of maternal obesity on birthweight and neonatal fat mass: a prospective clinical trial. PloS One 2017;12(7):e0181307.

[5] Owens LA, et al. Atlantic dip: the impact of obesity on pregnancy outcome in glucose-tolerant women. Diabetes Care 2010;33(3):577–9.

[6] Roland MC, et al. Fetal growth versus birthweight: the role of placenta versus other determinants. PloS One 2012;7(6):e39324.

[7] Wade GN, Schneider JE. Metabolic fuels and reproduction in female mammals. Neurosci Biobehav Rev 1992;16(2):235–72.
[8] Sidebottom DA, Kennedy R, Hildebrand WH. Class I MHC expression in the yellow baboon. J Immunol 2001;166(6):3983–93.
[9] Catalano PM, Hauguel-De Mouzon S. Is it time to revisit the Pedersen hypothesis in the face of the obesity epidemic? Am J Obstet Gynecol 2011;204(6):479–87.
[10] Di Cianni G, et al. Maternal triglyceride levels and newborn weight in pregnant women with normal glucose tolerance. Diabet Med 2005;22(1):21–5.
[11] Harmon KA, et al. Continuous glucose profiles in obese and normal-weight pregnant women on a controlled diet: metabolic determinants of fetal growth. Diabetes Care 2011;34(10):2198–204.
[12] Retnakaran R, et al. Effect of maternal weight, adipokines, glucose intolerance and lipids on infant birth weight among women without gestational diabetes mellitus. CMAJ (Can Med Assoc J) 2012;184(12):1353–60.
[13] Challier JC, et al. Obesity in pregnancy stimulates macrophage accumulation and inflammation in the placenta. Placenta 2008;29(3):274–81.
[14] Madan JC, et al. Maternal obesity and markers of inflammation in pregnancy. Cytokine 2009;47(1):61–4.
[15] Ramsay JE, et al. Maternal obesity is associated with dysregulation of metabolic, vascular, and inflammatory pathways. J Clin Endocrinol Metab 2002;87(9):4231–7.
[16] Roberts KA, et al. Placental structure and inflammation in pregnancies associated with obesity. Placenta 2011;32(3):247–54.
[17] Brynhildsen J, et al. Leptin and adiponectin in cord blood from children of normal weight, overweight and obese mothers. Acta Paediatr 2013;102(6):620–4.
[18] Catalano PM, et al. Fetuses of obese mothers develop insulin resistance in utero. Diabetes Care 2009;32(6):1076–80.
[19] de Toledo Baldi E, et al. Tumor necrosis factor-alpha levels in blood cord is directly correlated with the body weight of mothers. Obes Sci Pract 2016;2(2):210–4.
[20] Farah N, et al. Correlation between maternal inflammatory markers and fetomaternal adiposity. Cytokine 2012;60(1):96–9.
[21] Jones HN, Jansson T, Powell TL. Full-length adiponectin attenuates insulin signaling and inhibits insulin-stimulated amino Acid transport in human primary trophoblast cells. Diabetes 2010;59(5):1161–70.
[22] Rosario FJ, et al. Chronic maternal infusion of full-length adiponectin in pregnant mice down-regulates placental amino acid transporter activity and expression and decreases fetal growth. J Physiol 2012;590(6):1495–509.
[23] Leon-Garcia SM, et al. Maternal obesity and sex-specific differences in placental pathology. Placenta 2016;38:33–40.
[24] Mando C, et al. Sex specific adaptations in placental biometry of overweight and obese women. Placenta 2016;38:1–7.
[25] Brass E, Hanson E, O'Tierney-Ginn PF. Placental oleic acid uptake is lower in male offspring of obese women. Placenta 2013;34(6):503–9.
[26] O'Tierney-Ginn PF, et al. Maternal weight gain regulates omega-3 fatty acids in male, not female, neonates. Reprod Sci 2017;24(4):560–7.
[27] Goldspink G, Ward PS. Changes in rodent muscle fibre types during post-natal growth, undernutrition and exercise. J Physiol 1979;296:453–69.
[28] Thiebaud D, et al. The effect of graded doses of insulin on total glucose uptake, glucose oxidation, and glucose storage in man. Diabetes 1982;31(11):957–63.
[29] Du M, et al. Maternal obesity, inflammation, and fetal skeletal muscle development. Biol Reprod 2010;82(1):4–12.
[30] Bayol SA, et al. Evidence that a maternal "junk food" diet during pregnancy and lactation can reduce muscle force in offspring. Eur J Nutr 2009;48(1):62–5.

[31] Bucci M, et al. Resistance training improves skeletal muscle insulin sensitivity in elderly offspring of overweight and obese mothers. Diabetologia 2016;59(1):77–86.
[32] Beauchamp B, et al. Low birth weight is associated with adiposity, impaired skeletal muscle energetics and weight loss resistance in mice. Int J Obes 2015;39(4):702–11.
[33] Aguiari P, et al. High glucose induces adipogenic differentiation of muscle-derived stem cells. Proc Natl Acad Sci U S A 2008;105(4):1226–31.
[34] Zhu MJ, et al. AMP-activated protein kinase signalling pathways are down regulated and skeletal muscle development impaired in fetuses of obese, over-nourished sheep. J Physiol 2008;586(10):2651–64.
[35] Brumbaugh DE, et al. Intrahepatic fat is increased in the neonatal offspring of obese women with gestational diabetes. J Pediatr 2013;162(5):930–936 e1.
[36] Ayonrinde OT, et al. Infant nutrition and maternal obesity influence the risk of non-alcoholic fatty liver disease in adolescents. J Hepatol 2017;67(3):568–76.
[37] Puppala S, et al. Primate fetal hepatic responses to maternal obesity: epigenetic signalling pathways and lipid accumulation. J Physiol 2018;596(23):5823–37.
[38] Gidrewicz DA, Fenton TR. A systematic review and meta-analysis of the nutrient content of preterm and term breast milk. BMC Pediatr 2014;14:216.
[39] Andreas NJ, Kampmann B, Mehring Le-Doare K. Human breast milk: a review on its composition and bioactivity. Early Hum Dev 2015;91(11):629–35.
[40] Ballard O, Morrow AL. Human milk composition: nutrients and bioactive factors. Pediatr Clin 2013;60(1):49–74.
[41] Bzikowska-Jura A, et al. Maternal nutrition and body composition during breast-feeding: association with human milk composition. Nutrients 2018;10(10).
[42] Grote V, et al. Breast milk composition and infant nutrient intakes during the first 12 months of life. Eur J Clin Nutr 2016;70(2):250–6.
[43] Kugananthan S, et al. Associations between maternal body composition and appetite hormones and macronutrients in human milk. Nutrients 2017;9(3).
[44] De Luca A, et al. Higher concentrations of branched-chain amino acids in breast milk of obese mothers. Nutrition 2016;32(11–12):1295–8.
[45] McCormack SE, et al. Circulating branched-chain amino acid concentrations are associated with obesity and future insulin resistance in children and adolescents. Pediatr Obes 2013;8(1):52–61.
[46] Fleddermann M, et al. Role of selected amino acids on plasma IGF-I concentration in infants. Eur J Nutr 2017;56(2):613–20.
[47] Makela J, et al. Breast milk fatty acid composition differs between overweight and normal weight women: the STEPS Study. Eur J Nutr 2013;52(2):727–35.
[48] Panagos PG, et al. Breastmilk from obese mothers has pro-inflammatory properties and decreased neuroprotective factors. J Perinatol 2016;36(4):284–90.
[49] Storck Lindholm E, et al. Different fatty acid pattern in breast milk of obese compared to normal-weight mothers. Prostaglandins Leukot Essent Fatty Acids 2013;88(3):211–7.
[50] Innis SM. Impact of maternal diet on human milk composition and neurological development of infants. Am J Clin Nutr 2014;99(3). 734S-41S.
[51] Monthe-Dreze C, et al. Maternal pre-pregnancy obesity attenuates response to omega-3 fatty acids supplementation during pregnancy. Nutrients 2018;10(12).
[52] Yang LG, et al. Low n-6/n-3 PUFA ratio improves lipid metabolism, inflammation, oxidative stress and endothelial function in rats using plant oils as n-3 fatty acid source. Lipids 2016;51(1):49–59.
[53] Martin CR, Ling PR, Blackburn GL. Review of infant feeding: key features of breast milk and infant formula. Nutrients 2016;8(5).
[54] Valentine CJ, Wagner CL. Nutritional management of the breastfeeding dyad. Pediatr Clin 2013;60(1):261–74.

[55] Bravi F, et al. Impact of maternal nutrition on breast-milk composition: a systematic review. Am J Clin Nutr 2016;104(3):646–62.
[56] Ali MA, et al. Lower polyamine levels in breast milk of obese mothers compared to mothers with normal body weight. J Hum Nutr Diet 2013;26(Suppl. 1):164–70.
[57] Andreas NJ, et al. Effect of maternal body mass index on hormones in breast milk: a systematic review. PloS One 2014;9(12):e115043.
[58] Aydin S, et al. Ghrelin is present in human colostrum, transitional and mature milk. Peptides 2006;27(4):878–82.
[59] Chan D, et al. Adiponectin, leptin and insulin in breast milk: associations with maternal characteristics and infant body composition in the first year of life. Int J Obes 2018;42(1):36–43.
[60] Bonnet M, et al. Mammary leptin synthesis, milk leptin and their putative physiological roles. Reprod Nutr Dev 2002;42(5):399–413.
[61] Bautista CJ, et al. Changes in milk composition in obese rats consuming a high-fat diet. Br J Nutr 2016;115(3):538–46.
[62] Slupecka M, Romanowicz K, Wolinski J. Maternal high-fat diet during pregnancy and lactation influences obestatin and ghrelin concentrations in milk and plasma of wistar rat dams and their offspring. Internet J Endocrinol 2016;2016:5739763.
[63] Savino F, et al. Ghrelin and obestatin in infants, lactating mothers and breast milk. Horm Res Paediatr 2012;78(5–6):297–303.
[64] Ley SH, et al. Associations of prenatal metabolic abnormalities with insulin and adiponectin concentrations in human milk. Am J Clin Nutr 2012;95(4):867–74.
[65] Casabiell X, et al. Presence of leptin in colostrum and/or breast milk from lactating mothers: a potential role in the regulation of neonatal food intake. J Clin Endocrinol Metab 1997;82(12):4270–3.
[66] Sanchez J, et al. Leptin orally supplied to neonate rats is directly uptaken by the immature stomach and may regulate short-term feeding. Endocrinology 2005;146(6):2575–82.
[67] Bouret SG. Neurodevelopmental actions of leptin. Brain Res 2010;1350:2–9.
[68] Dawod B, Marshall JS. Cytokines and soluble receptors in breast milk as enhancers of oral tolerance development. Front Immunol 2019;10:16.
[69] Lucas A. Programming by early nutrition in man. Ciba Found Symp 1991;156:38–50. discussion 50-5.
[70] Lucas A. Programming by early nutrition: an experimental approach. J Nutr 1998;128(2 Suppl. l):401S–6S.
[71] Bayol SA, Farrington SJ, Stickland NC. A maternal 'junk food' diet in pregnancy and lactation promotes an exacerbated taste for 'junk food' and a greater propensity for obesity in rat offspring. Br J Nutr 2007;98(4):843–51.
[72] Boney CM, et al. Metabolic syndrome in childhood: association with birth weight, maternal obesity, and gestational diabetes mellitus. Pediatrics 2005;115(3):e290–6.
[73] Godfrey KM, et al. Influence of maternal obesity on the long-term health of offspring. Lancet Diabetes Endocrinol 2017;5(1):53–64.
[74] Lindberg SM, Adams AK, Prince RJ. Early predictors of obesity and cardiovascular risk among American Indian children. Matern Child Health J 2012;16(9):1879–86.
[75] Smith J, et al. Effects of maternal surgical weight loss in mothers on intergenerational transmission of obesity. J Clin Endocrinol Metab 2009;94(11):4275–83.
[76] Dabelea D, et al. Intrauterine exposure to diabetes conveys risks for type 2 diabetes and obesity: a study of discordant sibships. Diabetes 2000;49(12):2208–11.
[77] Hochner H, et al. Associations of maternal prepregnancy body mass index and gestational weight gain with adult offspring cardiometabolic risk factors: the Jerusalem Perinatal Family Follow-up Study. Circulation 2012;125(11):1381–9.

[78] Reynolds RM, et al. Maternal obesity during pregnancy and premature mortality from cardiovascular event in adult offspring: follow-up of 1 323 275 person years. BMJ 2013;347:f4539.
[79] Guo F, Jen KL. High-fat feeding during pregnancy and lactation affects offspring metabolism in rats. Physiol Behav 1995;57(4):681–6.
[80] Huang Y, et al. Maternal high-fat diet during pregnancy and lactation affects hepatic lipid metabolism in early life of offspring rat. J Biosci 2017;42(2):311–9.
[81] Ainge H, et al. A systematic review on animal models of maternal high fat feeding and offspring glycaemic control. Int J Obes 2011;35(3):325–35.
[82] Walker CD, et al. Perinatal maternal fat intake affects metabolism and hippocampal function in the offspring: a potential role for leptin. Ann N Y Acad Sci 2008;1144:189–202.
[83] Samuelsson AM, et al. Diet-induced obesity in female mice leads to offspring hyperphagia, adiposity, hypertension, and insulin resistance: a novel murine model of developmental programming. Hypertension 2008;51(2):383–92.
[84] Kubo A, et al. Associations between maternal obesity and pregnancy hyperglycemia and timing of puberty onset in adolescent girls: a population-based study. Am J Epidemiol 2018;187(7):1362–9.
[85] Ambrosetti V, et al. Increase in endogenous estradiol in the progeny of obese rats is associated with precocious puberty and altered follicular development in adulthood. Endocrine 2016;53(1):258–70.
[86] Day FR, et al. Puberty timing associated with diabetes, cardiovascular disease and also diverse health outcomes in men and women: the UK Biobank study. Sci Rep 2015;5:11208.
[87] Waddington CH. The epigenotype. Int J Epidemiol 1942;41(1):10–3. 2012.
[88] LaSalle JM, Powell WT, Yasui DH. Epigenetic layers and players underlying neurodevelopment. Trends Neurosci 2013;36(8):460–70.
[89] Cruz G, et al. Long-term effects of early-life exposure to environmental oestrogens on ovarian function: role of epigenetics. J Neuroendocrinol 2014;26(9):613–24.
[90] Zama AM, Uzumcu M. Epigenetic effects of endocrine-disrupting chemicals on female reproduction: an ovarian perspective. Front Neuroendocrinol 2010;31(4):420–39.
[91] Cantone I, Fisher AG. Epigenetic programming and reprogramming during development. Nat Struct Mol Biol 2013;20(3):282–9.
[92] Boland MJ, Nazor KL, Loring JF. Epigenetic regulation of pluripotency and differentiation. Circ Res 2014;115(2):311–24.
[93] Waterland RA. Epigenetic mechanisms affecting regulation of energy balance: many questions, few answers. Annu Rev Nutr 2014;34:337–55.
[94] Fan W, et al. Role of melanocortinergic neurons in feeding and the agouti obesity syndrome. Nature 1997;385(6612):165–8.
[95] Miltenberger RJ, et al. The role of the agouti gene in the yellow obese syndrome. J Nutr 1997;127(9):1902S–7S.
[96] Wolff GL, et al. Maternal epigenetics and methyl supplements affect agouti gene expression in Avy/a mice. Faseb J 1998;12(11):949–57.
[97] Tamashiro KL, et al. Cloned mice have an obese phenotype not transmitted to their offspring. Nat Med 2002;8(3):262–7.
[98] Elhamamsy AR. Role of DNA methylation in imprinting disorders: an updated review. J Assist Reprod Genet 2017;34(5):549–62.
[99] Ramsden SC, et al. Practice guidelines for the molecular analysis of Prader-Willi and Angelman syndromes. BMC Med Genet 2010;11:70.

[100] Gali Ramamoorthy T, et al. Maternal overnutrition programs epigenetic changes in the regulatory regions of hypothalamic Pomc in the offspring of rats. Int J Obes 2018;42(8):1431–44.
[101] Vucetic Z, et al. Maternal high-fat diet alters methylation and gene expression of dopamine and opioid-related genes. Endocrinology 2010;151(10):4756–64.
[102] McKee SE, et al. Methyl donor supplementation alters cognitive performance and motivation in female offspring from high-fat diet-fed dams. Faseb J 2017;31(6):2352–63.
[103] McKee SE, et al. Perinatal high fat diet and early life methyl donor supplementation alter one carbon metabolism and DNA methylation in the brain. J Neurochem 2018;145(5):362–73.
[104] Masuyama H, et al. The effects of high-fat diet exposure in utero on the obesogenic and diabetogenic traits through epigenetic changes in adiponectin and leptin gene expression for multiple generations in female mice. Endocrinology 2015;156(7):2482–91.
[105] Yang F, et al. [Effects of oils on lipid metabolism in obese C57BL/6J mice induced by a high fat diet]. Wei Sheng Yan Jiu 2013;42(6):901–6. 914.
[106] Liang X, et al. Maternal obesity epigenetically alters visceral fat progenitor cell properties in male offspring mice. J Physiol 2016;594(15):4453–66.
[107] Ding Y, et al. DNA hypomethylation of inflammation-associated genes in adipose tissue of female mice after multigenerational high fat diet feeding. Int J Obes 2014;38(2):198–204.
[108] Wankhade UD, et al. Enhanced offspring predisposition to steatohepatitis with maternal high-fat diet is associated with epigenetic and microbiome alterations. PloS One 2017;12(4):e0175675.
[109] Aagaard-Tillery KM, et al. Developmental origins of disease and determinants of chromatin structure: maternal diet modifies the primate fetal epigenome. J Mol Endocrinol 2008;41(2):91–102.
[110] Suter MA, et al. In utero exposure to a maternal high-fat diet alters the epigenetic histone code in a murine model. Am J Obstet Gynecol 2014;210(5):463 e1–463 e11.
[111] Zhou D, et al. Early-life exposure to high-fat diet may predispose rats to gender-specific hepatic fat accumulation by programming Pepck expression. J Nutr Biochem 2015;26(5):433–40.
[112] Strakovsky RS, et al. Gestational high fat diet programs hepatic phosphoenolpyruvate carboxykinase gene expression and histone modification in neonatal offspring rats. J Physiol 2011;589(Pt 11):2707–17.
[113] Benatti RO, et al. Maternal high-fat diet consumption modulates hepatic lipid metabolism and microRNA-122 (miR-122) and microRNA-370 (miR-370) expression in offspring. Br J Nutr 2014;111(12):2112–22.
[114] Zhang J, et al. Maternal high fat diet during pregnancy and lactation alters hepatic expression of insulin like growth factor-2 and key microRNAs in the adult offspring. BMC Genom 2009;10:478.
[115] Tsai WC, et al. MicroRNA-122 plays a critical role in liver homeostasis and hepatocarcinogenesis. J Clin Invest 2012;122(8):2884–97.
[116] Vidakovic AJ, et al. Body mass index, gestational weight gain and fatty acid concentrations during pregnancy: the Generation R Study. Eur J Epidemiol 2015;30(11):1175–85.
[117] Kawabata T, et al. Polyunsaturated fatty acid levels in maternal erythrocytes of Japanese women during pregnancy and after childbirth. Nutrients 2017;9(3).
[118] Cinelli G, et al. Influence of maternal obesity and gestational weight gain on maternal and foetal lipid profile. Nutrients 2016;8(6).

[119] Ortega-Senovilla H, et al. Gestational diabetes mellitus upsets the proportion of fatty acids in umbilical arterial but not venous plasma. Diabetes Care 2009;32(1):120–2.
[120] Donahue SM, et al. Prenatal fatty acid status and child adiposity at age 3 y: results from a US pregnancy cohort. Am J Clin Nutr 2011;93(4):780–8.
[121] Vidakovic AJ, et al. Maternal plasma PUFA concentrations during pregnancy and childhood adiposity: the Generation R Study. Am J Clin Nutr 2016;103(4):1017–25.
[122] Rytter D, et al. Fish oil supplementation during late pregnancy does not influence plasma lipids or lipoprotein levels in young adult offspring. Lipids 2011;46(12):1091–9.
[123] Rytter D, et al. No association between the intake of marine n-3 PUFA during the second trimester of pregnancy and factors associated with cardiometabolic risk in the 20-year-old offspring. Br J Nutr 2013;110(11):2037–46.
[124] Haghiac M, et al. Dietary omega-3 fatty acid supplementation reduces inflammation in obese pregnant women: a randomized double-blind controlled clinical trial. PloS One 2015;10(9):e0137309.
[125] Lager S, et al. Docosahexaenoic acid supplementation in pregnancy modulates placental cellular signaling and nutrient transport capacity in obese women. J Clin Endocrinol Metab 2017;102(12):4557–67.
[126] Much D, et al. Effect of dietary intervention to reduce the n-6/n-3 fatty acid ratio on maternal and fetal fatty acid profile and its relation to offspring growth and body composition at 1 year of age. Eur J Clin Nutr 2013;67:282.
[127] Krauss-Etschmann S, et al. Decreased cord blood IL-4, IL-13, and CCR4 and increased TGF-β levels after fish oil supplementation of pregnant women. J Allergy Clin Immunol 2008;121(2):464–70. e6.
[128] Mozurkewich EL, et al. Effect of prenatal EPA and DHA on maternal and umbilical cord blood cytokines. BMC Pregnancy Childbirth 2018;18(1):261.
[129] Al-Hinai M, et al. Maternal intake of omega-3 and omega-6 polyunsaturated fatty acids during mid-pregnancy is inversely associated with linear growth. J Dev Orig Health Dis 2018;9(4):432–41.
[130] Helland IB, et al. Supplementation of n-3 fatty acids during pregnancy and lactation reduces maternal plasma lipid levels and provides DHA to the infants. J Matern Fetal Neonatal Med 2006;19(7):397–406.
[131] Zhou SJ, et al. Fish-oil supplementation in pregnancy does not reduce the risk of gestational diabetes or preeclampsia. Am J Clin Nutr 2012;95(6):1378–84.
[132] Muhlhausler BS, et al. DHA supplementation during pregnancy does not reduce BMI or body fat mass in children: follow-up of the DHA to Optimize Mother Infant Outcome randomized controlled trial. Am J Clin Nutr 2016;103(6):1489–96.
[133] Wood K, et al. The effect of maternal DHA supplementation on body fat mass in children at 7 years: follow-up of the DOMInO randomized controlled trial. Prostaglandins Leukot Essent Fatty Acids 2018;39:49–54.
[134] Foster BA, et al. Randomized controlled trial of DHA supplementation during pregnancy: child adiposity outcomes. Nutrients 2017;9(6).
[135] Hidaka BH, et al. Intrauterine DHA exposure and child body composition at 5 y: exploratory analysis of a randomized controlled trial of prenatal DHA supplementation. Am J Clin Nutr 2018;107(1):35–42.
[136] van Dijk SJ, et al. Effect of prenatal DHA supplementation on the infant epigenome: results from a randomized controlled trial. Clin Epigenet 2016;8:114.
[137] Chu SY, et al. Maternal obesity and risk of gestational diabetes mellitus. Diabetes Care 2007;30(8):2070–6.
[138] Feig DS, Moses RG. Metformin therapy during pregnancy: good for the goose and good for the gosling too? Diabetes Care 2011;34(10):2329–30.

[139] Rowan JA, et al. Metformin versus insulin for the treatment of gestational diabetes. N Engl J Med 2008;358(19):2003–15.
[140] Ainuddin J, et al. Metformin versus insulin treatment in gestational diabetes in pregnancy in a developing country: a randomized control trial. Diabetes Res Clin Pract 2015;107(2):290–9.
[141] Syngelaki A, et al. Metformin versus placebo in obese pregnant women without diabetes mellitus. N Engl J Med 2016;374(5):434–43.
[142] Gregg BE, et al. Gestational exposure to metformin programs improved glucose tolerance and insulin secretion in adult male mouse offspring. Sci Rep 2018;8(1):5745.
[143] Salomaki H, et al. Prenatal metformin exposure in mice programs the metabolic phenotype of the offspring during a high fat diet at adulthood. PloS One 2013;8(2):e56594.
[144] Alvarez D, et al. Prenatal metformin treatment improves ovarian function in offspring of obese rats. J Endocrinol 2018;239(3):325–38.
[145] Rowan JA, et al. Metformin in gestational diabetes: the offspring follow-up (MiG TOFU): body composition at 2 years of age. Diabetes Care 2011;34(10):2279–84.
[146] Hanem LGE, et al. Metformin use in PCOS pregnancies increases the risk of offspring overweight at 4 Years of age: follow-up of two RCTs. J Clin Endocrinol Metab 2018;103(4):1612–21.

PART 2

Molecular biology of the cell

CHAPTER 10

"Molecular aspects of dietary polyphenols in pregnancy"

Carmela Santangelo, Roberta Masella
Italian National Institute of Health, Center for Gender-Specific Medicine, Rome, Italy

Contents

Introduction

Nutritional intervention is the first of the 39 World Health Organization (WHO) recommendations addressed to improve the quality of antenatal care and achieve a healthy pregnancy [1]. Maternal malnutrition that includes both undernutrition and overfeeding is a big concern worldwide as these conditions increase the morbidity and mortality both in mother and child [2,3]. The increasing number of studies highlighting an inverse relationship between fruit and vegetables intake and the risk of chronic diseases has prompted WHO to recommend at least 400 g/day (five portions) of fruit and vegetable consumption [4]. Plant-derived food has been indicated as key component of a balanced diet throughout pregnancy because of their protective effects [5—10]. Benefits of fruit and vegetables intake come from a wide variety of nutritive components including the bioactive compounds such as polyphenols that influence maternal and offspring outcomes also later in the life [5]. However, it should be

Molecular Nutrition
ISBN 978-0-12-813862-5
https://doi.org/10.1016/B978-0-12-813862-5.00010-4

considered that the possible deleterious effect of polyphenol-rich food on mother and developing fetus is still an unsolved issue that need to be taken into account [11,12].

Finally, the need to formulate appropriate nutritional advices in pregnancy requires also a deeper knowledge of the molecular mechanisms governing the activity of dietary polyphenols. To this end, the present review is aimed at summarizing the current knowledge on the mechanisms of action of these bioactive compounds throughout the gestational period discussing about the potential beneficial effects on pregnancy and offspring.

Dietary sources, structure, and bioavailability of polyphenols

Dietary polyphenols are nonnutritional bioactive compounds that occur in small and variable amounts in fruit, vegetables, cereals, legumes, nuts, chocolate, olive oil, in plant-derived beverages such as tea, coffee, wine, as well as in spices and algae [13,14]. Polyphenols are secondary metabolites synthesized by the plants during the normal development, as well as in response to different stimuli including stress and UV radiation [15]. These bioactive compounds may contain one or more phenol structural units and comprise a large range of molecules, such as the simple phenolic acids to the complex proanthocyanidin polymers; to date more than 8000 phenolic structures are known [13]. According to both the number of phenolic ring they contain and the structural elements that bind the rings, phenolics can be classified as flavonoids and nonflavonoids [13] (Fig. 10.1). It has long been known that polyphenols are strong antioxidant agents [16] with antiinflammatory [17], antidiabetic [10], antihypertensive [18], neuroprotective [19], anticancer [20], estrogen-like[21], and immunomodulatory [22] activities. These properties are determined by either the chemical structure or the capability of polyphenols to interact with many biological targets, including cellular membranes, receptors, enzymes, and transcription factors [23,24].

Flavonoids and phenolic acids are the most abundant polyphenols in the diet, mostly derived from coffee, tea, and fruit [25,26], even though it must be considered that each plant and plant-derived food contains a mixture of different amounts of phytochemicals that interact exerting synergistic or antagonistic effects [27,28].

Measuring polyphenol intake represents a big challenge because of the extreme variability of polyphenol content in food. However, to establish

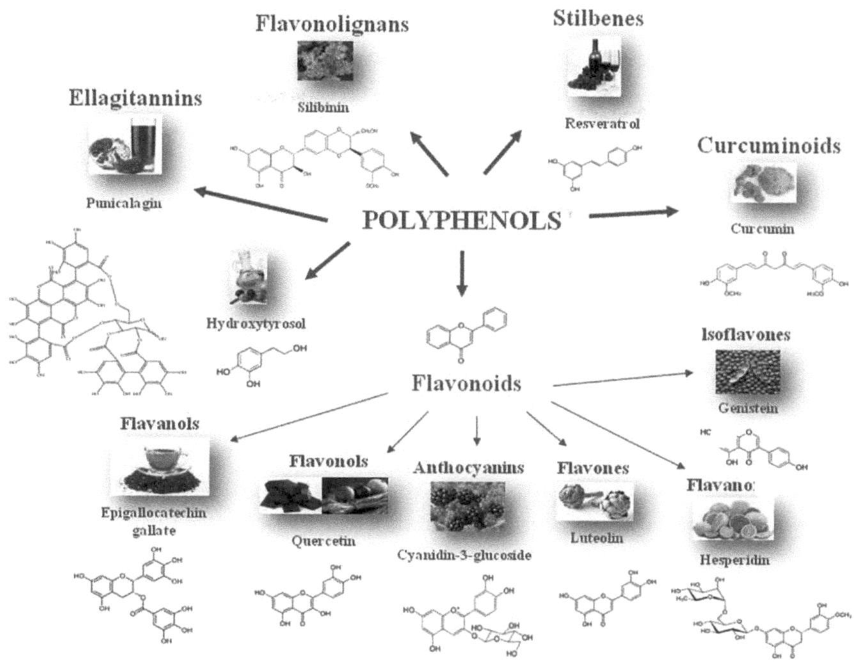

Figure 10.1 Classification, chemical structure, and representative dietary sources of selected polyphenols.

possible associations between polyphenol consumption and health outcomes, it is mandatory to calculate the intake of polyphenols through the diet [29]. To this end, over the time, researchers have built databases on polyphenols content in food, such as the USDA database on flavonoids [30] and isoflavones [31]; the Phenol-Explorer database that reports also the effects of cooking and food processing on polyphenol content [32]; and the eBASIS database that provides information on several bioactive compounds and their biological effects, together with a developing probabilistic model for intake estimation [33]. Scalbert and colleagues have estimated that human dietary intake of polyphenols is about 1 g/day [34]. Latest data obtained by using food composition databases indicate that a geographical difference exists in polyphenol intake ranging from 584 mg/day in Greek to 1626 mg/day in Denmark women [25], with a mean value of 801 mg/day in a large population recruited from the United States and Canada [26]. Therefore, these data indicate a large heterogeneity of phenolic intake across the countries.

The real effects of dietary polyphenols on human health depend not only on polyphenol intake but also mainly on their bioavailability [35]. The individual response to the ingested phenolic compounds - because of differences in genetics, gender, age, pregnancy, obesity, pathologies, and gut microbiota - as well as the food matrix and synergistic and/or antagonist effects among polyphenols contained in the diet greatly influences the bioavailability of polyphenols [28,35,36]. In general, dietary polyphenols are poorly bioavailable; their concentrations and that of the related metabolites in plasma and tissue are very low, reaching only nano- or micromolar concentrations [28,35,36].

However, dietary polyphenols, after oral ingestion and before reaching their cellular targets, are extensively modified through the gastrointestinal tract and liver [37]. The majority of polyphenols exists *in planta* as glycosides, esters, and polymers; they are absorbed in the stomach, small intestine, and colon after biochemical transformations by gut microbiota [37]. Thus, any single polyphenol will appear in the bloodstream, in target sites, and as excretion products in a chemical structure different from that existing in food [38]. Moreover, polyphenols strongly influence intestinal microbiome and in so doing may impact on health [39]. Indeed, gut disturbance (dysbiosis) is involved in several chronic disorders such as obesity and type 2 diabetes, and most importantly, maternal dietary intake influences the composition of the infant gut microbiota with consequences on offspring neurological and metabolic programming with long-lasting effects [22,40,41].

Flavonoids

Flavonoids share a basic structure (C6-C3-C6) consisting of two benzene rings linked through a heterocyclic pyrone C ring [13]. Depending on the hydroxylation, methoxylation, prenylation, glycosylation pattern, and variations in the C ring, flavonoids can be divided into different subclasses such as anthocyanins, flavanols, flavones, flavanones, flavonols, and isoflavones [13,42]; flavonoids are contained in fruit (e.g., berries, citrus, pomes, pomegranate, tropical fruits), in vegetables (e.g., cabbages, eggplants, tomatoes, beans, soy, spinaches, onions, oregano), spices (e.g., capers, cloves), and beverages (e.g., wine, tea, chocolate) [30,32] and contribute to the 40% - 60% of total polyphenol intake in European regions [25]. Dietary flavonoids have been shown to participate in several biological processes (e.g., inflammation, proliferation, apoptosis, hormonal, and gene regulation) by modulating intracellular signaling pathways, such as arachidonic acid and nitric oxide pathways, and the activity of transcriptions factors such as nuclear transcription factor kappa B (NF-κB), mitogen-activated protein kinases (MAPKs), phosphatidylinositol-3 kinases (PI3K)/Akt, peroxisome proliferator-activated receptor (PPARs), and nuclear factor E2-related factor 2 (Nrf2) [21,23,24,43].

Flavanols are a complex subclass of flavonoids, ranging from the simple catechin to complex structure such as proanthocyanidins, whose degree of polymerization influence bioavailability [32]. They are present in considerable amount in many kinds of fruit and vegetables and also in tea, coffee, wine, cocoa powder, and chocolate [30,32]. Epigallocatechin gallate (EGCG) is the most abundant flavanol found in tea representing about 31% of total polyphenols in green tea (range 9,12−26,16 mg/100 mL) [32]. After ingestion, EGCG is rapidly absorbed in the upper intestine, and it reaches plasma in various forms at a concentration <1 μmol/L [44]. The poor bioavailability together with the health benefits of EGCG and the absence of side effects have pushed researchers to study new EGCG delivery tools to enhance the therapeutic effects [45].

Flavones: Apigenin, luteolin, and nobiletin are the main flavones in fruit, vegetables, herbs, and olives [46]. High contents of apigenin are found in fresh oregano (3,50 mg/100g), black olives (8.18 mg/100g), and orange juice (5,53 mg/100g); luteolin is found in dried peppermint (1170,35 mg/100g), artichoke (42,10 mg/100g), thyme (39,50 mg/100g), and sage (33,40 mg/g) [32]. Flavones and derivatives are quickly absorbed and detected in human plasma at concentrations <1 μmol/L [46]. Increasing attention has been receiving fisetin, a flavone contained in fruit and vegetables such as strawberry, apple, grape, onion, and cucumber with the highest concentration in strawberry (160 μg/g) [47]. Fisetin possesses several health benefits [48], which is able to inhibit the expression of inflammatory molecules such as COX-2 and matrix metalloproteinases (MMPs) to activate the antioxidant transcription factor Nrf2 [49] and to preserve the cellular redox homeostasis [50]. It is rapidly absorbed and reaches maximum plasma concentration in a few minutes [48].

Flavanones: Citrus and citrus juices are the main sources of flavanones and their glycosides, whose beneficial effects as antioxidant, antiinflammatory, and cardioprotective are well known [51]. Different citrus species contain specific flavanones, e.g., naringenin (1,56 mg/100 mL), and its glycoside naringin (30,78−45,05 mg/100 mL) are contained in grapefruit; the highest concentration of hesperidin is present in orange blond juice (25,85−52,68 mg/100 mL) and in lemon juice (24,99 mg/100 mL) [32]. Naringenin and hesperidin are rapidly absorbed and metabolized with the maximum plasma peak at about 6 h and the urinary excretion within 48 h [52].

Flavonols are present in a wide variety of fruit and vegetables; among them, quercetin and kaempferol are the most studied flavonols [32]. Onions are the main source of quercetin and derivatives (3,21−44,23 mg/100 g depending on the cultivar) that are also contained in high amount in chicory (8−50 mg/100 g), black elderberries (42 mg/100 g), and dark chocolate (25 mg/100 g) [32]. Kaempferol and its derivatives are mainly found in cabbages (9,6−27 mg/g), common beans (39,88 mg/100 g), black tea (12,20mg/100 mL), and spices (e.g., capers 104,21 mg/100 g) [32]. Both of them are potent antiinflammatory and antioxidant compounds, even though they have a low bioavailability and are quickly metabolized [53−55].

Anthocyanins, a big subclass of flavonoids, are contained especially in berries [32]. The highest quantities of anthocyanins are found in black elderberry (1317 mg/100 g), black chokeberry (878 mg/100 g), and blackcurrant (592 mg/100 g). These group of compounds includes cyanidin, delphynin, peonin, malvidin, petunidin, and their glucosides; cyanidine-3-glucoside (C3G) represents the most common anthocyanidin [32]. Anthocyanins are rapidly metabolized; after consumption of 500 mg C3G, indeed, the maximum concentrations of 0.14 ± 0.05 mmol/L and 168 ± 0.18 μM, in serum and urine, respectively, have been found by 2 h in healthy adults [56]. However, the numerous anthocyanins gut-derived metabolites persist longer in plasma and tissue and account for the observed multiple protective effects [57,58].

Isoflavones are an interesting subclass of flavonoids that possess a weak estrogenic activity because of the chemical structure similar to the 17-β-estradiol (E2) that enables them to bind and activate the estrogen receptors ERα and ERβ [13,43]. They are principally contained in soy bean (about 200 mg/100 g) and soy-based products (e.g., soy flour 467 mg/100 g; soy yogurt 80 mg/100 g; miso 60−250 mg/100 g) and red clover (21 mg/100 g) [31,32]. Isoflavones intake varies greatly from Asian (30−50 mg/day) and non-Asian ($<$ 3 mg/day) consumers [59]; these compounds are rapidly metabolized and can be detected in plasma (concentration $<$ 1 μM) at 1−5 h after ingestion. Actually, it has been demonstrated that the ingestion of fermented soy milk containing daidzein and genistein may enhance their bioavailability in premenopausal women [60]. Genistein and daidzein are the most studied isoflavones [13], with promising antihypertensive properties as well [61].

Nonflavonoids

Nonflavonoid phenolics represent a heterogeneous group of compounds, ranging from the simple hydroxytyrosol to the complex punicalagin; they are found in fruit, vegetables, wine, olive oil, and spices. They have considerable importance in human nutrition because of their widespread diffusion and ability to exert a number of beneficial effects including estrogenic activities [13,32,43].

Stilbenes are polyphenols with a C6-C2-C6 structure [13]. Resveratrol (RSV), the most representative stilbene, is found in trace in red wine (range 0,28–1,34 mg/100 mL) as aglycones (trans- and cis-RSV), glucosides, and dimers [32]. RSV has been extensively studied in virtue of its capability to protect against CVD, cancer, metabolic, and neurodegenerative disorders because of its antiinflammatory, antiapoptotic, antioxidative, and anti-angiogenic activities [62].

Despite the aforementioned positive effects, RSV has a poor bioavailability; it is extensively and rapidly metabolized - highest plasma concentration reached around 1h after ingestion - [63] and it is present at very low concentration in the diet ("resveratrol paradox") [62]. Nevertheless, the multiple intracellular activities of RSV at molecular (e.g., the modulation of NF-κB, MMPs, COX-2, NOSs, Il-6, TNFα, and Nrf2) and epigenetic (e.g., sirtuin modulation) levels have promoted several studies addressed to improve the bioefficacy of RSV to use it as pharmacological tool [62,64,65].

Extra virgin olive oil (*EVOO*) major phenolic compounds are largely responsible for the multiple beneficial effects of EVOO, the main source of dietary lipids in the Mediterranean diet [22,66]. The phenolic fraction of EVOO is a complex mixture of phenolic compounds ranging from the simple phenols tyrosol and hydroxytytosol (HT) to complex polyphenols such as oleuropein, ligstroside, oleocanthal, flavonoids, and lignans [67]. All together, they are able to exert antiinflammatory, cardioprotective, antithrombotic, neuroprotective, immunomodulatory, and anticancer activities [22,67]. Phenolic concentration in EVOO ranges from 50 to 800 mg/kg depending on the cultivar, climate, ripeness of olives, and climate factors [68]. HT is a major polyphenol in olive fruits (66 mg/100 g black olives), with a concentration in EVOO ranging from 0,35 to 0,77 mg/100 g [32]. Many studies have shown the capability of HT to improve glucose homeostasis, cardiovascular dysfunctions, and dyslipidemia and to exert antioxidant and antiinflammatory actions by interacting with an increasing number of multiple cellular targets [69]. HT is absorbed in a dose-dependent manner, reaching a peak in plasma and urine at around 1 h after EVOO ingestion [70]. The useful effects of EVOO polyphenols have been recognized by the European Food Safety Authority (EFSA) that recommends a daily consumption of 5 mg of HT and its derivatives (per 20 g olive oil daily dose; two tablespoons) to protect blood lipids from oxidative damage [71].

Curcumin is a diarylheptanoid, belonging to curcuminoid group, derived from tumeric (*Curcuma longa*) that is accountable for the yellow color [72]. Dried tumeric contains 2213.57 mg/100 g curcumin that can be also detected in curry powder (285.26 mg/100 g), a mix of spices including turmeric [32]. Curcumin is a hydrophobic polyphenol with antiinflammatory, anticancer, antiangiogenic, and antioxidant activities exerted by modulating several signal transduction pathways including MAPK, ERK, SAPK/JNK, and NF-κB [72,73]. Even though curcumin exerts all these healthy effects in vitro, it is in vivo, poorly absorbed, and rapidly metabolized and excreted. Actually, several studies have shown that after the ingestion of more than 10 grams of curcumin, serum concentration is very low (a few ng or μg) and declines by a few hours [74]. Furthermore, 6-month ingestion of 1500 mg/day curcumin results in increased serum levels of adiponectin and decreased level of leptin, in association with an improvement of the lipid profile, in type 2 diabetes patients [75].

Flavonolignans, also called "nonconventional lignans," have been found in vegetables belonging to different plant families. Milk thistle (*Silybum marianum*) represents the richest plant source of flavonolignans; its extract, silymarin, contains a mixture of flavonolignans (i.e., silybin A and B, isosilybin A and B, silydianin, and silychristina, and flavonoids taxifolin and quercetin), of which silibinin (or silybin) is the main active compound [76]. In the last decades, silymarin has received much attention in virtue of its antiinflammatory and antioxidant activity in liver disorders [76]. In particular, it has been demonstrated that silymarin participates in the regulation of the antioxidant system by modulating several transcription factors including Nrf2 and NF-κB [77] and modulates inflammatory processes by reducing the expression of inflammatory molecules such as COX-2, IL-6, IL-1β, and also in gestational tissues [78]. According to European Pharmacopoeia, milk thistle dry extract contains 30%–65% silymarin [79]; however, even if consumed in high doses (>1500 mg/day) that have been shown to be safe in humans, silymarin components have a poor bioavailability and absorption, are rapidly metabolized by phase I and phase II enzymes in the liver, and are excreted in bile and urine [80]. In consideration of the evident benefits of this compound, different kinds of approaches to improve silymarin bioavailability have been studied [80]. Moreover, a recent online survey on breastfeeding mothers has reinforced the galactagogues effect of silymarin, reporting an increased milk supply after silymarin ingestion [27,81].

Ellagitannins are a family of hydrolysable tannins found in fruit including pomegranate and red raspberries [13,82]. Pomegranate fruit (*Punica granatum* L.) besides to contain several flavonoids is rich in punicalagin, gallic, and ellagic acid. Punicalagin (2,3-hexahydroxydiphenoyl-gallagyl-d-glucose) is the major ellagitannin isolated from pomegranate fruit that appears to exert antiinflammatory [83], antioxidant [84], and antiapoptotic activities [85] by modulating several cell signaling pathways, including Nrf2, NF-κB, MAPK, and ERKs, and by reducing inflammatory (e.g., NO, PGE2, IL-6, TNFα) [83,86] and apoptotic molecules (e.g., p52, p21, MDM1) [85]. Pomegranate juice contains 135,31 mg/100 mL punicalagin [32]. This compound has high bioavailability; it is hydrolyzed into smaller phenolic compounds such as ellagic acid that is found in blood. In addition, following metabolism by gut microbiota, punicalagin is transformed in urolithin A and B that circulate into the blood and is excreted in the urine [87].

Polyphenols intake in pregnancy

Maternal diet deeply influences pregnancy outcomes, and a healthy diet containing fruit and vegetables appears to reduce the risk of maternal and fetal complications also later in life [5,10] (Fig. 10.2). Although well-

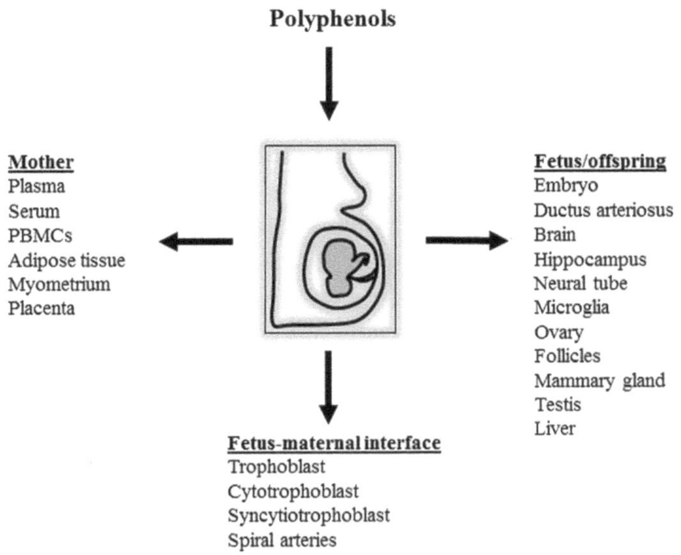

Figure 10.2 Maternal intake of dietary polyphenols differently influences mother and offspring health. The amount and kind of ingested polyphenols affect fetus development depending on the gestational period of exposition and in an organ-specific manner.

defined dietary recommendations have not been provided, the known benefits of dietary polyphenols have led researchers to test them during pregnancy both in animals and humans. In humans, it has been observed that the intake of fruit, vegetables, nuts, whole grains, and key components of Mediterranean dietary pattern during pregnancy associates with reduced cardiometabolic markers [8] and GDM risk [88] and decreases the risk of preeclampsia (PE) [89] and the incidence of preterm birth (PTB) [90]. Furthermore, Mediterranean diet seems to influence gestational weight gain [91] and to protect the fetus against the development of metabolic syndrome throughout life [92].

Regular ingestion ($\geq$1−3 servings/week) of a polyphenol-rich food such as chocolate greatly reduces risk of PE; time of exposure indicates that the intake during the first or third trimester is equally protective against PE [89]. On the contrary, a maternal diet rich in polyphenols [93,94] in the third trimester of healthy pregnancy causes intrauterine fetal ductus arteriosus constriction with potential severe consequences on neonatal pulmonary arterial hypertension [12]. Moreover, excessive consumption of fruit (mean 419 g/d), also with a moderate or high glycemic index such as tropical and citrus fruit, during the second trimester may be associated with an increased likelihood of GDM [95]. These findings suggest that antiinflammatory effects of polyphenols might not be positive in late pregnancy and attention must be paid to pregnancy diet (Fig. 10.2).

To this end, and to shed light on the role of specific phenolic compounds, several nutritional intervention studies in animal models have been performed.

It has been observed that maternal ingestion of high doses of epicatechin (8000 mg):catechin (2000 mg) in a ratio of 4:1 reflecting the ratio in cocoa-containing products [30] before getting pregnant, during pregnancy, and lactation does not have deleterious effects on fetal growth in mice [96]. On the contrary, consumption of grape seed procyanidins (25 mg/kg of body weight) containing gallic acid (1.8%), epicatechin (5.5%), epicatechin gallate (5.5%), and catechin (9.1%), as well as dimeric (18.4%) and trimeric (2.8%) procyanidins, corresponding to the average of the human daily ingested procyanidin (240−450 mg), during pregnancy and lactation, negatively modifies lipid profile, increasing TG and reducing HDL-cholesterol, thus resulting in a CVD-prone phenotype in rat offspring [97].

Neural defects induced by hyperglycemia can be counteracted by the maternal ingestion of EGCG (10 μM) in diabetic pregnant mice at embryonic day 5.5 [98]. Likewise, C3G (10 mg/kg) administration ameliorates malformations of the central nervous system as a consequence of fetal alcohol exposure in a rat model of ethanol neurotoxicity [99].

Daily administration of RSV (20 mg/kg body weight) in pregnant rats decreases maternal and offspring oxidative stress [100]. RSV supplementation (0.2% dry feed) during pregnancy increases energy expenditure in mice feed a high fat diet, thus protecting the offspring against obesity and insulin resistance later in life [65]. Quercetin administration (50, 100, or 200 mg/kg body weight) during pregnancy improves insulin sensitivity and lipid metabolism and reduces birth weight and the weight gain in offspring and in obese rats [101]. Hydroxytyrosol supplementation in pregnancy appears to improve pre- and early postnatal development of offspring also in the presence of risk of intrauterine growth restriction as demonstrated in an animal model receiving 1.5 mg of HT/kg/day starting from gestational day 35 until delivery [102]. Timing of exposure to hesperidin and naringin appears to negatively influence bone development. Maternal consumption of diet supplemented with 0.5% hesperidin and 0.25% naringin before and during pregnancy results in a transient detrimental effect on skeletal integrity in female offspring. Specifically, female offspring fed at weaning a control diet recovers integrity at 6 months of age [103]. Genistein (20 mg/kg) administered to dams from gestational day 14 to parturition induces an increased IgE production in young adults mice. These findings indicate that exposure to high levels of isoflavones during a sensitive period for the immune system development may increase allergic sensitization [104]. High levels of genistein (100 μg/g body weight/day) administered from day 11 of gestation to day 8 postpartum induce alterations of estrogen-dependent adult behaviors influencing anxiety-related behaviors, in male mice. The increasing use of soy-based food raises the need of further studies to assess the role of phytoestrogens during pregnancy [105].

Potential mechanisms on pregnancy

Antioxidant/antiinflammatory activity

Pregnancy is a physiological condition characterized by considerable immunological, hormonal, and metabolic changes of the body aimed at accept, maintain, and accommodate fetus growth [106], as well as to dispose fetus delivery [107]. Changes in immune response, by following specific temporal patterns, with the involvement of Th1 (cell-mediated immunity) and Th2 (humoral immunity) cytokines, account for normal pregnancy outcome [106,107]. In addition, reactive oxygen species (ROS) regulate physiological gene transcription and downstream activities such as trophoblast proliferation, invasion, and angiogenesis [108,109]. Excessive ROS production and altered inflammatory responses, including altered arachidonic acid pathway, increased inflammatory cytokines levels, and dysregulated activity of numerous transcription factors, are involved in several pregnancy disorders leading to adverse pregnancy outcomes [106,110].

Dietary polyphenols exert antiinflammatory and antioxidant effects by modulating the expression of several genes and most of the cell signaling pathways, including NFkB, MAPKs, and JNK [16,17]. Polyphenols can influence endogenous defense systems by influencing enzymatic, such as superoxide dismutase (SOD), catalase (CAT), glutathione peroxidase (GPx), glutathione reductase (GR), glutathione S-transferase (GST), and nonenzymatic antioxidants, such as glutathione (GSH) and heme oxygenase-1 (HO-1) [16,111]. The redox-sensitive transcription factor Nrf2 is able to modulate gene expression by binding the antioxidant responsive elements detected in the promoter region of detoxifying and antioxidant enzymes and inflammatory genes as well. This transcription factor in its inactive form is bound to Kelch-like ECH-associated protein (Keap1). Stressors such as ROS modify the Nrf2–Keap1 complex, resulting in the nuclear translocation of Nrf2 and upregulation of the expression of target genes [16]. Nfr2 shows antiinflammatory action by targeting several molecules and by binding to other transcription factors such as NF-κB in human fetal membranes [112]. Polyphenols by activating Nrf2 signaling pathway appear to mitigate oxidative stress–related pregnancy disorders [113]. Oxidative stress is associated with PTB, and Nfr2 appears to regulate several pathways involved in PTB susceptibility. It has been observed that the placenta from $Nrf2^{-/-}$mice express high levels of proinflammatory molecules involved in PTB, including NF-κB, IL-6, and TNF-α [114] (Fig. 10.3).

In utero exposure to quercetin (302 mg/kg) and genistein (270 mg/kg) potentiates the antioxidant defense system in the liver of adult mice. Specifically, this occurs by the activation of the Nfr2 pathway, which leads to increased expression of the antioxidant Ho-1, Cat, and Gpx3 genes. In addition, ingestion of flavonoids associates with a reduction of DNA damage induced by oxidative stress in the liver of adult offspring. Overall, these data highlight the long-lasting effects of these phenolic compounds on the antioxidant status [53]. Interestingly, quercetin is able to counteract the adverse effects of air pollution exposure in dams exposed to fine particulate matter 2.5 (PM2.5). Specifically, in pregnant mice, the treatment with

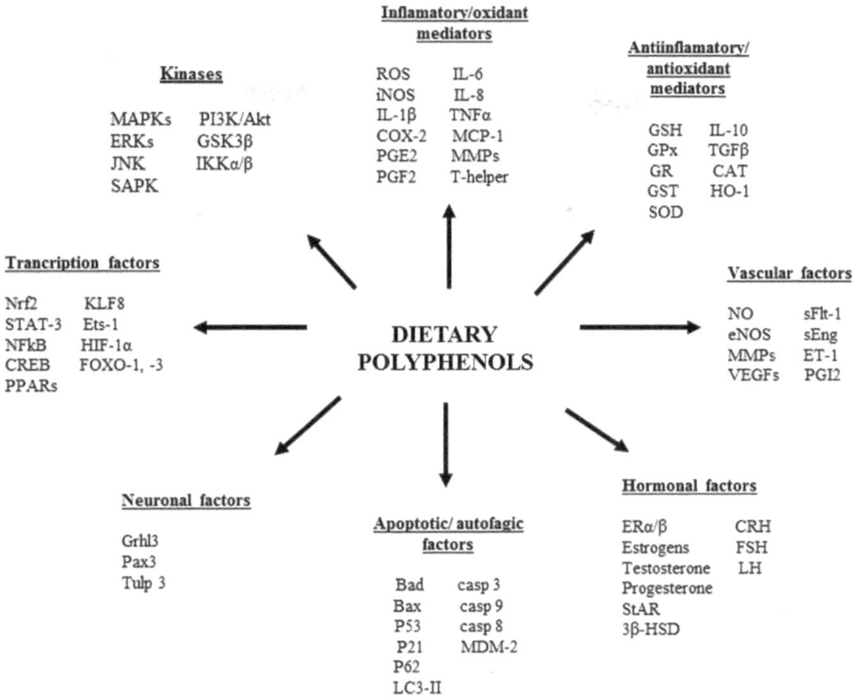

Figure 10.3 Schematic representation of the major cellular mediators influenced by dietary polyphenols in pregnancy. Phenolic compounds are able to modulate at different points the complex network of signaling pathways accountable for fetus development and mother health.

100 mg/kg quercetin from day 0 to day 17 gestation reduces the number of CD3+CD4+ and CD3+CD8+ T lymphocytes and serum levels of IL-6 and IL-8 and increases serum concentration of CAT and HO-1. Considering the constant exposure to different mixture of PM2.5, a dietary supplementation with quercetin may be appropriate to potentiate maternal immunity [115]. The increased ROS production observed in human preeclamptic placental trophoblast is significantly reduced by genistein. Specifically, 2 μM genistein incubation attenuates lipid hydroperoxide, 4-hydroxy-2-nanenol, and NO^{2-} levels, in preeclamptic trophoblast, most likely by increasing the total antioxidant capacity of the cells by enhancing GPx expression [116]. Thus, the capability of genistein to modify oxidant—antioxidant status indicates a possible role of this phytoestrogen in the management of PE.

Lappas and colleagues have evaluated the effects of different phenolic compounds such as nobiletin (200 μM) [117], luteolin (20 μM), kaempferol

(100 μM) [54], apigenin (20 μM), naringenin (400 μM), and curcumin (60 μM) [118] in human gestational tissues. The obtained data show the capability of these compounds to counteract the increased expression of the proinflammatory cytokines TNF-α, IL-1β, IL-6, and IL-8 in fetal membranes and placentas and COX-2, MMP-9, PGE2, and PGF2α secretion in myometrium, stimulated with LPS or IL-1β. NFkB binding activity is reduced after luteolin and kaempferol incubation.

Of note, incubation of fetal membrane from spontaneous PTB with nobiletin results in reduction of the above prolabor mediators, thus supporting the benefits of fruit ingestion [117].

Dissecting the molecular mechanisms of curcumin action, it has been observed that this compound (30 μM) reduces the production of IL-6 in human and rodent uterine stromal/decidual cells. This occurs via NFkB and by the inactivation of IKKα/β and STAT-3 [73]. The chemiopreventive and proapoptotic effects of polyphenols in cancer cells are well known [119]. In human placental choriocarcinoma cells (JAR and JEG3), curcumin reduces proliferation and migration of transformed cells in a dose-dependent manner. Curcumin (50 μM) induces strong apoptosis in both cell lines by activating different signaling pathways. By studying the apoptotic pathway, it has been shown that curcumin acts via mitochondria - loss of MMP - upregulating the proapoptotic molecules such as Bad, bak, and bax in JAR, by activating caspase-9 and increasing ERK1/2 and JNK phosphorylation in both cell lines [72].

The intake of pomegranate juice (8 oz ≈ 237 mL/day) from 35 to 38 wk gestation until delivery reduces oxidative stress and apoptosis in human placentas obtained from healthy women. Specifically, incubation with pomegranate juice and punicalagin (33.8 μM) decreases both spontaneous and stimulated apoptosis in syncytiotrophoblasts, in vitro [84]. This effect occurs by downregulating the mRNA expression of p53, the major regulator of stress-induced apoptosis, in cells cultured in hypoxic conditions. Moreover, it has shown that punicalagin decreases the expression of two p53 target genes, p21 and MDM2, as well as mRNA and protein expression of the transcription factor hypoxia-inducible factor 1 alpha (HIF1α). Punicalagin protects human trophoblasts against apoptosis by promoting autophagy, as demonstrated by the reduced levels of the autophagy markers LC3-II and p62 and increased number of lysosomes in syncytiotrophoblasts [120]. Punicalagin appears to exert its protective action in a complex manner by modulating several signaling pathways.

RSV counteracts inflammation in human tissues obtained from healthy women undergoing elective caesarean. RSV (200 μM) significantly reduces IL-1β, IL-6, and IL-8 mRNA expression and secretion in IL-1β–stimulated placentas and decreases the aforementioned proinflammatory cytokines also in omental adipose tissue treated with TNF-α, IL-1β, or LPS. In addition, RSV restores insulin signaling in TNF-α or LPS-treated skeletal muscle [121]. RSV seems to have a role also in reducing inflammation and oxidative stress in PE. Human cytotrophoblasts, from term caesarean section placentas, when incubated with 100 μM RSV show a reduced mRNA expression of the inflammatory molecules IL-6, IL-1β, and NF-κB and secrete only IL-6 and TNF-α. In addition, RSV improves the p-eNOS/eNOS ratio in an in vitro model of endothelial dysfunction (HUVECs treated with TNF-α) [122]. All together, these findings suggest that RSV may be a useful therapeutic agent in different pathological conditions.

Silibinin (200 μM) also reduces inflammation induced by LPS and IL-1β in human gestational tissues. An in vivo study shows that silibinin downregulates IL-8 mRNA expression in fetal brain and does not modify inflammatory parameters, such as IL-6, IL-8, IL-1β, COX-2, and MMP-9, in the placenta and myometrium isolated from mice injected with LPS [78]. Of note, silibinin (50 μM) reverts the high spontaneous levels of O_2, H_2O_2, and TNF-α and the lower levels of IL-10 and TGF-β observed in monocytes [123] and counteracts the increases in the endogenous activation of NF-κB and IL-1β release in peripheral blood mononuclear cells [124] obtained from preeclamptic women compared with normotensive pregnant.

Endocrine effects

Several studies indicate that a diet rich in isoflavones ameliorates menopausal symptoms including hot flushes, osteoporosis, obesity, cancers, and cardiovascular disorders promoted by the reduced secretion of ovarian estrogen [125]. As a result, the EFSA stated that isoflavones intake, from supplements, does not adversely affect mammary gland, uterus, and thyroid in peri- and postmenopausal women [126,127]. Also, Food and Drug Administration (FDA) established that "soy protein included in a diet low in saturated fat and cholesterol may reduce the risk of CHD by lowering blood cholesterol levels" [128]. Following ingestion of 20–133 g/d soy protein (for 3 weeks to 1 year), indeed, a reduction of LDL-cholesterol ranging from 7.9% to 10.3% has been demonstrated [129]. Despite the multiple potential benefits of dietary isoflavones [43,59,125], these compounds rise many concerns because of their estrogenic activity, and they should be considered as endocrine disruptors [130]. It is known that throughout gestational period, hormonal pathway, in which estrogens, progesterone, and human chorionic gonadotropin (hCG) are the major players, exerts fundamental actions to establish and maintain pregnancy and to develop mammary glands [131]. However, even though the function of each hormone in different stage of pregnancy is not completely understood, an accurate hormonal regulation is necessary to have a successful pregnancy [131]. However, timing of exposure, form, and doses of phytoestrogens as well as age, health status, and gut microbiota of individuals influence the estrogen-like activity of isoflavones [132] (Fig. 10.3).

To this regard, it has been observed that consumption of soy protein containing low or high concentration of isoflavones (1.64 ± 0.19 mg or 61.7 ± 7.35 mg/day; for 8 wk) does not affect semen quality in a sample of healthy adult men [133]. On the contrary, data obtained from pregnant animals studies show deleterious effects of isoflavones exposure on parturition and fertility in both male and female offspring.

Co-administration of genistein and LPS (40, 200, and 400 mg/kg/day from day 13 to day 17 gestation) alters the hormonal regulation related to parturition and rises the incidence of early delivery in mice. These effects associate with increased levels of corticotropin-releasing hormone (CRH) both in the plasma and placenta (mRNA) and reduced plasma progesterone concentration, favoring preterm delivery [134]. Low doses of genistein (2, 20, or 100 mg/kg) injected in pregnant rat during the critical period of reproductive organs development (days 12–19 of gestation) modify reproductive organs, by altering fertility (i.e., steroidogenesis and spermatogenesis) in adult male rats [135]. Specifically, the altered spermatogenesis is associated with reduced testosterone and increased FSH and LH plasma levels [135]. A study carried out in in vitro organ cultures has shown that 10^{-8} and 10^{-6} M genistein incubation determined, in a dose-dependent manner, a strong reduction of testosterone secretion in mice fetal testis (day 12.5 of gestation); and this effect associated with a significant downregulation (40%–50%) of key genes of steroidogenesis such as steroidogenic acute regulatory protein (*StAR*), 17alpha-hydroxylase-C17-20 lyase (*p450C17*), and 3beta hydroxysteroid dehydrogenase (*3β-HSD*). Moreover, by using (*ERα−/−*) and (*ERβ−/−*) knockout mice, it has been demonstrated that genistein, by mimicking estrogen action, exerts its inhibitory effect through an *ERα*-

dependent mechanism [136]. Exposure to low dose of genistein (1 mg/kg-d) during pregnancy modifies mammary gland development with increased proliferation and ductal hyperplasia in rat female offspring [137]. Maternal ingestion of higher doses of genistein (150 mg/kg) negatively modifies oviduct mucosa layer and consequently the future fertilization processes in murine offspring [138].

In addition, maternal administration of daidzein (5 or 60 mg/kg) on 6–21 gestational days negatively influences follicologenesis in adult female rat offspring with effects similar to that of 17α-ethinyl estradiol administration during the same period. Daidzein reduces ovarian surface epithelial cell height and the number of secondary and tertiary follicles, and increases the number of atretic follicles [139]. The ability of DZ to bind estrogen receptors may account for these deleterious effects.

Daidzein (0.1–1 μM) and genistein (0.1–1 μM) treatments reduce progesterone and increase estrogen secretion in a dose-dependent manner in cytotrophoblast cells obtained from term human placentae. These data indicate possible harmful consequences for the pregnancy as reduced progesterone might negatively influence the maintenance and development of the fetus [140]. Offspring hypospadias appear to be associated with maternal consumption of soy food (i.e., isoflavones) [141]. Actually, most of these mothers followed a vegetarian and vegan diets; thus, it is hypothesized that the lack of fish and meat is responsible for the increased hypospadias risk [142,143].

Establishing the real concentration of isoflavones in soy-derived foods is a crucial point to understand better the phytoestrogens/isoflavones activities. Soybeans, soy protein isolate, or isoflavones, in fact, should not be considered equivalent because of the numerous other constituents with bioactive capacity (e.g., high-quality proteins and polyunsaturated fatty acids) contained in soybeans [59,144]. In addition, soy-derived food obtained from modern processes retains a higher and underestimated amount of isoflavones compared with that maintained with the traditional cooking practices [130].

Whether and when isoflavones have beneficial or detrimental effects on human health is an open question that requires further studies.

Vasculature activity

Maternal vascular dysfunction, in which concur genetic, metabolic, and environmental factors, influences pregnancy outcome [145]. Appropriate development of placental vascular network is fundamental for positive pregnancy outcomes. Fetal growth restriction, PE, and fetal death represent some of the pathological conditions resulting from altered placental angiogenesis [146]. Maternal lifestyle, diet, obesity, and metabolic factors influence the correct balance among specific transcription factors including Krüppel-like factor 8 (KLF8), E26 transformation specific oncogene homolog 1 (Ets-1), NF-κB, STAT-3, and Nrf2 [146]; circulating molecules including VEGFs, fms-like tyrosine kinase 1 (sFlt-1), soluble endoglin (sEng), IL-6, TNFα, HIF-1; and vascular targets such as NO, HO-1, MMPs, and PGI2, which all are involved in the placental vascular development and function [147]. Regarding the role of diet, the adherence to a healthful dietary pattern associates with a reduced risk of developing hypertension among women with a history of gestational diabetes [148]. Dietary polyphenols improve endothelial dysfunction and exert vasodilation, antihypertensive, and antiplatelet activities by positively modulating several cellular mechanisms/molecules including activation of PI3K/Akt and ERK kinases leading to eNOS phosphorylation and consequent increased NO bioavailability [18,61]. Virtually, they can modulate all of the actors involved in pathophysiological angiogenesis in pregnancy, as observed in in vitro and in rodents studies [149] (Fig. 10.3). In particular, cocoa polyphenols appear to lower blood pressure and improve vascular function, in both healthy subjects and patients with risk factors. Although not completely understood, the mechanisms responsible of these effects seem to be an increased NO availability, the inhibition of angiotensin-converting enzyme, and a reduced inflammation [150]. On the basis of results from several clinical trials, EFSA suggests "to consume 200 mg of cocoa flavanols per day, provided by 2.5 g of high-flavanol cocoa powder or 10 g of high-flavanol dark chocolate, in the context of a balanced diet" to improve endothelial function and lower blood pressure [151].

However, the benefits observed in adults following cocoa polyphenols ingestion appear to be detrimental in the third trimester of pregnancy because of the interference with fetal DA dynamics [93]. Ingestion of a diet rich in polyphenol (3100 mg/day) during late pregnancy induces fetal DA constriction, decrease in serum NO levels, and increase in GPx and catalase activity in pregnant sheep [152]. Worth of note, a reversal of fetal ductal constriction occurs when the daily intake of polyphenols decreased from 1277 to 126 mg for a period of 2 weeks or more in the third trimester of pregnancy women. This effect appears to associate with a significant increase in plasma PGE2 levels, supporting the antiinflammatory activity of polyphenols [153,154].

All data show the need of paying attention to diet in the last period of pregnancy.

A recent prospective study (3142 participants) provided evidence on the benefits of dietary intake of isoflavone-rich food, including soy and soy products in reducing systolic blood pressure [155]. Specifically, among the other biological properties, genistein exerts antithrombotic, antiatherosclerotic, and vasodilating activities [61]. The inverse association between genistein intake and risk of developing PE observed in healthy pregnant women could be also because of hypotensive effects of this isoflavone [156]. However, phytoestrogens inhibit gene expression and activity of aromatase with consequent reduction of testosterone levels [43]. This inhibitory activity should be taken in consideration when studying PE as aromatase levels are lower in the placentas obtained from patients with PE in comparison with healthy placentas [157]. RSV also appears to be therapeutic in PE by reducing secretion of antiangiogenic factors. It has been observed that human cytotrophoblast, from healthy placentas, incubated with 100 μM RSV results in the reduction of sFlt-1 and sEng secretion and decreases endothelin-1 (ET-1) secretion in HUVECs treated with TNF-α [122].

Among the activities of curcumin, the capability of positively influencing vascular functions exists. Curcumin administration appears to improve vascular health by modulating arterial structural proteins, inflammation, oxidative stress, and NO bioavailability [158]. In a PE-like rat model (0.5 mg/kg LPS on GD 5), curcumin administration (0.36 mg/kg) until day 18 gestation ameliorates LPS-induced high blood pressure. Moreover, curcumin improves trophoblast invasion and spiral artery remodeling, reduces IL-6 and MCP-1 levels both in serum and placenta, and influences toll-like receptor 4 (TLR4) signaling by diminishing TLR4 and NF-kB expression in the placenta, thus counteracting the harmful effects of cross-talk between LPS and TLR4 [159]. Similarly, curcumin abolishes LPS-induced hypertension in mice by reducing the levels of the proinflammatory cytokines TNFα, IL-1β, IL-6, and chemokines MCP-1 and MIP in association with increased Akt phosphorylation in the placentas [160]. These studies provide additional evidences on the ability of curcumin to prevent and mitigate inflammation in pregnancy complications.

Neuroprotective activity

Maternal inflammation and obesity have deleterious effects on neurodevelopment of the embryo. In addition, maternal dysbiosis significantly participates in disturbing neurologic function in murine offspring in a sex-specific manner [41] and with long-term effects.

Dietary polyphenols in virtue of their antiinflammatory and antioxidant effects have shown to possess neuroprotective effects in neurodegenerative disorders such as Alzheimer's and Parkinson's disease, by influencing neuronal survival, growth, and functions by modulating several signaling pathways including NFkB, MAPK, JAK/STAT, PI3Kinase/Akt, CREB, and Nfr2 [19,22,161] (Fig. 10.3).

Some polyphenols such as those contained in tea (i.e., catechin) appear to have harmful effects on neuronal development probably because of the ability in interfering with the absorption of fundamental micronutrient such as folic acid [162].

The neural tube closure is a complex and sophisticated process not completely understood yet. Neural tube defects (NTDs) are disastrous birth defects [163]. In diabetic pregnant mice, quercetin (100 mg/kg) administrated from day 7.5 to day 10.5 gestation strongly reduces apoptosis in the neural tissues of the dorsal region as confirmed by reduced expression of caspase-3. Moreover, quercetin reduces oxidative stress by diminishing iNOS expression - implicated in diabetic embryopathy - and by increasing the antioxidative enzymes SOD2 and SOD3 [164]. This flavonol inhibits inflammatory response in LPS-treated murine BV-2 microglial cells. Quercetin (0−10 μM) reduces LPS-induced NO production and induces HO-1 protein expression by activating Nrf2, ERK1/2, and p38MAPK [165]. Punicalagin has protective effects under high glucose conditions. Specifically mouse embryos (embryonic day 8.5) cultured in high glucose media and in presence of punicalagin (20 μM) present a significant NTD and endoplasmatic reticulum stress reduction associated with reduced lipid peroxidation. In addition, punicalagin decreases apoptosis and caspase-3 and 8 activation [86]. Similarly, curcumin reduces NTD by modifying all the above tested molecules induced by high glucose in a mouse model [166]. EGCG (10 μM) given to diabetic pregnant mice at embryonic day 5.5 until day 8.75 reduces NTD and diminishes the global DNA methylation levels in embryos induced by maternal diabetes. In particular, EGCG attenuates DNA hypermethylation in specific genes related to tube neural closure such as CpG islands of *Grhl3*, *Pax3*, and *Tulp3* genes. Thus, EGCG is able to reactivate essential genes, repressed by hyperglycemia, by modulating epigenetic modifications [98]. On the contrary, similar doses of EGCG (5-10 μM) disturb cell migration by altering cell adhesion in human neural progenitor cells (NPCs; gestational week 16−29) in vitro. These effects occur because of the capability of EGCG to bind to the extracellular matrix glycoprotein laminin and to impede NPC adhesion, thus altering neurodevelopment [167]. These in vitro results indicate that EGCG neurotoxicity on human fetal nervous system development is an issue that need further investigation, also in vivo, to avoid inappropriate dietary intake in pregnancy.

Cyanidin-3-glucoside (C3G) counteracts alcohol-induced damage in rat developing brain. Administration of C3G (10 mg/kg) reduces neurodegeneration by decreasing microglia activation, lipid peroxidation, and the activation of the serine/threonine kinase glycogen synthase kinase 3beta (GSK3β) involved in the alcohol-induced neurotoxicity [99]. An in vitro study has showed that C3G reduces, in a dose dependent-manner (ranging to 25 μM), LPS or IFNγ-induced ROS production, in bv-2 microglia cells [168]. In utero exposure to methyl mercury (MeHg) causes neurotoxicity in offspring. Simultaneous administration of MeHg and fisetin (10 and 50 mg/kg) from gestational day 5 until parturition significantly reduces Hg accumulation in the brain of offspring (PND 25). Fisetin counteracts the MeHg-induced oxidative stress by diminishing the levels of lipid peroxidation and by preserving the enzymatic and nonenzymatic antioxidants levels as well as the activities of Na^+-K^+ ATPase in specific brain regions of the offspring. All these effects indicate that fisetin is able to reduce cellular and functional damages induced by MeHg in rats [50].

Olive oil polyphenols appear to have neuroprotective effects by modulating neurotrophins levels [161]. Hydroxytyrosol ingestion (10 and 50 mg/kg/day) during pregnancy ameliorates neurogenesis and cognitive functions in rats exposed to prenatal restraint stress. Maternal administration of HT increases BDNF expression, improves function and mitochondrial DNA copy number, ameliorates oxidative stress, and increases SOD2 and HO-1 expression by activating the transcriptor factors Nrf2 and FOXO-1 and -3 in hippocampus of stressed offspring. It is possible to conclude that HT may be useful in managing the stress as well [169].

Conclusions

An adequate nutrition is required to have the best pregnancy outcomes. Fruit, vegetables, and plant-derived foods are key elements of a healthy diet, also because of the high amount of polyphenols they provide.

Several studies have established that these bioactive compounds have protective effects against several chronic diseases by reducing the risk of developing pregnancy-related disorders. Nevertheless, the intake of polyphenol-rich foods in pregnancy has raised concerns on their potential harmful effects.

The adaptive changes characterized by an accurate succession of events occurring in pregnancy are deeply influenced by maternal diet. The antiinflammatory, antioxidant, and estrogen-like activities of polyphenols that appear to be favorable under specific conditions seem to disturb the fetal growth and development (i.e., reproductive, immunological, and nervous systems), at certain times of gestation. Even though it is recognized that women of child-bearing age should consume a balanced diet rich in fruit and vegetables, there are not specific advises for dietary intake of polyphenols.

Consequently, to evaluate the real polyphenols contribution in pregnancy, it is overwhelming to design appropriate studies to accurately evaluate phenol composition of plant food, to estimate their metabolites (food metabolome) in human samples, and to test safety and or toxicity of polyphenols.

Further investigation, by using new technological methods, on polyphenols bioavailability enhancement and gut microbiota stability will provide additional information to shed light on the complex interaction among polyphenols and their metabolites, other dietary components, and cellular macromolecules and may help us make specific nutritional recommendation throughout pregnancy.

References

[1] World Health Organization. WHO recommandations on antenatal care for a positive pregnancy experience. 2017. Geneva, Switzerland, http://www.who.int/reproductivehealth.

[2] Black RE, Victora CG, Walker SP, Bhutta ZA, Christian P, de Onis M, et al. Maternal and child undernutrition and overweight in low-income and middle-income countries. Lancet 2013;382(9890):427–51.

[3] Shin D, Lee KW, Song WO. Pre-pregnancy weight status is associated with diet quality and nutritional biomarkers during pregnancy. Nutrients 2016;8(3):162.

[4] Diet, nutrition and the prevention of chronic diseases: report of a joint WHO/FAO expert consultation. WHO technical report series. Geneva: WHO; 2003. No.916.

[5] Santangelo C, Vari R, Scazzocchio B, Filesi C, Masella R. Management of reproduction and pregnancy complications in maternal obesity: which role for dietary polyphenols? Biofactors 2014;40(1):79–102.

[6] Santangelo C, Filesi C, Vari R, Scazzocchio B, Filardi T, Fogliano V, et al. Consumption of extra-virgin olive oil rich in phenolic compounds improves metabolic control in patients with type 2 diabetes mellitus: a possible involvement of reduced levels of circulating visfatin. J Endocrinol Invest 2016;39(11):1295–301.

[7] Skreden M, Bere E, Sagedal LR, Vistad I, Overby NC. Changes in fruit and vegetable consumption habits from pre-pregnancy to early pregnancy among Norwegian women. BMC Pregnancy and Childbirth 2017;17(1):107.
[8] Martin CL, Siega-Riz AM, Sotres-Alvarez D, Robinson WR, Daniels JL, Perrin EM, et al. Maternal dietary patterns are associated with lower levels of cardiometabolic markers during pregnancy. Paediatr Perinat Epidemiol 2016;30(3):246–55.
[9] Murphy MM, Stettler N, Smith KM, Reiss R. Associations of consumption of fruits and vegetables during pregnancy with infant birth weight or small for gestational age births: a systematic review of the literature. Int J Wom Health 2014;6:899–912.
[10] Santangelo C, Zicari A, Mandosi E, Scazzocchio B, Mari E, Morano S, et al. Could gestational diabetes mellitus be managed through dietary bioactive compounds? Current knowledge and future perspectives. Br J Nutr 2016;115(7):1129–44.
[11] Barenys M, Masjosthusmann S, Fritsche E. Is intake of flavonoid-based food supplements during pregnancy safe for the developing child? A literature review. Curr Drug Targets 2017;18(2):196–231.
[12] Hahn M, Baierle M, Charao MF, Bubols GB, Gravina FS, Zielinsky P, et al. Polyphenol-rich food general and on pregnancy effects: a review. Drug Chem Toxicol 2017;40(3):368–74.
[13] Crozier A, Jaganath IB, Clifford MN. Dietary phenolics: chemistry, bioavailability and effects on health. Nat Prod Rep 2009;26(8):1001–43.
[14] Fernando IP, Kim M, Son KT, Jeong Y, Jeon YJ. Antioxidant activity of marine algal polyphenolic compounds: amechanistic approach. J Med Food 2016;19(7):615–28.
[15] Naczk M, Shahidi F. Extraction and analysis of phenolics in food. J Chromatogr A 2004;1054(1–2):95–111.
[16] Masella R, Di Benedetto R, Vari R, Filesi C, Giovannini C. Novel mechanisms of natural antioxidant compounds in biological systems: involvement of glutathione and glutathione-related enzymes. J Nutr Biochem 2005;16(10):577–86.
[17] Santangelo C, Vari R, Scazzocchio B, Di Benedetto R, Filesi C, Masella R. Polyphenols, intracellular signalling and inflammation. Annali dell'Istituto superiore di sanita 2007;43(4):394–405.
[18] Hugel HM, Jackson N, May B, Zhang AL, Xue CC. Polyphenol protection and treatment of hypertension. Phytomed Int J Phytother Phytopharmacol 2016;23(2):220–31.
[19] Moosavi F, Hosseini R, Saso L, Firuzi O. Modulation of neurotrophic signaling pathways by polyphenols. Drug Design, Develop Therapy 2016;10:23–42.
[20] Rothwell JA, Knaze V, Zamora-Ros R. Polyphenols: dietary assessment and role in the prevention of cancers. Curr Opin Clin Nutr Metab Care 2017;20(6):512–21.
[21] Nie Q, Xing M, Hu J, Hu X, Nie S, Xie M. Metabolism and health effects of phytoestrogens. Crit Rev Food Sci Nutr 2017;57(11):2432–54.
[22] Santangelo C, Vari R, Scazzocchio B, De Sanctis P, Giovannini C, D'Archivio M, et al. Anti-inflammatory activity of extra virgin olive oil polyphenols: which role in the prevention and treatment of immune-mediated inflammatory diseases? Endocrine. Metabol Immune Disord Drug Targets 2018;18(1):36–50.
[23] Fraga CG, Galleano M, Verstraeten SV, Oteiza PI. Basic biochemical mechanisms behind the health benefits of polyphenols. Mol Aspect Med 2010;31(6):435–45.
[24] Chen L, Teng H, Jia Z, Battino M, Miron A, Yu Z, et al. Intracellular signaling pathways of inflammation modulated by dietary flavonoids: the most recent evidence. Crit Rev Food Sci Nutr 2017:1–17.
[25] Zamora-Ros R, Knaze V, Rothwell JA, Hemon B, Moskal A, Overvad K, et al. Dietary polyphenol intake in Europe: the European prospective investigation into cancer and nutrition (EPIC) study. Eur J Nutr 2016;55(4):1359–75.

[26] Burkholder-Cooley N, Rajaram S, Haddad E, Fraser GE, Jaceldo-Siegl K. Comparison of polyphenol intakes according to distinct dietary patterns and food sources in the Adventist Health Study-2 cohort. Br J Nutr 2016;115(12):2162–9.
[27] Dietz BM, Hajirahimkhan A, Dunlap TL, Bolton JL. Botanicals and their bioactive phytochemicals for women's health. Pharmacol Rev 2016;68(4):1026–73.
[28] Phan MAT, Paterson J, Bucknall M, Arcot J. Interactions between phytochemicals from fruits and vegetables: effects on bioactivities and bioavailability. Crit Rev Food Sci Nutr 2016:1–20.
[29] Burkholder-Cooley NM, Rajaram SS, Haddad EH, Oda K, Fraser GE, Jaceldo-Siegl K. Validating polyphenol intake estimates from a food-frequency questionnaire by using repeated 24-h dietary recalls and a unique method-of-triads approach with 2 biomarkers. Am J Clin Nutr 2017;105(3):685–94.
[30] USDA. Database for the flavonoid content of selected foods. 2015. https://www.ars.usda.gov.
[31] USDA. Database for the isoflavone content of selected foods. 2015. https://www.ars.usda.gov.
[32] Rothwell JA, Perez-Jimenez J, Neveu V, Medina-Remon A, M'Hiri N, Garcia-Lobato P, et al. Phenol-Explorer 3.0: a major update of the Phenol-Explorer database to incorporate data on the effects of food processing on polyphenol content. Database J Biol Databases Curat 2013. https://doi.org/10.1093/database/bat070. 2013:bat070.
[33] Plumb J, Pigat S, Bompola F, Cushen M, Pinchen H, Norby E, et al. eBASIS (bioactive substances in food information systems) and bioactive intakes: major updates of the bioactive compound composition and beneficial bioeffects database and the development of a probabilistic model to assess intakes in Europe. Nutrients 2017;9(4).
[34] Scalbert A, Williamson G. Dietary intake and bioavailability of polyphenols. J Nutr 2000;130(8S Suppl. l). 2073S-85S.
[35] Bohn T. Dietary factors affecting polyphenol bioavailability. Nutr Rev 2014;72(7):429–52.
[36] D'Archivio M, Filesi C, Vari R, Scazzocchio B, Masella R. Bioavailability of the polyphenols: status and controversies. Int J Mol Sci 2010;11(4):1321–42.
[37] Espin JC, Gonzalez-Sarrias A, Tomas-Barberan FA. The gut microbiota: a key factor in the therapeutic effects of (poly)phenols. Biochem Pharmacol 2017;139:82–93.
[38] Williamson G, Clifford MN. Role of the small intestine, colon and microbiota in determining the metabolic fate of polyphenols. Biochem Pharmacol 2017;139:24–39.
[39] Ozdal T, Sela DA, Xiao J, Boyacioglu D, Chen F, Capanoglu E. The reciprocal interactions between polyphenols and gut microbiota and effects on bioaccessibility. Nutrients 2016;8(2):78.
[40] Mulligan CM, Friedman JE. Maternal modifiers of the infant gut microbiota: metabolic consequences. J Endocrinol 2017;235(1):R1–12.
[41] Bruce-Keller AJ, Fernandez-Kim SO, Townsend RL, Kruger C, Carmouche R, Newman S, et al. Maternal obese-type gut microbiota differentially impact cognition, anxiety and compulsive behavior in male and female offspring in mice. PloS One 2017;12(4). e0175577.
[42] Xiao J. Dietary flavonoid aglycones and their glycosides: which show better biological significance? Crit Rev Food Sci Nutr 2017;57(9):1874–905.
[43] Lephart ED. Modulation of aromatase by phytoestrogens. Enzym Res 2015;2015:594656.

[44] Williamson G, Dionisi F, Renouf M. Flavanols from green tea and phenolic acids from coffee: critical quantitative evaluation of the pharmacokinetic data in humans after consumption of single doses of beverages. Mol Nutr Food Res 2011;55(6):864–73.

[45] Granja A, Frias I, Neves AR, Pinheiro M, Reis S. Therapeutic potential of epigallocatechin gallate nanodelivery systems. BioMed Research International 2017;2017:5813793.

[46] Hostetler GL, Ralston RA, Schwartz SJ. Flavones: food sources, bioavailability, metabolism, and bioactivity. Advan nutr 2017;8(3):423–35.

[47] Kimira M, Arai Y, Shimoi K, Watanabe S. Japanese intake of flavonoids and isoflavonoids from foods. J Epidemiol 1998;8(3):168–75.

[48] Khan N, Syed DN, Ahmad N, Mukhtar H. Fisetin: a dietary antioxidant for health promotion. Antioxi Redox Signal 2013;19(2):151–62.

[49] Wu PY, Lyu JL, Liu YJ, Chien TY, Hsu HC, Wen KC, et al. Fisetin regulates Nrf2 expression and the inflammation-related signaling pathway to prevent UVB-induced skin damage in hairless mice. Int J Mol Sci 2017;18(10).

[50] Jacob S, Thangarajan S. Effect of gestational intake of fisetin (3,3',4',7-tetrahydroxyflavone) on developmental methyl mercury neurotoxicity in F1 generation rats. Biol Trace Elem Res 2017;177(2):297–315.

[51] Barreca D, Gattuso G, Bellocco E, Calderaro A, Trombetta D, Smeriglio A, et al. Flavanones: citrus phytochemical with health-promoting properties. Biofactors 2017;43(4):495–506.

[52] Brett GM, Hollands W, Needs PW, Teucher B, Dainty JR, Davis BD, et al. Absorption, metabolism and excretion of flavanones from single portions of orange fruit and juice and effects of anthropometric variables and contraceptive pill use on flavanone excretion. Br J Nutr 2009;101(5):664–75.

[53] Vanhees K, van Schooten FJ, van Waalwijk van Doorn-Khosrovani SB, van Helden S, Munnia A, Peluso M, et al. Intrauterine exposure to flavonoids modifies antioxidant status at adulthood and decreases oxidative stress-induced DNA damage. Free Radical Biol Med 2013;57:154–61.

[54] Wall C, Lim R, Poljak M, Lappas M. Dietary flavonoids as therapeutics for preterm birth: luteolin and kaempferol suppress inflammation in human gestational tissues in vitro. Oxidat med cellul longevity 2013:485201. 2013.

[55] Chen AY, Chen YC. A review of the dietary flavonoid, kaempferol on human health and cancer chemoprevention. Food Chem 2013;138(4):2099–107.

[56] Czank C, Cassidy A, Zhang Q, Morrison DJ, Preston T, Kroon PA, et al. Human metabolism and elimination of the anthocyanin, cyanidin-3-glucoside: a (13)C-tracer study. Am J Clin Nutr 2013;97(5):995–1003.

[57] Masella R, Santangelo C, D'Archivio M, Li Volti G, Giovannini C, Galvano F. Protocatechuic acid and human disease prevention: biological activities and molecular mechanisms. Curr Med Chem 2012;19(18):2901–17.

[58] Kay CD, Pereira-Caro G, Ludwig IA, Clifford MN, Crozier A. Anthocyanins and flavanones are more bioavailable than previously perceived: areview of recent evidence. Annual rev food sci technol 2017;8:155–80.

[59] Messina M. Soy and health update: evaluation of the clinical and epidemiologic literature. Nutrients 2016;8(12).

[60] Nagino T, Kano M, Masuoka N, Kaga C, Anbe M, Miyazaki K, et al. Intake of a fermented soymilk beverage containing moderate levels of isoflavone aglycones enhances bioavailability of isoflavones in healthy premenopausal Japanese women: a double-blind, placebo-controlled, single-dose, crossover trial. Biosci microbiota, food and health 2016;35(1):9–17.

[61] Sureda A, Sanches Silva A, Sanchez-Machado DI, Lopez-Cervantes J, Daglia M, Nabavi SF, et al. Hypotensive effects of genistein: from chemistry to medicine. Chem Biol Interact 2017;268:37−46.
[62] Dvorakova M, Landa P. Anti-inflammatory activity of natural stilbenoids: a review. Pharmacol Res 2017;124:126−45.
[63] Wenzel E, Somoza V. Metabolism and bioavailability of trans-resveratrol. Mol Nutr Food Res 2005;49(5):472−81.
[64] Biasutto L, Mattarei A, Azzolini M, La Spina M, Sassi N, Romio M, et al. Resveratrol derivatives as a pharmacological tool. Ann N Y Acad Sci 2017;1403(1):27−37.
[65] Zou T, Chen D, Yang Q, Wang B, Zhu MJ, Nathanielsz PW, et al. Resveratrol supplementation of high-fat diet-fed pregnant mice promotes brown and beige adipocyte development and prevents obesity in male offspring. J Physiol 2017;595(5):1547−62.
[66] Buckland G, Gonzalez CA. The role of olive oil in disease prevention: a focus on the recent epidemiological evidence from cohort studies and dietary intervention trials. Br J Nutr 2015;113(Suppl. 2):S94−101.
[67] Martin-Pelaez S, Covas MI, Fito M, Kusar A, Pravst I. Health effects of olive oil polyphenols: recent advances and possibilities for the use of health claims. Mol Nutr Food Res 2013;57(5):760−71.
[68] Vissers MN, Zock PL, Katan MB. Bioavailability and antioxidant effects of olive oil phenols in humans: a review. Eur J Clin Nutr 2004;58(6):955−65.
[69] Peyrol J, Riva C, Amiot MJ. Hydroxytyrosol in the prevention of the metabolic syndrome and related disorders. Nutrients 2017;9(3).
[70] Miro-Casas E, Covas MI, Farre M, Fito M, Ortuno J, Weinbrenner T, et al. Hydroxytyrosol disposition in humans. Clin Chem 2003;49(6 Pt 1):945−52.
[71] Panel EN. Scientific Opinion on the substantation of health claims related to polyphenols in olive and protection of LDL particles from oxidative damage. EFSA J 2019;9:P2033.
[72] Lim W, Jeong M, Bazer FW, Song G. Curcumin suppresses proliferation and migration and induces apoptosis on human placental choriocarcinoma cells via ERK1/2 and SAPK/JNK MAPK signaling pathways. Biol Reprod 2016;95(4):83.
[73] Devi YS, DeVine M, DeKuiper J, Ferguson S, Fazleabas AT. Inhibition of IL-6 signaling pathway by curcumin in uterine decidual cells. PloS One 2015;10(5). e0125627.
[74] Anand P, Kunnumakkara AB, Newman RA, Aggarwal BB. Bioavailability of curcumin: problems and promises. Mol Pharm 2007;4(6):807−18.
[75] Chuengsamarn S, Rattanamongkolgul S, Phonrat B, Tungtrongchitr R, Jirawatnotai S. Reduction of atherogenic risk in patients with type 2 diabetes by curcuminoid extract: a randomized controlled trial. J Nutr Biochem 2014;25(2):144−50.
[76] Federico A, Dallio M, Loguercio C. Silymarin/silybin and chronic liver disease: amarriage of many years. Molecules 2017;22(2).
[77] Surai PF. Silymarin as a natural antioxidant: an overview of the current evidence and perspectives. Antioxidants 2015;4(1):204−47.
[78] Lim R, Morwood CJ, Barker G, Lappas M. Effect of silibinin in reducing inflammatory pathways in in vitro and in vivo models of infection-induced preterm birth. PloS One 2014;9(3):e92505.
[79] European Pharmacopoeia, Council of Europe. European directorate for the quality of medicines and healthcare. Assessment report on Silybum marianum (L.) Gaertn., fructus. 7th edition 2010. https://www.ema.europa.eu/en/documents/herbal-report/draft-assessment-report-silybum-marianum-l-gaertn-fructus_en.pdf.

[80] Javed S, Kohli K, Ali M. Reassessing bioavailability of silymarin. Alternative Med Rev AJ Clin Therap 2011;16(3):239–49.
[81] Bazzano AN, Cenac L, Brandt AJ, Barnett J, Thibeau S, Theall KP. Maternal experiences with and sources of information on galactagogues to support lactation: a cross-sectional study. Int J Wom Health 2017;9:105–13.
[82] Clifford MN, Scalbert A. Ellagitannins - nature, occurrence and dietary burden. J Sci Food Agric 2000;80(7):1118–25.
[83] Xu X, Li H, Hou X, Li D, He S, Wan C, et al. Punicalagin induces Nrf2/HO-1 expression via upregulation of PI3K/AKT pathway and inhibits LPS-induced oxidative stress in RAW264.7 macrophages. Mediat Inflamm 2015:380218. 2015.
[84] Chen B, Tuuli MG, Longtine MS, Shin JS, Lawrence R, Inder T, et al. Pomegranate juice and punicalagin attenuate oxidative stress and apoptosis in human placenta and in human placental trophoblasts. Am J Physiol Endocrinol Metab 2012;302(9):E1142–52.
[85] Chen B, Longtine MS, Nelson DM. Punicalagin, a polyphenol in pomegranate juice, downregulates p53 and attenuates hypoxia-induced apoptosis in cultured human placental syncytiotrophoblasts. Am J Physiol Endocrinol Metab 2013;305(10):E1274–80.
[86] Zhong J, Reece EA, Yang P. Punicalagin exerts protective effect against high glucose-induced cellular stress and neural tube defects. Biochem Biophys Res Commun 2015;467(2):179–84.
[87] Seeram NP, Henning SM, Zhang Y, Suchard M, Li Z, Heber D. Pomegranate juice ellagitannin metabolites are present in human plasma and some persist in urine for up to 48 hours. J Nutr 2006;136(10):2481–5.
[88] Tryggvadottir EA, Medek H, Birgisdottir BE, Geirsson RT, Gunnarsdottir I. Association between healthy maternal dietary pattern and risk for gestational diabetes mellitus. Eur J Clin Nutr 2016;70(2):237–42.
[89] Saftlas AF, Triche EW, Beydoun H, Bracken MB. Does chocolate intake during pregnancy reduce the risks of preeclampsia and gestational hypertension? Ann Epidemiol 2010;20(8):584–91.
[90] Martin CL, Sotres-Alvarez D, Siega-Riz AM. Maternal dietary patterns during the second trimester are associated with preterm birth. J Nutr 2015;145(8):1857–64.
[91] Hrolfsdottir L, Schalkwijk CG, Birgisdottir BE, Gunnarsdottir I, Maslova E, Granstrom C, et al. Maternal diet, gestational weight gain, and inflammatory markers during pregnancy. Obesity 2016;24(10):2133–9.
[92] Lorite Mingot D, Gesteiro E, Bastida S, Sanchez-Muniz FJ. Epigenetic effects of the pregnancy Mediterranean diet adherence on the offspring metabolic syndrome markers. J Physiol Biochem 2017;73(4):495–510.
[93] Zielinsky P, Martignoni FV, Vian I. Deleterious effects of maternal ingestion of cocoa upon fetal ductus arteriosus in late pregnancy. Front Pharmacol 2014;5:281.
[94] Rakha S. Excessive maternal orange intake - areversible etiology of fetal premature ductus arteriosus constriction: acase report. Fetal Diagnosis and Therapy 2017;42(2):158–60.
[95] Huang WQ, Lu Y, Xu M, Huang J, Su YX, Zhang CX. Excessive fruit consumption during the second trimester is associated with increased likelihood of gestational diabetes mellitus: a prospective study. Sci Rep 2017;7:43620.
[96] Lesser MNR, Keen CL, Lanoue L. Reproductive and developmental outcomes, and influence on maternal and offspring tissue mineral concentrations, of (-)-epicatechin, (+)-catechin, and rutin ingestion prior to, and during pregnancy and lactation in C57BL/6J mice. Toxicol reports 2015;2:443–9.

[97] Del Bas JM, Crescenti A, Arola-Arnal A, Oms-Oliu G, Arola L, Caimari A. Intake of grape procyanidins during gestation and lactation impairs reverse cholesterol transport and increases atherogenic risk indexes in adult offspring. J Nutr Biochem 2015;26(12):1670–7.
[98] Zhong J, Xu C, Reece EA, Yang P. The green tea polyphenol EGCG alleviates maternal diabetes-induced neural tube defects by inhibiting DNA hypermethylation. Am J Obstet Gynecol 2016;215(3):368 e1–e10.
[99] Ke Z, Liu Y, Wang X, Fan Z, Chen G, Xu M, et al. Cyanidin-3-glucoside ameliorates ethanol neurotoxicity in the developing brain. J Neurosci Res 2011;89(10):1676–84.
[100] Vega CC, Reyes-Castro LA, Rodriguez-Gonzalez GL, Bautista CJ, Vazquez-Martinez M, Larrea F, et al. Resveratrol partially prevents oxidative stress and metabolic dysfunction in pregnant rats fed a low protein diet and their offspring. J Physiol 2016;594(5):1483–99.
[101] Wu Z, Zhao J, Xu H, Lyv Y, Feng X, Fang Y, et al. Maternal quercetin administration during gestation and lactation decrease endoplasmic reticulum stress and related inflammation in the adult offspring of obese female rats. Eur J Nutr 2014;53(8):1669–83.
[102] Vazquez-Gomez M, Garcia-Contreras C, Torres-Rovira L, Pesantez JL, Gonzalez-Anover P, Gomez-Fidalgo E, et al. Polyphenols and IUGR pregnancies: maternal hydroxytyrosol supplementation improves prenatal and early-postnatal growth and metabolism of the offspring. PloS One 2017;12(5). e0177593.
[103] Sacco SM, Saint C, LeBlanc PJ, Ward WE. Maternal consumption of hesperidin and naringin flavanones exerts transient effects to tibia bone structure in female CD-1 offspring. Nutrients 2017;9(3).
[104] Guo TL, Meng AH. In: Utero exposure to genistein enhanced intranasal house dust mite allergen-induced respiratory sensitization in young adult B6C3F1 mice. Toxicology letters, vol. 253; 2016. p. 17–26.
[105] Rodriguez-Gomez A, Filice F, Gotti S, Panzica G. Perinatal exposure to genistein affects the normal development of anxiety and aggressive behaviors and nitric oxide system in CD1 male mice. Physiol Behav 2014;133:107–14.
[106] Challis JR, Lockwood CJ, Myatt L, Norman JE, Strauss 3rd JF, Petraglia F. Inflammation and pregnancy. Reprod Sci 2009;16(2):206–15.
[107] Choi SJ, Oh S, Kim JH, Roh CR. Changes of nuclear factor kappa B (NF-kappaB), cyclooxygenase-2 (COX-2) and matrix metalloproteinase-9 (MMP-9) in human myometrium before and during term labor. Eur J Obstet Gynecol Reprod Biol 2007;132(2):182–8.
[108] Wu F, Tian FJ, Lin Y. Oxidative stress in placenta: health and diseases. BioMed Research International 2015:293271. 2015.
[109] Duhig K, Chappell LC, Shennan AH. Oxidative stress in pregnancy and reproduction. Obstet Med 2016;9(3):113–6.
[110] Boyle AK, Rinaldi SF, Norman JE, Stock SJ. Preterm birth: inflammation, fetal injury and treatment strategies. J Reprod Immunol 2017;119:62–6.
[111] Yuan L, Liu J, Zhen J, Xu Y, Chen S, Halm-Lutterodt NV, et al. Vegetable and fruit juice enhances antioxidant capacity and regulates antioxidant gene expression in rat liver, brain and colon. Genet Mol Biol 2017;40(1):134–41.
[112] Lim R, Barker G, Lappas M. The transcription factor Nrf2 is decreased after spontaneous term labour in human fetal membranes where it exerts anti-inflammatory properties. Placenta 2015;36(1):7–17.
[113] Hussain T, Tan B, Liu G, Murtaza G, Rahu N, Saleem M, et al. Modulatory mechanism of polyphenols and Nrf2 signaling pathway in LPS challenged pregnancy disorders. Oxidat med cellul longevity 2017:8254289. 2017.

[114] Sussan TE, Sudini K, Talbot Jr CC, Wang X, Wills-Karp M, Burd I, et al. Nrf2 regulates gene-environment interactions in an animal model of intrauterine inflammation: implications for preterm birth and prematurity. Sci Rep 2017;7:40194.
[115] Liu W, Zhang M, Feng J, Fan A, Zhou Y, Xu Y. The influence of quercetin on maternal immunity, oxidative stress, and inflammation in mice with exposure of fine particulate matter during gestation. Int J Environ Res Publ Health 2017;14(6).
[116] Ekambaram P, Balan C, Susai CJ. Genistein attenuates oxidative damage in preeclamptic placental trophoblast. Hypertens Pregnancy 2016;35(2):250−63.
[117] Morwood CJ, Lappas M. The citrus flavone nobiletin reduces pro-inflammatory and pro-labour mediators in fetal membranes and myometrium: implications for preterm birth. PloS One 2014;9(9):e108390.
[118] Lim R, Barker G, Wall CA, Lappas M. Dietary phytophenols curcumin, naringenin and apigenin reduce infection-induced inflammatory and contractile pathways in human placenta, foetal membranes and myometrium. Mol Hum Reprod 2013;19(7):451−62.
[119] Giovannini C, Scazzocchio B, Vari R, Santangelo C, D'Archivio M, Masella R. Apoptosis in cancer and atherosclerosis: polyphenol activities. Annali dell'Istituto superiore di sanita 2007;43(4):406−16.
[120] Wang Y, Chen B, Longtine MS, Nelson DM. Punicalagin promotes autophagy to protect primary human syncytiotrophoblasts from apoptosis. Reproduction 2016;151(2):97−104.
[121] Tran HT, Liong S, Lim R, Barker G, Lappas M. Resveratrol ameliorates the chemical and microbial induction of inflammation and insulin resistance in human placenta, adipose tissue and skeletal muscle. PloS One 2017;12(3):e0173373.
[122] Hannan NJ, Brownfoot FC, Cannon P, Deo M, Beard S, Nguyen TV, et al. Resveratrol inhibits release of soluble fms-like tyrosine kinase (sFlt-1) and soluble endoglin and improves vascular dysfunction - implications as a preeclampsia treatment. Sci Rep 2017;7(1):1819.
[123] Cristofalo R, Bannwart-Castro CF, Magalhaes CG, Borges VT, Peracoli JC, Witkin SS, et al. Silibinin attenuates oxidative metabolism and cytokine production by monocytes from preeclamptic women. Free Radic Res 2013;47(4):268−75.
[124] Giorgi VS, Peracoli MT, Peracoli JC, Witkin SS, Bannwart-Castro CF. Silibinin modulates the NF-kappab pathway and pro-inflammatory cytokine production by mononuclear cells from preeclamptic women. J Reprod Immunol 2012;95(1−2):67−72.
[125] Rietjens I, Louisse J, Beekmann K. The potential health effects of dietary phytoestrogens. Br J Pharmacol 2017;174(11):1263−80.
[126] Aguilar F, Crebelli R, Di Domenico A, Dusemund B, Frutos MJ, Galtier P, et al. Risk assessment for peri- and post-menopausal women taking food supplements containing isolated isoflavones. Efsa J 2015;13(10).
[127] Panel of Foos Additives and nutrient sources added to Food Scientific opinion on the risk assessment for peri- and post-mrnopausal women taking food supplements containing isolated isoflavones. EFSA J 2015;13:4246.
[128] Food labeling: health claims; soy protein and coronary heart disease. Food and Drug Administration, HHS. Final rule. Fed Regist 1999;64(206):57700−33.
[129] Jenkins DJ, Mirrahimi A, Srichaikul K, Berryman CE, Wang L, Carleton A, et al. Soy protein reduces serum cholesterol by both intrinsic and food displacement mechanisms. J Nutr 2010;140(12). 2302S-11S.
[130] Fernandez-Lopez A, Lamothe V, Delample M, Denayrolles M, Bennetau-Pelissero C. Removing isoflavones from modern soyfood: why and how? Food Chemistry 2016;210:286−94.
[131] Costa MA. The endocrine function of human placenta: an overview. Reprod Biomed Online 2016;32(1):14−43.

[132] Patisaul HB, Jefferson W. The pros and cons of phytoestrogens. Front Neuroendocrinol 2010;31(4):400–19.
[133] Beaton LK, McVeigh BL, Dillingham BL, Lampe JW, Duncan AM. Soy protein isolates of varying isoflavone content do not adversely affect semen quality in healthy young men. Fertil Steril 2010;94(5):1717–22.
[134] Huang H, Li L, Wang Y, Tang LY, Wang CC, Leung LK. Genistein upregulates placental corticotropin-releasing hormone expression in lipopolysaccharide-sensitized mice. Placenta 2011;32(10):757–62.
[135] Meena R, Supriya C, Pratap Reddy K, Sreenivasula Reddy P. Altered spermatogenesis, steroidogenesis and suppressed fertility in adult male rats exposed to genistein, a non-steroidal phytoestrogen during embryonic development. Food Chem Toxicol : An Int J Pub British Indus Biol Res Associ 2017;99:70–7.
[136] Lehraiki A, Chamaillard C, Krust A, Habert R, Levacher C. Genistein impairs early testosterone production in fetal mouse testis via estrogen receptor alpha. Toxicol Vitro : An Int J Pub Assoc BIBRA 2011;25(8):1542–7.
[137] El Sheikh Saad H, Meduri G, Phrakonkham P, Berges R, Vacher S, Djallali M, et al. Abnormal peripubertal development of the rat mammary gland following exposure in utero and during lactation to a mixture of genistein and the food contaminant vinclozolin. Reprod Toxicol 2011;32(1):15–25.
[138] Lofamia EA, Ramos GB, Mamon MA, Salido FM, Su GS, de Vera MP. Isoflavone maternal-supplemetation during periconception period: inflence on the reproductive organs of the first generation (F1) murine weanling-stage offspring. Asian Pacific J Reprod 2014;3(4):268–74.
[139] Talsness C, Grote K, Kuriyama S, Presibella K, Sterner-Kock A, Poca K, et al. Prenatal exposure to the phytoestrogen daidzein resulted in persistent changes in ovarian surface epithelial cell height, folliculogenesis, and estrus phase length in adult Sprague-Dawley rat offspring. J Toxicol Environ Health Part A 2015;78(10):635–44.
[140] Richter DU, Mylonas I, Toth B, Scholz C, Briese V, Friese K, et al. Effects of phytoestrogens genistein and daidzein on progesterone and estrogen (estradiol) production of human term trophoblast cells in vitro. Gynecol Endocrinol : The Offici J Int Soci Gynecol Endocrinol 2009;25(1):32–8.
[141] Carmichael SL, Cogswell ME, Ma C, Gonzalez-Feliciano A, Olney RS, Correa A, et al. Hypospadias and maternal intake of phytoestrogens. Am J Epidemiol 2013;178(3):434–40.
[142] Akre O, Boyd HA, Ahlgren M, Wilbrand K, Westergaard T, Hjalgrim H, et al. Maternal and gestational risk factors for hypospadias. Environ Health Perspect 2008;116(8):1071–6.
[143] Pistollato F, Sumalla Cano S, Elio I, Masias Vergara M, Giampieri F, Battino M. Plant-based and plant-rich diet patterns during gestation: beneficial effects and possible shortcomings. Advanc nutr 2015;6(5):581–91.
[144] Cederroth CR, Zimmermann C, Nef S. Soy, phytoestrogens and their impact on reproductive health. Mol Cell Endocrinol 2012;355(2):192–200.
[145] Ganss R. Maternal metabolism and vascular adaptation in pregnancy: the PPAR link. Trends Endocrinol Metabol: TEM (Trends Endocrinol Metab) 2017;28(1):73–84.
[146] Pereira RD, De Long NE, Wang RC, Yazdi FT, Holloway AC, Raha S. Angiogenesis in the placenta: the role of reactive oxygen species signaling. BioMed Res Int 2015:814543. 2015.
[147] Shah DA, Khalil RA. Bioactive factors in uteroplacental and systemic circulation link placental ischemia to generalized vascular dysfunction in hypertensive pregnancy and preeclampsia. Biochem Pharmacol 2015;95(4):211–26.

[148] Li S, Zhu Y, Chavarro JE, Bao W, Tobias DK, Ley SH, et al. Healthful dietary patterns and the risk of hypertension among women with a history of gestational diabetes mellitus: aprospective cohort study. Hypertension 2016;67(6):1157–65.
[149] Diniz C, Suliburska J, Ferreira I. New insights into the antiangiogenic and proangiogenic properties of dietary polyphenols. Mol Nutr Food Res 2017;61(6).
[150] Ludovici V, Barthelmes J, Nagele MP, Enseleit F, Ferri C, Flammer AJ, et al. Cocoa, blood pressure, and vascular function. Front in nutr 2017;4:36.
[151] Panel EN. Scientific opinion on the substantiation of a health claim related to cocoa flavanols and maintenance of normal endothelium-dependent vasodilation pursuant to Article 13 (5) of Regulation (EC) No 1924/2006. EFSA J 2012;10:2809. https://doi.org/10.2903/j.efsa.2012.2809.
[152] Bubols GB, Zielinsky P, Piccoli Jr AL, Nicoloso LH, Vian I, Moro AM, et al. Nitric oxide and reactive species are modulated in the polyphenol-induced ductus arteriosus constriction in pregnant sheep. Prenat Diagn 2014;34(13):1268–76.
[153] Zielinsky P, Piccoli Jr AL, Vian I, Zilio AM, Naujorks AA, Nicoloso LH, et al. Maternal restriction of polyphenols and fetal ductal dynamics in normal pregnancy: an open clinical trial. Arq Bras Cardiol 2013;101(3):217–25.
[154] Vian I, Zielinsky P, Zilio AM, M.I.S., Brum C, Lampert KV, et al. Increase of prostaglandin E2 in the reversal of ductal constriction after polyphenol restriction. Ultrasound Obstet Gynecol : The Offici J Int Soci Ultraso Obstet Gynecol 2018;52(5):617–22.
[155] Richardson SI, Steffen LM, Swett K, Smith C, Burke L, Zhou X, et al. Dietary total isoflavone intake is associated with lower systolic blood pressure: the coronary artery risk development in young adults (CARDIA) study. J Clin Hypertens 2016;18(8):778–83.
[156] Fernandez AR, Omar SZ, Husain R. Role of genistein in preeclampsia: acase-control study. J Reprod Med 2016;61(1–2):47–51.
[157] Perez-Sepulveda A, Monteiro LJ, Dobierzewska A, Espana-Perrot PP, Venegas-Araneda P, Guzman-Rojas AM, et al. Placental aromatase is deficient in placental ischemia and preeclampsia. PloS One 2015;10(10). e0139682.
[158] Campbell MS, Fleenor BS. The emerging role of curcumin for improving vascular dysfunction: a review. Crit Rev Food Sci Nutr 2017:1–10.
[159] Gong P, Liu M, Hong G, Li Y, Xue P, Zheng M, et al. Curcumin improves LPS-induced preeclampsia-like phenotype in rat by inhibiting the TLR4 signaling pathway. Placenta 2016;41:45–52.
[160] Zhou J, Miao H, Li X, Hu Y, Sun H, Hou Y. Curcumin inhibits placental inflammation to ameliorate LPS-induced adverse pregnancy outcomes in mice via upregulation of phosphorylated Akt. Inflamm Res 2017;66(2):177–85.
[161] Carito V, Ceccanti M, Tarani L, Ferraguti G, Chaldakov GN, Fiore M. Neurotrophins' modulation by olive polyphenols. Curr Med Chem 2016;23(28):3189–97.
[162] Yazdy MM, Tinker SC, Mitchell AA, Demmer LA, Werler MM. Maternal tea consumption during early pregnancy and the risk of spina bifida. Birth Defects Res Part A, Clin and Molecul Teratol 2012;94(10):756–61.
[163] Wilde JJ, Petersen JR, Niswander L. Genetic, epigenetic, and environmental contributions to neural tube closure. Annu Rev Genet 2014;48:583–611.
[164] Cao L, Tan C, Meng F, Liu P, Reece EA, Zhao Z. Amelioration of intracellular stress and reduction of neural tube defects in embryos of diabetic mice by phytochemical quercetin. Sci Rep 2016;6:21491.
[165] Sun GY, Chen Z, Jasmer KJ, Chuang DY, Gu Z, Hannink M, et al. Quercetin attenuates inflammatory responses in BV-2 microglial cells: role of MAPKs on the Nrf2 pathway and induction of heme oxygenase-1. PloS One 2015;10(10). e0141509.

[166] Wu Y, Wang F, Reece EA, Yang P. Curcumin ameliorates high glucose-induced neural tube defects by suppressing cellular stress and apoptosis. Am J Obstet Gynecol 2015;212(6). 802 e1-8.
[167] Barenys M, Gassmann K, Baksmeier C, Heinz S, Reverte I, Schmuck M, et al. Epigallocatechin gallate (EGCG) inhibits adhesion and migration of neural progenitor cells in vitro. Arch Toxicol 2017;91(2):827–37.
[168] Simonyi A, Chen Z, Jiang J, Zong Y, Chuang DY, Gu Z, et al. Inhibition of microglial activation by elderberry extracts and its phenolic components. Life Sci 2015;128:30–8.
[169] Zheng A, Li H, Cao K, Xu J, Zou X, Li Y, et al. Maternal hydroxytyrosol administration improves neurogenesis and cognitive function in prenatally stressed offspring. J Nutr Biochem 2015;26(2):190–9.

CHAPTER 11

Maternal overnutrition and mitochondrial function

Marloes Dekker Nitert[1], Sue Maye Siow[2], Olivia Holland[2]
[1]School of Chemistry and Molecular Biosciences, The University of Queensland, St. Lucia, QLD, Australia; [2]School of Medical Science, Griffith University, Gold Coast Campus, Southport, QLD, Australia

Contents

Introduction

Overweight and obesity is on the rise worldwide in the adult population, and also in women of child-bearing age. Globally, the proportion of women of reproductive age who are overweight or obese is between 20% and 40%, but reaches as high as ~70% in parts of the Caribbean and the Middle East [1] (Fig. 11.1). Overweight and obesity are associated with

Molecular Nutrition
ISBN 978-0-12-813862-5
https://doi.org/10.1016/B978-0-12-813862-5.00011-6

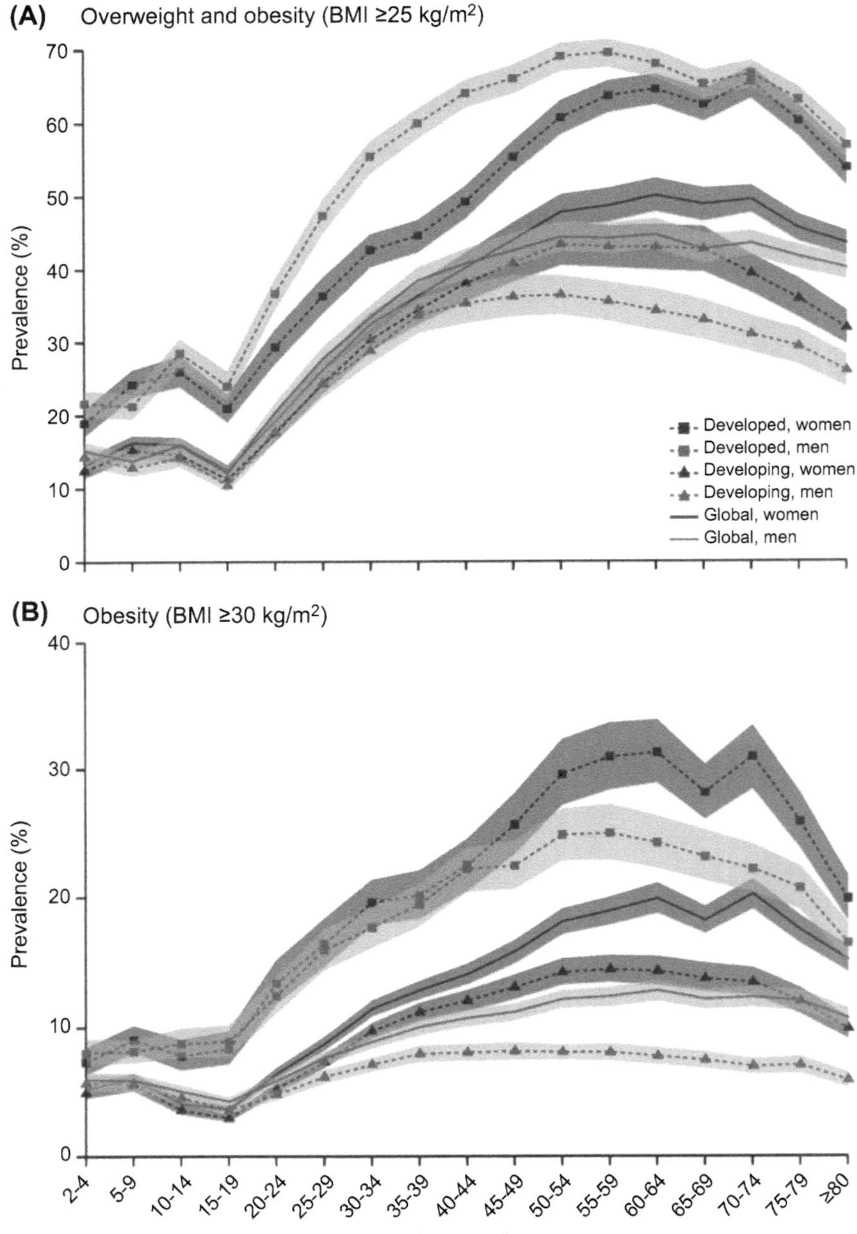

Figure 11.1 Prevalence of overweight and obesity and obesity alone in developed and developing countries, by age and sex, 2013. *BMI*, body mass index. *(Reproduced with permission from Ng M, Fleming T, Robinson M, Thomson B, Graetz N, Margono C, et al. Global, regional, and national prevalence of overweight and obesity in children and adults during 1980–2013: a systematic analysis for the Global Burden of Disease Study 2013. Lancet 2014;384(9945):766–81.)*

increased risk of pregnancy complications for the mother including gestational diabetes mellitus (GDM), preeclampsia, and instrumental delivery or delivery by Caesarean section [2]. For the fetus, maternal overweight is associated with a higher risk of being born large for gestational age and birth trauma. Maternal complications such as GDM and preeclampsia are also associated with adverse outcomes for the baby. The risk of adverse health effects do not end at birth, with increased risk of future metabolic and cardiovascular disease for both mother and offspring.

The increased risk of poor health that is associated with overweight and obesity is modified by factors such as ethnicity, age, genetic background, and physical activity. Weight gain during gestation can also contribute to the risk of developing pregnancy complications, since excessive gestational weight gain is associated with adverse outcomes for mother and baby [3]. Therefore, the prevention of pregnancy complications that are associated with maternal overnutrition is instrumental to reduce short-term and long-term poor health sequelae for mother and offspring. There are currently no highly successful strategies to prevent these complications: diet and physical activity interventions have had conflicting results. The successful trials usually are time- and labor-intensive, which limits their implementation into the wider community. In order to identify new targets for the prevention and/or treatment of pregnancy complications, a deeper understanding of the pathogenesis of these complications and how they are influenced by high adiposity is required.

In this chapter, we will focus on the metabolic changes in healthy pregnancy, and pregnancy affected by maternal overnutrition. We specifically explore the role of mitochondria in healthy pregnancy and pregnancy complications that are often associated with maternal overnutrition, e.g., GDM and preeclampsia. Mitochondria play a central role in the regulation of metabolism and redox state in cells and thereby are likely important both in the maintenance of healthy pregnancy and in pregnancy complications.

Part I mitochondrial function in healthy pregnancy

Mitochondria

Mitochondria are at the center of metabolic processes and are critical to cellular and organ function [4] Structurally, mitochondria consist of an encapsulating outer membrane, and an inner membrane folded into cristae that increase the surface area (Fig. 11.2A). The mitochondrial electron transport chain (ETC) functions to produce cellular energy through

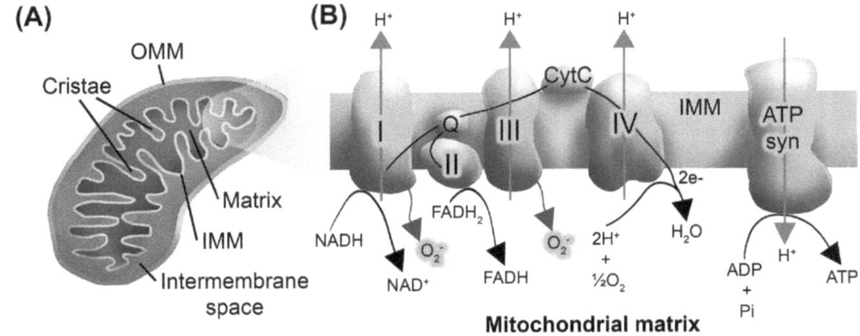

Figure 11.2 Mitochondrial structure and the electron transport chain. (A) Mitochondria have a double membrane structure, with an outer mitochondrial membrane (*OMM*) and an inner mitochondrial membrane (*IMM*). The IMM is folded into cristae that function to increase the internal surface area of the mitochondria also have structural roles. (B) The electron transport chain (*ETC*) is composed of complexes I to IV as well as coenzyme Q (*Q*) and cytochrome c (*CytC*). Reducing equivalents (nicotinamide adenine dinucleotide; NADH and flavin adenine dinucleotide; $FADH_2$) enter the ETC at complex I (*NADH*) or II (*$FADH_2$*) and are passed through the chain with oxygen as the final electron acceptor. The passage of electrons through the ETC leads to the passage of protons (*H^+*) into the intermembrane space and the establishment of an electrochemical gradient. This electrochemical gradient is used by ATP synthase (*ATP syn*) to generate adenosine triphosphate (*ATP*) from adenosine diphosphate (*ADP*) phosphate (*Pi*). Passage of electrons through the ETC also produces a variable amount of superoxide (O_2^-), a reactive oxygen species.

oxidation and reduction reactions (oxidative phosphorylation, or OXPHOS) and is found on the inner mitochondrial membrane (IMM). The ETC is a multiprotein system composed of four respiratory chain complexes (CI—CIV) that oxidize reducing equivalents fed into the ETC from the tricarboxylic acid cycle (TCA) and other sources, with oxygen as the last acceptor of electrons. The final part of the ETC is adenosine triphosphate (ATP) synthase (sometimes referred to as complex V), which uses the proton gradient created by the other complexes to generate ATP, the main source of cellular energy (Fig. 11.2B) [5]. In addition to energy generation, mitochondria have many other critical functions and are vital in intracellular signaling and metabolism. Cells can respond to metabolic challenges by altering the mitochondrial content, morphology, and substrate use. A large amount of evidence places mitochondria as central to the regulation of the cell's response to stress, and mitochondria have important roles in both cell death and survival [4].

Mitochondrial energetic functions involve the management of vast amounts of oxygen, as well as coping with the potentially damaging

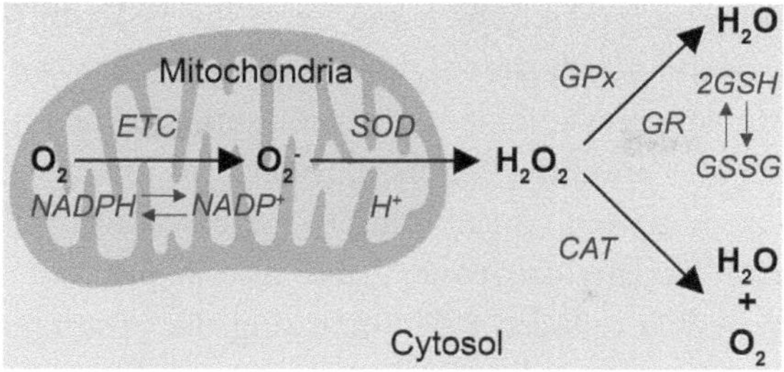

Figure 11.3 Reactive oxygen species generation and elimination. The mitochondrial electron transport chain (*ETC*) can generate the reactive oxygen species superoxide (O_2^-). Superoxide dismutases (*SODs*) are a group of antioxidants found in both mitochondria and the cytosol that convert superoxide into another reactive oxygen species, hydrogen peroxide (H_2O_2), which can then be further processed by antioxidant systems such as catalase (*CAT*) or glutathione peroxidase (GPx). *GR*, glutathione reductase; *GSH*, glutathione; *GSSH*, glutathione disulfide; *NADP*$^+$, nicotinamide adenine dinucleotide phosphate.

reactive oxygen species (ROS) produced as by-products of the ETC (Fig. 11.2B). These ROS are crucial in cellular signaling, influencing numerous systems including energy metabolism, stress response, redox balance, and cell migration/adhesion. ROS can also cause damage through the oxidation of proteins and lipids, and mitochondrial depolarization (the breakdown of the mitochondrial proton gradient). ROS levels are balanced by antioxidant networks, which scavenge and process ROS into less damaging or non-harmful products (Fig. 11.3, see also sections on skeletal muscle function in pregnancy; liver function in GDM and placental function in preeclampsia). However, an imbalance of ROS production and the antioxidants that counter them can lead to dysfunction. Mitochondrial dysfunction and the oxidative stress that occurs with excessive ROS production are associated with many pathophysiological conditions, including during pregnancy. Pregnancy itself is characterized by low grade oxidative stress, which is increased in many gestational complications [6,7].

Metabolic changes during pregnancy

Metabolism in early pregnancy is characterized by an increase in anabolic processes, leading to increased fat storage, which may serve as an energy supply in late pregnancy. This results in more visceral fat accumulation in pregnancy [8]. In late pregnancy, metabolism undergoes a shift toward catabolic processes with maternal metabolism deriving energy from lipid metabolism, reducing maternal lipid stores [9] and thereby enabling fetal growth to be driven by glucose. This shift is associated with a large increase in maternal insulin resistance, which can be in the order of 50% [10]. The maternal insulin resistance creates a glucose gradient between maternal and fetal blood that guarantees sufficient glucose supply to the fetus (Fig. 11.4). In addition, hepatic insulin resistance results in increased endogenous hepatic glucose production, contributing to increased availability of glucose for fetal growth. In late pregnancy, the insulin-induced repression of whole-body lipolysis is reduced [11], increasing the postprandial excursion in free fatty acids [12]. These free fatty acids are mainly used by the mother to fulfill her energy requirements with a smaller proportion of the free fatty acids transported to the fetus.

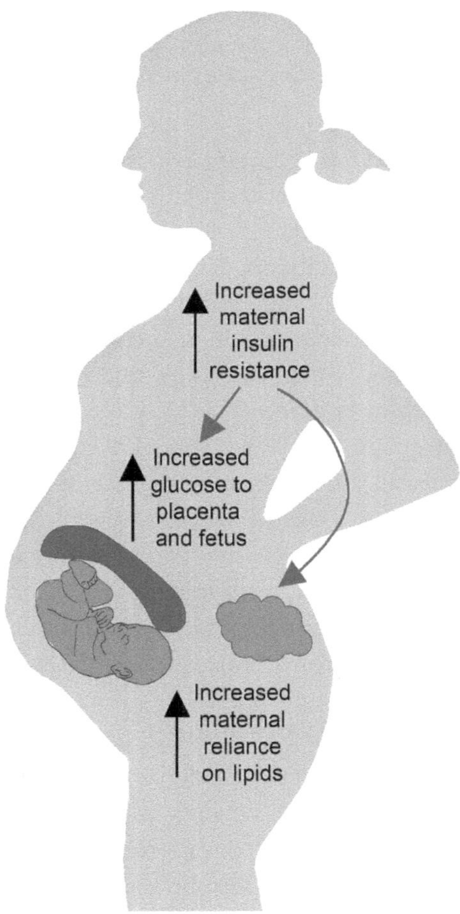

Figure 11.4 Metabolic changes during late pregnancy. In late pregnancy, maternal systems utilize more fatty acid/lipids as a fuel source. This, and increased maternal insulin resistance, leads to adequate glucose being supplied to the placental/fetal unit.

Maternal fasting blood glucose levels usually decrease slightly in pregnancy which is caused partially by the increase in blood volume, partially by increased utilization, and partially by reduced overall endogenous glucose production [13]. Maternal circulating glucose levels are not only determined by maternal factors but also appear to be regulated by fetal sex. In early pregnancy, women carrying a male fetus have higher insulin secretion as measured by the homeostatic model assessment of beta cell function (HOMA-B) index [14]. At the beginning of the third trimester, fasting blood glucose levels are slightly higher in women carrying a male fetus than in women carrying a female fetus [15]. In one study, higher maternal blood glucose values were seen throughout the oral glucose tolerance test in women carrying a male fetus, whereas in another study, the differences were restricted to the fasting glucose values [15,16]. Additionally, the initial insulin peak (first-phase insulin response) is lower in women carrying a male fetus as is the HOMA-B index [14,15]. However, no differences in postprandial insulin responses or the index of homeostatic model assessment of insulin resistance (HOMA-IR) were observed between women carrying male and female infants. It is unclear how the sex of the fetus affects maternal glucose concentrations but the placenta, which is fetal in origin, may differentially secrete hormones affecting maternal glucose control.

The importance of insulin resistance for adequate fetal growth becomes apparent in women with unexplained fetal growth retardation, e.g., fetal growth retardations that are not associated with genetic or placental dysfunction, who are less insulin resistant than their counterparts with normal weight infants [17]. In addition to lower insulin resistance, women with unexplained fetal growth retardation also show higher beta-cell function, which may further contribute to the growth retardation of the baby [18]. Therefore, in healthy pregnancy, a delicate balance between sufficient but not excessive insulin resistance needs to be maintained in the presence of sufficient beta cell reserve to increase insulin secretion in response to the physiological increase in insulin resistance. We will now discuss changes to metabolism and mitochondrial function in the most important organs regulating maternal metabolism in pregnancy: pancreatic beta cells, skeletal muscle, adipose tissue, liver, and the placenta.

Pancreatic beta cells

Beta cell mass. Insulin secretion from the pancreatic beta cells safeguards maternal glucose supply in the setting of the physiological insulin resistance of pregnancy by increasing insulin release in response to meals.

Increased insulin supply can arise from either an increase in the absolute number of pancreatic beta cells or from an increase in the amount of insulin released by each beta cell or a combination thereof. In rodents, pancreatic beta cell mass in dams expands mainly by mitosis from existing beta cells in response to the release of lactogens from the pituitary and placenta in pregnancy [19]. It is less clear what happens in human pregnancy, given the lack of data on beta cell mass at different time points in pregnancy for obvious practical and ethical reasons. Studies of the effects of lactogen stimulation on isolated human pancreatic beta cells have yielded conflicting results with some studies reporting similar increases in proliferation as in rodent beta cells, whereas others have not [19].

Insulin secretion. Basal insulin secretion, e.g., insulin release during fasting or between meals, is lower in pregnancy, with the majority of the glucose taken up by the maternal brain, the placenta, and the fetus [20]. In response to a meal, the amount of insulin secreted is increased as compared with the nonpregnant state, especially the first-phase insulin response [21]. The lactogens secreted by the placenta elicit serotonin signaling in the beta cells which not only potentially affects proliferation but also affects insulin secretion [19]. Lactogens increase the production of serotonin. Binding of serotonin to the Htra3 receptor, which is a cationic ion channel, causes an influx of Na^+ ions into the mouse beta cell, resulting in plasma membrane depolarization and thereby lowering the threshold for the closing of K_{ATP} channels in response to ATP released from the mitochondria after metabolism of glucose [19]. In addition, greater intercellular coupling between beta cells allows for electrical coupling of pancreatic beta cells, increasing insulin secretion in response to glucose [19]. Insulin secretion in pregnancy is also regulated through higher expression and activity of glucokinase, which catalyzes the rate-limiting first step of glycolysis in pancreatic beta cells and in the liver. In addition, increases in cyclic AMP (cAMP) levels are seen; cAMP serves as an important second messenger that can result in increased insulin secretion. Higher levels of some of the proteins that are critically important in the docking of insulin granules to the plasma membrane, the SNARE proteins, have also been reported [22]. A larger number of docked insulin granules could result in the increased first-phase insulin response reported in pregnancy.

Effects of fetal sex. The difference in maternal fasting glucose levels between women carrying a male versus female fetus suggests that there is a difference in pancreatic beta-cell sensitivity rather than insulin resistance. Indeed, there is some evidence to suggest that while measures of insulin resistance are similar between women carrying a male versus female fetus, those carrying a female fetus have better beta cell function at the start of the third trimester of pregnancy [16]. This could potentially be due to differential hormone secretion by the placenta, although not of leptin, since leptin signaling inhibits insulin secretion from pancreatic beta cells [23].

Skeletal muscle cells

In healthy individuals, almost all (90%) insulin-dependent glucose uptake from the circulation occurs in skeletal muscle. Therefore, insulin resistance in skeletal muscle cells, which is ubiquitous in pregnancy, is critically important for ensuring sufficient glucose supply to the fetus. The insulin resistance in skeletal muscle occurs through reduced signaling through the insulin receptor pathway [24], this likely results in reduced transport of the GLUT4 glucose transporter to the plasma membrane on the skeletal muscle cell or reduced activity of the GLUT4 transporters thereby reducing glucose uptake from the circulation. Outside pregnancy, insulin resistance in skeletal muscle is characterized by increased oxidative stress and decreased mitochondrial metabolism. Oxidative stress results from mitochondrial production of ROS (Fig. 11.2B), often in situations where the energy supply exceeds mitochondrial capacity (e.g., in obesity) [25]. Oxidative stress can be counteracted by antioxidant enzymes (Fig. 11.3) but if it exceeds antioxidant capacity, it can cause cellular damage [26].

Adipose tissue

Insulin resistance. White adipocytes are critical in regulating whole-body lipid metabolism. In adipocytes, insulin suppresses lipolysis through activation of phosphodiesterases which inhibit the action of the intracellular lipase, hormone-sensitive lipase. The physiological rise in insulin resistance in healthy pregnancy reduces the inhibition of hormone-sensitive lipase contributing to the increased release of free fatty acids into the circulation. However, in healthy pregnancy, the exact mechanisms behind insulin resistance in adipose tissue are not entirely clear. The mechanisms may depend on the location and type of the fat depot. For subcutaneous adipose tissue, there appear to be no changes to the gene and protein expression of insulin signaling proteins, which could suggest that any insulin resistance in subcutaneous fat is due to altered protein activity [12]. In contrast, in omental (visceral) adipocytes, downregulation of insulin receptor substrate-1 (IRS-1) has been reported [27]. These differences may represent differences in the response to pregnancy between subcutaneous and visceral adipose tissue.

Fatty acid uptake. In pregnancy, transport of the fatty acid translocase/CD36 was increased on the surface of epicardial white adipocytes of mice compared to that in virgin female mice [28]. However, in humans, CD36 expression was actually decreased in white adipocytes from visceral fat in pregnancy [27], indicating that the expression may be different for different fat deposition sites, pregnancy stage (not specified in the murine study) or species. Nevertheless, altered CD36 expression may reflect the greater flux in lipids during pregnancy and/or the greater maternal reliance on fat metabolism. It may also reflect the higher circulating insulin levels since insulin and obesity are known to stimulate CD36 gene expression and transport to the plasma membrane [29], which increases fatty acid uptake outside pregnancy.

Mitochondrial function. In addition to changes to the insulin signaling pathway, it is possible that altered mitochondrial function could play a role in conducing some of the changes to adipocyte metabolism. A recent study showed that in the mouse adipocyte, there are changes to the mitochondrial membrane potential of the cell in addition to changes to the phenotype of the mitochondria during pregnancy [28]. The changes again are dependent on the location and type of the fat depot with the membrane potential being less depolarized in brown adipocytes of pregnant dams compared with brown adipocytes of male mice. This may be a result of differential expression of the uncoupling proteins, which are highly expressed in brown adipocytes. In midpregnancy in rats (E13), brown adipocyte mitochondrial DNA (mtDNA) content is reduced and the mitochondrial proton gradient is more uncoupled than in nonpregnant rats, probably in response to an increase in estrogen and progesterone levels [30]. This would result in less energy being used for thermogenesis at a time where energy needs to preserved for the growth and development of the fetus.

Liver function

The liver is the main integrator of metabolism and its function is affected by changes in metabolism to other organs. In the third trimester of pregnancy, hepatic insulin resistance causes an increase in endogenous glucose production of up to 30% [10]. Late in pregnancy, the liver produces approximately 955 μmol glucose/min, and whole-body glycerol production (from lipolysis occurring in adipose tissue and the liver) is approximately 235 μmol glycerol/min [31]. The glycerol can be used to generate energy through entry into the TCA and oxidative phosphorylation; it can serve as a substrate for hepatic endogenous glucose production but can also bind to free fatty acids to form triglycerides. The production of glucose and glycerol are highly correlated even though only endogenous glucose production was correlated to maternal insulin concentrations (or insulin resistance) [31]. This indicates that maternal glycerol production likely is affected by other factors than the lack of repression by insulin alone. Indeed, the rates of glucose and glycerol production are strongly positively correlated with maternal weight, fat mass, and fat-free mass, as well as resting energy expenditure, but not with circulating glucose levels. This suggests that maternal fat mass may be an important determinant of the rates of glycerol and glucose production, which only partially can be explained by increased insulin resistance.

Hepatic glucose and glycerol production rates are also strongly positively correlated with estimated fetal weight, independently of maternal weight, fat mass, and measures of glucose control. This suggests that fetal growth in late pregnancy is not solely determined by maternal glucose availability but also by maternal lipid metabolism. In late pregnancy, the fetus accrues fat mass [32] and transport of glycerol and fatty acids over the placenta perhaps become more important over gestation.

Mitochondrial function in the liver in pregnancy has not been studied in great detail in humans. This is due to the difficulties of obtaining samples from this tissue. Animal models could be useful in this area but hepatic mitochondrial function in response to pregnancy is an underexplored area of research.

Placental metabolism and mitochondrial function

The placenta functions in the shift of maternal metabolism to a greater reliance on fatty acids as a fuel source (Fig. 11.4) through the secretion of leptin and adiponectin [33,34], and in altering maternal insulin resistance and beta cell function through the secretion of placental lactogen, prolactin, placental growth hormone, and adipokines [35,36]. Mitochondria in the placenta play an important role at all stages of pregnancy, with key functions in ATP production, steroidogenesis, regulation of apoptosis, interactions with other organelles, and regulation of protein folding [37–39].

Mitochondria of cytotrophoblasts and the syncytiotrophoblast. Two of the main functional cell types of the human placenta, the cytotrophoblasts and the syncytiotrophoblast, contain mitochondria with vastly different structures and functions (Fig. 11.5). Mononuclear cytotrophoblasts are the progenitor cells of the multinuclear syncytiotrophoblast, the outer layer of the human placenta. The mitochondria of cytotrophoblasts are classical in both structure and function, having typical lamellar cristae in an orthodox

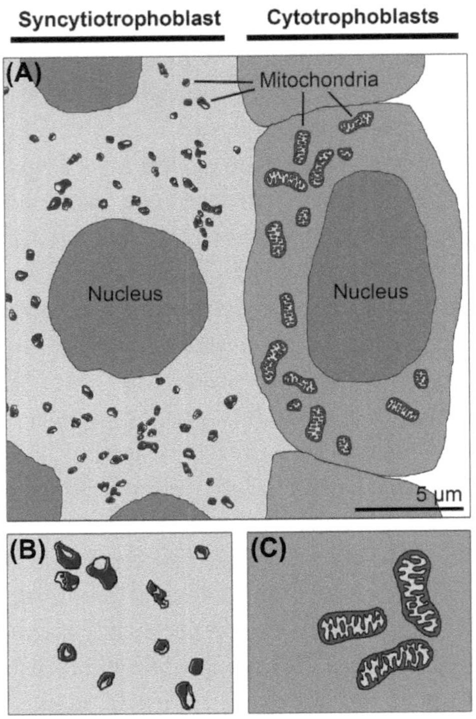

Figure 11.5 Syncytiotrophoblast and cytotrophoblast mitochondria. (A) Cartoon depicting general structural features of mitochondria from the syncytiotrophoblast and cytotrophoblasts. (B) Mitochondria with the syncytiotrophoblast are small and have a nonclassical vesicular cristae structure and dense matrix. (C) Mitochondria with cytotrophoblasts are relatively larger than syncytiotrophoblast mitochondria and have a more typical cristae structure. *(Reproduced with permission from Holland O, Dekker Nitert M, Gallo LA, Vejzovic M, Fisher JJ, Perkins AV. Review: placental mitochondrial function and structure in gestational disorders. Placenta 2016.)*

configuration and functioning primarily in ATP generation [37]. In contrast, the mitochondria of the syncytiotrophoblast are smaller and lose their lamellar cristae configuration when differentiating from cytotrophoblasts. Instead, syncytiotrophoblast mitochondria have heterogeneous, vesicular cristae that are thought to aid in one of the major functions of the placenta, steroid production [40]. The syncytiotrophoblast plays a large role in steroidogenesis; progesterone is a key hormone that maintains pregnancy and is produced by the mitochondria of the syncytiotrophoblast, taking over from the maternal corpus luteum from the end of the first trimester [41]. Syncytiotrophoblast mitochondria have an abundance of the cholesterol side-chain cleavage enzyme (P450scc), which is present only in negligible amounts in the mitochondria of cytotrophoblasts[42]. Syncytiotrophoblast mitochondria synthesize pregnenolone from cholesterol via the P450scc enzyme system [37,41]. Similar to the mitochondrial ETC (Fig. 11.2B), normal functioning of P450scc can also generate ROS in the form of the superoxide anion, a highly reactive free radical. ROS such as superoxide contribute to apoptosis that is important for normal placental development, but may also be involved in the pathophysiology of pregnancy-related diseases when produced in excess [40]. The presence of 3β—OH—steroid-dehydrogenase-Δ5-6isomerase (3HSD) in the inner membrane of the mitochondria allows the conversion of pregnenolone synthesized by P450scc to progesterone [37]. This system differs to steroidogenesis in other tissues such as the adrenal glands, where steroidogenic acute regulatory protein (StAR) activity plays a key role in production of pregnenolone from cholesterol [43]. As placental mitochondria do not possess StAR, synthesis of pregnenolone is thought to occur at a slower rate than in other steroidogenic tissues, and the unusual structure of syncytiotrophoblast may aid in the diffusion of cholesterol to the IMM [41,42].

Apoptosis. In the placenta, apoptotic processes may be important for normal turnover of villous trophoblasts; *i.e.*, the differentiation of cytotrophoblasts and the formation then shedding of the syncytiotrophoblast [44—46]. Mitochondria are key mediators in regulating apoptosis, with proapoptotic structural changes including the mitochondrial outer membrane permeabilization pore (MOMP), cristae remodeling, and mitochondrial fission, as well as antiapoptotic-related process such as mitochondrial fusion, and B-cell lymphoma 2 (BCL2) or B-cell lymphoma extra-large (BCL-xL) recruitment [38,47]. The responses to stimuli such as ROS can trigger MOMP [48], which leads to the release of IMM proteins such as cytochrome c [47] that activate caspase 3, an end-stage signaling molecule in apoptosis [49]. Proapoptotic signaling may also be driven by the presence of ROS independent of these pathways [49]. This apoptotic cascade can be limited by the recruitment of BCL2 or BCL-xL from the cytoplasm to the mitochondria, which then functions to prevent the release of IMM proteins. In normal pregnancies, apoptosis appears to originate in cytotrophoblasts but is completed when the cell becomes part of the syncytiotrophoblast [50]. There is evidence that the initiation of the apoptotic cascade is important in the fusion of cytotrophoblasts into the syncytiotrophoblast, and also that mitochondria are involved in limiting the full progression of apoptosis, with increased levels of the mitochondrial-linked antiapoptotic members of the BCL2 family in the syncytiotrophoblast compared to cytotrophoblasts [45,51]. Further, BCL2 and another antiapoptotic protein, induced myeloid leukemia cell differentiation protein (MCL-1), have been reported to be reduced around syncytial knots [52,53]. BCL2 is expressed in cytoplasm of the syncytiotrophoblast throughout gestation but may be absent from nontrophoblast (i.e., mesenchymal and endothelial) placental cells [46,54]. Bcl2-associated X protein (BAX) is a proapoptotic member of the BCL2 family that is involved in the release of IMM proteins and loss of mitochondrial membrane potential. BAX has been reported to be expressed in first trimester cytotrophoblasts and third trimester syncytiotrophoblasts, and to be associated with areas of placental degradation [46].

Mitochondrial dynamics and interactions with the endoplasmic reticulum. Mitochondria exist in the reticular network that is in a constant state of flux via the opposing processes of mitochondrial fission and fusion, where fission functions to break apart the network and fusion to join mitochondria together. Fission is important for mitochondrial biogenesis and to isolate damaged mitochondria that can then be disposed of via autophagy, whereas fusion can salvage damaged mitochondria by joining them to more highly functioning parts of the reticular network [38,55,56]. Mitochondrial fusion is associated with increasing mitochondrial membrane potential, intracellular ATP levels, and oxygen consumption capacity. Fusion and fission are important for maintaining optimal mitochondrial function. Unregulated fission leads to an accumulation of dysfunctional cells, while unregulated fusion leads to a lack of coordination of mitochondrial function [57]. Several reports have demonstrated that trophoblasts possess the intracellular machinery required for mitochondrial fission and fusion, and that these proteins are important for placental function [58–61]. In mice, knockout of the mitofusins Mfn1 or Mfn2 is embryonically lethal at midgestation due to placental dysfunction, with evidence that each mitofusin has distinct roles in specific placental cell types [59]. In humans, decreased fusion/increased fission is associated with preeclampsia and unexplained miscarriage [58,60], but little is currently known about how fission and fusion function in the healthy placenta, or how these processes are regulated in the unique environment of the syncytiotrophoblast. However, mitochondrial fusion and fission regulators, in particular optic atrophy 1 (OPA1), have been linked to the remodeling and steroidogenic ability of mitochondria in syncytializing BeWo trophoblast-like cells [61]. Together, these results indicate that mitochondrial dynamics are likely to be central to many placental functions.

Mitochondria closely interact with other organelles, in particular the endoplasmic reticulum (ER), communicating via mitochondria-associated ER membranes to regulate numerous functions including mitochondrial fusion and fission, calcium (Ca^{2+}) transfer, and autophagy [39,62]. The syncytiotrophoblast possesses large amounts of ER, which is the site of protein synthesis and processing [39]. The regulation of protein folding is potentially also mediated by the mitochondria in the placenta [39]. The unfolded protein response (UPR) is a regulatory response to disruptions to the homeostasis of ER function and is activated when misfolded proteins accumulate in the lumen [63]. A similar UPR pathway appears to exist in the mitochondria, where the presence of abnormal proteins triggers a signal to be transmitted to the nucleus resulting in the expression of genes encoding specific proteases to remove the proteins and restore homeostasis [39]. The UPR is important during placental development and the activation of UPR signaling pathways has been shown to be altered in preeclampsia [64]. Interactions of the ER and mitochondria also play a role in autophagy as a protective mechanism against syncytiotrophoblast senescence, which may be triggered by increased stress arising from increased fetal nutritional demands exceeding maternal perfusion [39,62]. Additionally, trophoblastic autophagy is important in normal pregnancy, being higher in the low oxygen conditions that characterize early pregnancy and also potentially functioning in trophoblast invasion of the uterus in the establishment of the placenta [65,66].

Part II mitochondrial function in obesity and gestational diabetes mellitus

Overall metabolic changes in women with overweight and/or GDM

Overweight and obese women often have preexisting insulin resistance which is exacerbated by the physiological increase in insulin resistance in pregnancy. In GDM, insulin's ability to repress whole-body lipolysis is reduced further than in healthy pregnancy, which leads to even larger excursions in free fatty acids postprandially [12,67] (Fig. 11.6). Higher circulating free fatty acid levels could affect whole-body metabolism through increasing gluconeogenesis in the liver, reducing insulin secretion from pancreatic beta cells, and further increasing insulin resistance. Larger adipose tissue mass leads to low level inflammation outside pregnancy.

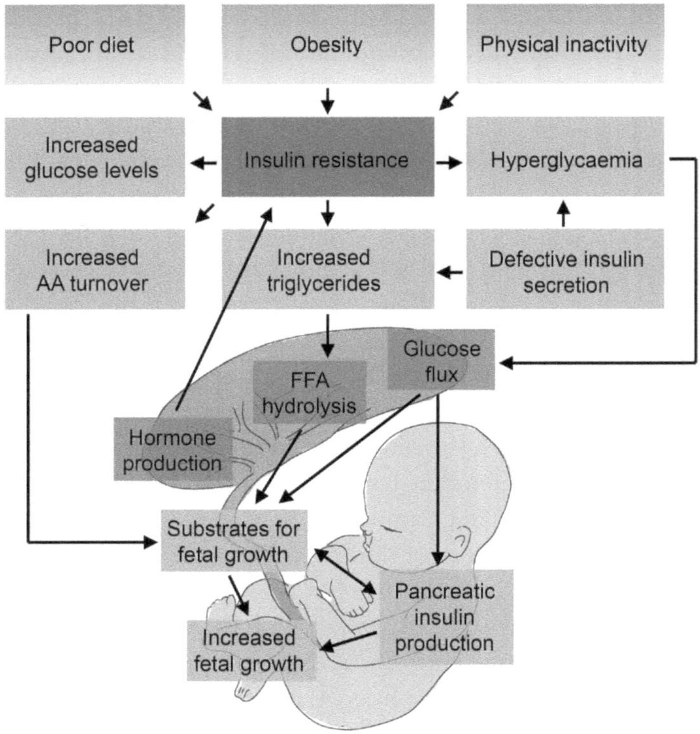

Figure 11.6 Overview of changes in metabolism in pregnancy affected by gestational diabetes mellitus. *AA*, amino acids; *FFA*, free fatty acids.

In overweight and obese pregnant women with or without GDM, levels of proinflammatory cytokines are higher in the circulation than in healthy pregnant women [68]. In monocytes and macrophages of obese women with GDM, mitochondrial size is increased compared with those of lean controls and ROS production is almost doubled [69], which may cause the release of proinflammatory cytokines by these cells. Proinflammatory cytokines are known to increase insulin resistance in GDM.

Carrying a male infant is associated with higher risk of developing GDM and is independent of other risk factors [16]. It is unclear if this is due to differences in sex hormone changes as compared to female infants or other factors, but it is likely to have similar causes to the higher blood glucose levels in mothers carrying a male fetus in healthy pregnancy. We will now discuss the metabolic and mitochondrial changes in metabolic target organs in obesity and GDM.

Pancreatic beta cells

Pancreatic beta cell function (and perhaps mass) increases markedly during pregnancy. Pancreatic beta cell function is an important determinant of circulating glucose levels throughout the day in obese, nondiabetic, African-American pregnant women [70]. BMI is positively associated with postprandial glucose concentrations independent of the carbohydrate content of the meal but this is partially due to lower insulin secretion in more obese women [70]. In fact, compared to lean, normoglycemic women, obese women display reduced capacity to upregulate insulin secretion from pancreatic beta cells throughout gestation [71]. Lower insulin secretion could be due to beta cell exhaustion in the face of continuously higher glucose and lipid levels in the circulation (glucolipotoxicity). High fat intake is associated with higher glucose levels supporting the hypothesis that hyperlipidemia may reduce insulin secretion [70]. Alternatively, an inhibitory effect on insulin secretion could be due to high leptin levels [72]; obese pregnant women have very high circulating leptin levels [73]. In obese women who develop GDM, circulating insulin levels are much increased in late pregnancy compared to overweight/obese normoglycemic controls [71], indicating that the difference may not be due to lower insulin secretion but rather insulin sensitivity. Lower insulin sensitivity would reduce glucose clearance from the circulation by skeletal muscle and adipose tissue. It may be further exacerbated by the relative lack of inhibition of endogenous hepatic glucose production in women with GDM [71], which would further increase circulating glucose levels.

Skeletal muscle

In women with GDM, insulin resistance is increased, and the late pregnancy shift to maternal lipid metabolism is less pronounced [71]. Skeletal muscle tissue plays an important role in determining circulating glucose concentrations. In skeletal muscle of obese pregnant women, decreased activity of mitochondrial complex II and coupled complex II+III has been reported, and this is independent of GDM and of mitochondrial protein content [74]. This may result in less efficient mitochondrial function and thus higher levels of oxidative stress. Indeed, in obese pregnant women, the levels of oxidative stress in skeletal muscle tissue are higher than those of lean women [74]. This is likely due to decreased activity of antioxidant proteins including manganese superoxide dismutase (MnSOD) and catalase [74]. Obese women with GDM tend to have lower mtDNA content in skeletal muscle than matched normoglycemic women, even though the expression of activators of mitochondrial biogenesis is similar [75]. In these women, oxidative phosphorylation is reduced in skeletal muscle as compared with obese women without GDM: this is due to lower expression of several proteins in complex I (NDUFV2; NDUFS3; and NDUFS8) of the ETC [75]. In addition to changes in protein amounts, the enzyme activity of complex I and III is significantly reduced in skeletal muscle of women with GDM, with a trend to lower complex IV activity [75]. This suggests that mitochondrial function is impacted in skeletal muscle by GDM independent of any effect of obesity. In addition, calcium signaling in skeletal muscle cells is altered in obese women with GDM [75]. Disruptions in calcium signaling are associated with cellular and mitochondrial stress, which is thought to be increased in women with GDM. High intracellular calcium levels may inhibit phosphorylation of the cellular energy marker protein AMPK. Phosphorylation levels of AMPK are also lower in skeletal muscle of obese women with GDM [75]. Together, this suggests that many aspects of skeletal muscle metabolism are affected by GDM. Lipid metabolism in skeletal muscle is one of the affected functions in GDM. The abundance of the fatty acid transporter CD36 was higher in skeletal muscle samples from obese women with GDM as compared with obese women with normal glucose tolerance [75]. This may result from higher levels of insulin resistance in obese women with GDM, given that insulin stimulates CD36 expression, and could also be in response to higher circulating lipid levels in women with GDM [76].

Adipose tissue

The main lipid storage site in pregnancy has been hypothesized to be different in obese women: shifting from predominantly lower-body fat tissue to more central storage [77]. This may be due to the lower-body fat depots already being replete in obesity, making the central fat depot the obvious choice for storage in pregnancy. Lower-body fat stores are more insulin-sensitive than central fat stores. In white adipose tissue of women with GDM, there are changes to the expression of mediators of insulin signaling. Expression of IRS-1, PPARγ, and lipoprotein lipase as well as the mitochondrial uncoupling protein 2 (UCP2) is reduced and this may give rise to greater insulin resistance in adipocytes which may contribute to the lower suppression of lipolysis in GDM [12]. While it can function as an uncoupling protein, UCP2 can also act as a regulator of ATP synthesis and

ROS, as well as stimulate free fatty acid uptake in adipocytes [78]. Reduced UCP2 expression in GDM could thus contribute to the increase in circulating free fatty acid levels observed in GDM [79]. It could also be a factor in the increase in oxidative stress that is a hallmark of adipose tissue in obesity and diabetes.

Liver

Given its role as a metabolic integrator, the increased dyslipidemia observed in obese pregnancy with or without GDM leads to higher concentrations of fatty acids in the circulation [80]. These fatty acids are thus available for incorporation into triglycerides in the liver (and in adipocytes). In the liver, fatty acids can also be incorporated in cholesterol particles especially VLDL lipoproteins. The proportion of lipids carried as triglycerides in VLDL, IDL, small LDL, and small and medium HDL cholesterol particles is indeed higher in women with GDM compared to lean non-GDM women [80].

In women with GDM, circulating levels of gamma-glutamyl transferase (GGT), which is a marker of liver damage, are increased [80]. In healthy pregnancy, GGT levels decrease or do not change [81]. GGT transfers a glutamyl residue from glutathione to an acceptor molecule such as amino acids or peptides, yielding cysteinyl glycine. GGT often serves to take apart glutathione at the plasma membrane to transport the amino acids across the plasma membrane and reconstitute glutathione intracellularly [81]. Glutathione serves as an antioxidant and when oxidative stress increases and the requirement for antioxidants rises (Fig. 11.3). The increased levels of GGT in women with GDM may therefore be a result of higher oxidative stress in the liver [81]. However, glutathione and GGT action can also cause the production of ROS in the extracellular space, especially when iron and copper are available [81], thereby potentially worsening the oxidative damage in women with GDM.

Placenta

The mitochondria in the placentas of women with GDM are often swollen with ridge deprivation and vacuolization [82]. In obesity, placental mitochondrial function is decreased [83]. In women with GDM who required pharmacological treatment, placental trophoblast expression of complexes I, II, III, and IV are reduced, whereas in those with GDM treated with diet only (*e.g.*, less severe GDM), the expression is not different from normoglycemic, BMI-matched controls [84]. The reduction in expression of complexes in the ETC is associated with lower placental levels of the mitochondrial biogenesis coactivator PGC1α [84]. In diet-treated GDM, similar reductions in PGC1α can be observed [84], indicating that some placental mitochondrial dysfunction is common to all forms of GDM. In the trophoblasts of women with GDM requiring pharmacological intervention, the likely reduction in energy production caused by reduced expression of proteins involved in oxidative phosphorylation may be compensated for by increased expression of regulatory enzymes of the glycolytic pathway including hexokinase, phosphofructokinase, and lactate dehydrogenase [84]. This may be due to the coordinated effect of reduced miR-143 expression on the activation of glycolytic and mitochondrial gene expression in trophoblasts of placentas of women affected by GDM who require pharmacological treatment for glucose control [84].

Increases in mitochondrial DNA (mtDNA) are associated with increased placental DNA oxidative stress [85], which itself is associated with pregnancy complications. In maternal obesity, placental mtDNA content is reduced, with lower activity of complex I and II but not of the other complexes as well as higher ROS formation [86]. However, placental mtDNA quantity does not seem to be affected by GDM compared with BMI-matched controls [85], whereas in type 1 diabetes, complex I and III activity is reduced in placenta, and ROS formation is increased; and in type 2 diabetes, there is decreased activity of complex II and III but no difference in ROS formation [86]. These results indicate that mitochondrial function in the placenta is often decreased by maternal metabolic perturbations, but that the mechanism behind the decrease is specific to the underlying condition.

The placenta can metabolize fatty acids through fatty acid oxidation. In the placenta of women with GDM, triglyceride content is increased and fatty acid oxidation is decreased compared with women of similar BMIs [87]. However, this is not due to a reduction in the number of mitochondria present but rather seems to result from glucose-related inhibition of carnitine palmitoyltransferase I (CPT I) activity, which is the mitochondrial enzyme that enables the transport of a fatty acid into the mitochondrion for beta-oxidation by adding an acyl group to a fatty acid to improve solubility. Reduced CPT I activity thus inhibits fatty acid oxidation and therefore activates storage of lipid in the form of triglycerides instead [87]. The high levels of triglyceride storage in the placenta in GDM may elicit the release of inflammatory cytokines and thus alter placental function.

Effects on offspring

Maternal obesity and GDM have long-term consequences for the metabolic health of the offspring. In lymphocytes obtained from umbilical cord blood of offspring of women with GDM, there is increased phosphorylation of pyruvate dehydrogenase, the enzyme catalyzing the conversion of pyruvate to acetyl-CoA in the mitochondrion [88]. Phosphorylation inhibits the function of pyruvate dehydrogenase. In a mouse model of diabetes in pregnancy, the offspring displays increased hepatic phosphorylation of pyruvate dehydrogenase and impaired glucose tolerance [88]. This suggests that aberrant mitochondrial function may not be limited to the mother but also affect the fetus/offspring.

In mice, offspring of dams fed a high fat diet during pregnancy show increased epididymal fat mass, and this is exacerbated in those individuals also fed a high fat diet after weaning [89]. However, heart morphology and function in the offspring does not seem to be affected by maternal high fat feeding but only by high fat feeding postweaning [89]. This extends to mitochondrial morphology and function, with only maternal and post-weaning high fat fed offspring showing damaged mitochondria with a lower mitochondrial membrane potential. However, given that mouse pups are born at the equivalent of the start of the third trimester of human pregnancy, it is possible that a high fat diet in humans during the relatively longer gestation would damage the cardiac mitochondria in offspring. In a rabbit model of maternal diabetes, maximal mitochondrial oxygen consumption in fetal brown adipocytes was significantly increased in those whose mothers had mild diabetes (comparable to GDM) but decreased in those whose mothers had severe diabetes (comparable to preexisting diabetes) [90]. The difference may be due to differences in insulin levels. The mildly diabetic rabbits did not show hyperinsulinemia, and the increased oxygen consumption may reflect increased lipolysis. The severely diabetic mothers, however, displayed hyperinsulinemia; this may have inhibited lipolysis in the brown adipocytes and thereby reduced oxygen consumption. It is also possible that mitochondrial ultrastructure or number was affected by the severe hyperglycemia and that this resulted in the decreased oxygen consumption [90].

Hepatic mtDNA copy number is reduced in the offspring of rat dams fed a high fat diet [91], and this may be tracked back to lower mtDNA copy numbers in oocytes from obese female rats, which could limit mtDNA copy number in all cells descending from the oocyte (*i.e.*, embryonic and placental). It is likely that mtDNA copy number would be similarly affected in other (metabolically active) tissues, which may result in a higher predisposition of the offspring to metabolic disease.

It is not clear if these changes observed in animal models are present in human offspring of mothers with obesity and/or GDM. Metabolic tissues are not readily accessible and the time frames for developing symptoms are quite extended. It is also unclear if the changes are associated with adverse metabolic outcomes in humans. These gaps in our knowledge can only be filled by prospective cohort studies.

Part III mitochondrial function in preeclampsia

Preeclampsia

Excessive caloric intake, as occurs with overnutrition, can cause mitochondrial dysfunction leading to effects on metabolism [92]. Excessive energy substrates can increase ROS production, causing cell damage, and ROS also reduce oxygen consumption and block fatty acid oxidation in adipocytes [93]. High levels of insulin resistance, such as those observed in overweight and obese women, are also associated with higher risk of developing preeclampsia. Preeclampsia is characterized by new-onset maternal hypertension, proteinuria, and endothelial cell dysfunction. These maternal symptoms are thought to be due to placental dysfunction secondary to poor placentation, especially in the early-onset (prior to 34 weeks gestation) severe form of preeclampsia. The shallow trophoblast invasion of the maternal uterine spiral arteries that is characteristic of early-onset preeclampsia is thought to lead to inadequate perfusion of the placenta, resulting in hypoxia-reoxygenation (H/R) injuries. H/R can cause increased ROS generation, primarily from the mitochondrial ETC (Fig. 11.2B) due to a lack of oxygen to accept electrons during the hypoxic period. Endogenous antioxidants counter ROS production (Fig. 11.3), but when their capacity is exceeded this results in oxidative stress [94]. Placental and maternal oxidative stress increases in preeclampsia, and this may lead to the release of mediators from the placenta that trigger a systemic inflammatory response affecting many maternal organs [95].

Placental dysfunction is central to preeclampsia, and placental mitochondrial dysfunction has been identified as potentially important in disease pathogenesis [96–98]. Preeclamptic placentae have increased lipid peroxidation and increased susceptibility to oxidation [99], and there is evidence of increased ETC activity correlated with the release of preeclampsia-associated antiangiogenic factors from the placenta [100]. Placental mitochondria from preeclamptic pregnancies show evidence of swelling, vacuolation, and a loss of cristae [95,101], as well as greater levels superoxide [99]. Structural changes, including less defined cristae and the presences of vacuoles, are also found in mitochondria in skeletal muscle of obese individuals, and may impair mitochondrial bioenergetic capacity [92,102]. Mitochondrial damage in the placenta, and associated effects on other organelles such as ER as well as the production of ROS, are likely to have a central role in metabolic changes that may drive disease progression. Dysfunction in placental mitochondria is often suggested to occur secondary to the primary etiology of preeclampsia, resulting from the insult of H/R caused by shallow trophoblast invasion of uterine vessels that supply the placenta. However, dysfunctional placental mitochondria could also be a primary cause of preeclampsia, as the placenta may be more prone to harboring mitochondria with defective genomes [103].

Antioxidants counter ROS production, and reduced antioxidant function is linked to oxidative stress. However, the relationship between antioxidants and ROS is complex, and ROS are important in cellular signaling and mitochondrial adaptations to environmental conditions. In preeclamptic placentae, the activity of the antioxidant enzymes superoxide dismutase (SOD), glutathione peroxidase (GPx), thioredoxin reductase, thioredoxin, and catalase has been observed to decrease [104,105], suggesting that dysfunction in these placentae may be linked to inadequate antioxidant response. However, an animal model of preeclampsia has shown protective effects from the inactivation of the antioxidant nuclear factor erythroid-derived 2-like 2 (Nrf2), and in humans, increased placental Nrf2 has been associated with preeclampsia and fetal growth restriction [106–108]. The increase in Nrf2 levels in these placentae suggests that ROS-mediated signaling may be important in the placental response to stress. Indeed, the placenta experiences large variations in oxygen levels over the course of normal gestation that have effects on placental mitochondrial function and antioxidant levels [109–111], and ROS signaling may be important in placental vasculature development [107]. Further, oxidative stress can influence the expression of angiogenesis transcription factors [107]. In the human placenta, increased Nrf2 also occurs in association with decreased expression of the angiogenic regulator vascular endothelial growth factor [112], and Nrf2 has been shown to regulate angiogenesis in response to ischemia in other tissue [113], although the role of this antioxidant system in preeclampsia itself is still unclear [108]. Further, the antioxidant protein peroxiredoxin III is increased in preeclampsia, and this may be another example of a protective response to oxidative stress [114]. The application of exogenous antioxidants in clinical trials for the treatment of preeclampsia has been generally unsuccessful [115,116], and this may in part be due to the complexities of ROS-mediated signaling and mitochondrial responses.

Mitochondria can adapt to environmental changes such as oxidative stress in several ways, and one key adaptive mechanism is changing the mitochondrial content of a cell, with both increases and decreases in mitochondrial content seen in response to stress. Placental mitochondrial content has been observed to be altered in preeclampsia, but there is no clear consensus on the effect of preeclampsia, with studies showing both increases and decreases, or no change [96]. Preeclampsia has a wide range of symptoms, and the variability in results may be due to different forms of the disorder. Indeed, mitochondrial content and fission/fusion processes have been shown to be differentially disrupted in early-onset (preeclampsia that develops before 34 weeks of gestation, often with more severe symptoms) versus late-onset preeclampsia, with increased markers of mitochondrial content and fission in early-onset preeclampsia [101].

In preeclampsia, placental mitochondria may also have changes to their substrate preferences; reduced fatty acid oxidation and lower levels of proteins regulating fatty acid oxidation have been observed in preeclampsia [98,117]. Further, increased levels of circulating free fatty acids have been reported in preeclampsia [104], and fetal fatty acid oxidation disorders are associated with an increased incidence of preeclampsia [118,119]. Elevated free fatty acids can lead to increased ROS and also affect mitochondria through the induction of proinflammatory cytokines [120–122]. High adiposity is a strong risk factor for the development of preeclampsia, and similar mitochondrial changes to those observed in preeclampsia are also found in overweight and obese pregnancies [123]. In placentae from obese women, there are also increases in the production of proinflammatory cytokines [121], which may damage mitochondria. There is evidence that in obese pregnancies, protective mechanisms may counter oxidative stress to a degree, but also that other free radicals (*i.e.*, reactive nitrogen species) are increased [124]. Therefore, excessive energy substrates can cause increased ROS production resulting in changes to mitochondrial energy substrate metabolism.

Most studies into preeclampsia have investigated whole placental tissue (largely made up of epithelial trophoblasts) or isolated primary trophoblasts. However, placental endothelial cells have also been shown to have increased oxidant production, lipid peroxidation, protein oxidation, and nitrative stress, as well as decreased activity of the antioxidants SOD and GPx, linked to markers of decreased mitochondrial function in preeclampsia [125]. This suggests that antioxidant systems in these cells are unable to cope with the production of ROS in preeclampsia, although, as seen with Nrf2 and peroxiredoxin III in trophoblasts [108,114], the additional protective mechanism of heat shock protein 70 (HSP70) recruitment to the mitochondria may help in the maintenance of mitochondrial integrity [125]. Further, mitochondrial-generated superoxide may be important in oxidative stress that occurs in the placenta and endothelial cells [99,126].

There is also evidence of changes in the preeclamptic uterus, with mitochondria of the myometrium showing evidence of damage in preeclampsia that may indicate a systemic metabolic disorder [127]. Additionally, maternal circulating factors show mitochondrial-related changes in preeclampsia; many factors are released from the placenta into the maternal circulation, and increased mtDNA copy number (a marker of mitochondrial content) in maternal serum has been associated with preeclampsia [128]. In maternal leukocytes from healthy pregnancies, mtDNA copy number was positively correlated with telomere length (a marker of cellular senescence), indicating a potential association between oxidative stress, cellular senescence, and mitochondrial dysfunction in pregnancy [129].

Conclusions

Metabolic changes in the mother are critically important for ensuring adequate nutrient supply to the fetus and the successful completion of a healthy pregnancy. With their central role in controlling cellular metabolism, mitochondria contribute to these changes in metabolically active organs during pregnancy. In maternal overnutrition, mitochondrial dysfunction is often already present prior to pregnancy, and the pregnancy-associated demands on changes to mitochondrial function predispose overweight and obese women to the development of pregnancy complications, including some of the most important and dangerous, GDM, and preeclampsia.

References

[1] Ng M, Fleming T, Robinson M, Thomson B, Graetz N, Margono C, et al. Global, regional, and national prevalence of overweight and obesity in children and adults during 1980–2013: a systematic analysis for the Global Burden of Disease Study 2013. Lancet 2014;384(9945):766–81.
[2] Dempsey JC, Ashiny Z, Qiu CF, Miller RS, Sorensen TK, Williams MA. Maternal pre-pregnancy overweight status and obesity as risk factors for cesarean delivery. J Matern Fetal Neonatal Med 2005;17(3):179–85.
[3] Dodd JM, Crowther CA, Robinson JS. Dietary and lifestyle interventions to limit weight gain during pregnancy for obese or overweight women: a systematic review. Acta Obstet Gynecol Scand 2008;87(7):702–6.
[4] Scheffler I. Mitochondria. Hoboken, NJ: John Wiley & Sons; 2007.
[5] Alison W, Scheffler I. Mitochondrial function, Part A mitochondrial electron transport complexes and reactive oxygen species. Burlington, VT: Elsevier Science; 2009.
[6] Belo L, Caslake M, Santos-Silva A, Castro EM, Pereira-Leite L, Quintanilha A, et al. LDL size, total antioxidant status and oxidised LDL in normal human pregnancy: a longitudinal study. Atherosclerosis 2004;177(2):391–9.
[7] Williamson RD, McCarthy C, McCarthy FP, Kenny LC. Oxidative stress in pre-eclampsia; have we been looking in the wrong place? Pregnancy Hypertens 2017;8:1–5.
[8] Kinoshita T, Itoh M. Longitudinal variance of fat mass deposition during pregnancy evaluated by ultrasonography: the ratio of visceral fat to subcutaneous fat in the abdomen. Gynecol Obstet Invest 2006;61(2):115–8.
[9] Taggart NR, Holliday RM, Billewicz WZ, Hytten FE, Thomson AM. Changes in skinfolds during pregnancy. Br J Nutr 1967;21(2):439–51.
[10] Catalano PM, Tyzbir ED, Wolfe RR, Calles J, Roman NM, Amini SB, et al. Carbohydrate metabolism during pregnancy in control subjects and women with gestational diabetes. Am J Physiol Endocrinol Metab 1993;264(1):E60–7.
[11] Sivan E, Homko CJ, Chen X, Reece EA, Boden G. Effect of insulin on fat metabolism during and after normal pregnancy. Diabetes 1999;48(4):834–8.
[12] Catalano PM, Nizielski SE, Shao J, Preston L, Qiao L, Friedman JE. Downregulated IRS-1 and PPARγ in obese women with gestational diabetes: relationship to FFA during pregnancy. Am J Physiol Endocrinol Metab 2002;282(3):E522–33.
[13] Lain KY, Catalano PM. Metabolic changes in pregnancy. Clin Obstet Gynecol 2007;50(4):938–48.
[14] Walsh JM, Segurado R, Mahony RM, Foley ME, McAuliffe FM. The effects of fetal gender on maternal and fetal insulin resistance. PLoS One 2015;10(9). e0137215.
[15] Geng X, Geng L, Zhang Y, Lu H, Shen Y, Chen R, et al. Fetal sex influences maternal fasting plasma glucose levels and basal β-cell function in pregnant women with normal glucose tolerance. Acta Diabetol 2017;54(12):1131–8.
[16] Retnakaran R, Kramer CK, Ye C, Kew S, Hanley AJ, Connelly PW, et al. Fetal sex and maternal risk of gestational diabetes mellitus: the impact of having a boy. Diabetes Care 2015;38(5):844.
[17] Khouzami VA, Ginsburg DS, Daikoku NH, Johnson JWC. The glucose tolerance test as a means of identifying intrauterine growth retardation. Am J Obstet Gynecol 1981;139(4):423–6.
[18] Dalfrà MG, Pacini G, Parretti E, Ragazzi E, Mello G, Lapolla A. Elevated insulin sensitivity and β-cell function during pregnancy in mothers of growth-restricted newborns. Am J Physiol Endocrinol Metab 2011;301(1):E25–30.
[19] Baeyens L, Hindi S, Sorenson RL, German MS. β-cell adaptation in pregnancy. Diabetes Obes Metabol 2016;18(S1):63–70.

[20] Nolan CJ, Proietto J. The feto-placental glucose steal phenomenon is a major cause of maternal metabolic adaptation during late pregnancy in the rat. Diabetologia 1994;37(10):976–84.
[21] Gradmark A, Pomeroy J, Renström F, Steiginga S, Persson M, Wright A, et al. Physical activity, sedentary behaviors, and estimated insulin sensitivity and secretion in pregnant and non-pregnant women. BMC Pregnancy Childbirth 2011;11(1):44.
[22] Cunha DA, Amaral ME, Carvalho CP, Collares-Buzato CB, Carneiro EM, Boschero AC. Increased expression of SNARE proteins and synaptotagmin IV in islets from pregnant rats and in vitro prolactin-treated neonatal islets. Biol Res 2006;39:555–66.
[23] Cantley J. The control of insulin secretion by adipokines: current evidence for adipocyte-beta cell endocrine signalling in metabolic homeostasis. Mamm Genome 2014;25(9):442–54.
[24] Friedman JE, Ishizuka T, Shao J, Huston L, Highman T, Catalano P. Impaired glucose transport and insulin receptor tyrosine phosphorylation in skeletal muscle from obese women with gestational diabetes. Diabetes 1999;48(9):1807–14.
[25] Koves TR, Ussher JR, Noland RC, Slentz D, Mosedale M, Ilkayeva O, et al. Mitochondrial overload and incomplete fatty acid oxidation contribute to skeletal muscle insulin resistance. Cell Metabol 2008;7(1):45–56.
[26] Anderson EJ, Lustig ME, Boyle KE, Woodlief TL, Kane DA, Lin C-T, et al. Mitochondrial H_2O_2 emission and cellular redox state link excess fat intake to insulin resistance in both rodents and humans. J Clin Invest 2009;119(3):573–81.
[27] Ogunyemi D, Xu J, Mahesan AM, Rad S, Kim E, Yano J, et al. Differentially expressed genes in adipocytokine signaling pathway of adipose tissue in pregnancy. J Diabetes Mellitus 2013;3(2):86–95.
[28] Boumelhem BB, Assinder SJ, Bell-Anderson KS, Fraser ST. Flow cytometric single cell analysis reveals heterogeneity between adipose depots. Adipocyte 2017;6(2):112–23.
[29] Schwenk RW, Luiken JJFP, Bonen A, Glatz JFC. Regulation of sarcolemmal glucose and fatty acid transporters in cardiac disease. Cardiovasc Res 2008;79(2):249–58.
[30] Frontera M, Pujol E, Rodríguez-Cuenca S, Català-Niell A, Roca P, García-Palmer FJ, et al. Rat Brown adipose tissue thermogenic features are altered during mid-pregnancy. Cell Physiol Biochem 2005;15(5):203–10.
[31] Diderholm B, Beardsall K, Murgatroyd P, Lees C, Gustafsson J, Dunger D. Maternal rates of lipolysis and glucose production in late pregnancy are independently related to foetal weight. Clin Endocrinol 2017;87(3):272–8.
[32] Haggarty P. Fatty acid supply to the human fetus. Annu Rev Nutr 2010;30:237–55.
[33] Ashworth CJ, Hoggard N, Thomas L, Mercer JG, Wallace JM, Lea RG. Placental leptin. Rev Reprod 2000;5(1):18–24.
[34] Chen J, Tan B, Karteris E, Zervou S, Digby J, Hillhouse EW, et al. Secretion of adiponectin by human placenta: differential modulation of adiponectin and its receptors by cytokines. Diabetologia 2006;49(6):1292–302.
[35] Brelje TC, Scharp DW, Lacy PE, Ogren L, Talamantes F, Robertson M, et al. Effect of homologous placental lactogens, prolactins, and growth hormones on islet B-cell division and insulin secretion in rat, mouse, and human islets: implication for placental lactogen regulation of islet function during pregnancy. Endocrinology 1993;132(2):879–87.
[36] Barbour LA, Shao J, Qiao L, Pulawa LK, Jensen DR, Bartke A, et al. Human placental growth hormone causes severe insulin resistance in transgenic mice. Am J Obstet Gynecol 2002;186(3):512–7.

[37] Martinez F, Milan R, Flores-Herrera O, Olvera-Sanchez S, Gomez-Chang E, Espinosa-Garcia MT. The role of mitochondria in syncytiotrophoblast cells: bioenergetics and steroidogenesis. In: Recent Advances in Research on the Human Placenta: InTech; 2012.
[38] Kasahara A, Scorrano L. Mitochondria: from cell death executioners to regulators of cell differentiation. Trends Cell Biol 2014;24(12):761–70.
[39] Burton GJ, Yung HW, Murray AJ. Mitochondrial–Endoplasmic reticulum interactions in the trophoblast: stress and senescence. Placenta 2017;52:146–55.
[40] Bustamante J, Ramírez-Vélez R, Czerniczyniec A, Cicerchia D, De Plata AA, Lores-Arnaiz S. Oxygen metabolism in human placenta mitochondria. J Bioenerg Biomembr 2014;46(6):459–69.
[41] Papadopoulos V, Miller WL. Role of mitochondria in steroidogenesis. Best Pract Res Clin Endocrinol Metabol 2012;26(6):771–90.
[42] Martinez F, Kiriakidou M, Strauss III JF. Structural and functional changes in mitochondria associated with trophoblast differentiation: methods to isolate enriched preparations of syncytiotrophoblast mitochondria. Endocrinology 1997;138(5):2172–83.
[43] Uribe A, Strauss III JF, Martınez F. Contact sites from human placental mitochondria: characterization and role in progesterone synthesis. Arch Biochem Biophys 2003;413(2):172–81.
[44] Huppertz B, Kingdom JC. Apoptosis in the trophoblast—role of apoptosis in placental morphogenesis. J Soc Gynecol Invest 2004;11(6):353–62.
[45] Huppertz B, Kadyrov M, Kingdom JC. Apoptosis and its role in the trophoblast. Am J Obstet Gynecol 2006;195(1):29–39.
[46] Heazell AE, Crocker IP. Live and let die - regulation of villous trophoblast apoptosis in normal and abnormal pregnancies. Placenta 2008;29(9):772–83.
[47] Detmer SA, Chan DC. Functions and dysfunctions of mitochondrial dynamics. Nat Rev Mol Cell Biol 2007;8(11):870.
[48] Kroemer G. Mitochondrial control of apoptosis: an introduction. Biochem Biophys Res Commun 2003;304(3):433–5.
[49] Cai J, Yang J, Jones D. Mitochondrial control of apoptosis: the role of cytochrome c. Biochim Biophys Acta Bioenerg 1998;1366(1–2):139–49.
[50] Smith SC, Baker PN, Symonds EM. Placental apoptosis in normal human pregnancy. Am J Obstet Gynecol 1997;177(1):57–65.
[51] LeBrun DP, Warnke RA, Cleary ML. Expression of bcl-2 in fetal tissues suggests a role in morphogenesis. Am J Pathol 1993;142(3):743–53.
[52] Huppertz B, Frank HG, Kingdom JC, Reister F, Kaufmann P. Villous cytotrophoblast regulation of the syncytial apoptotic cascade in the human placenta. Histochem Cell Biol 1998;110(5):495–508.
[53] Ishihara N, Matsuo H, Murakoshi H, Laoag-Fernandez JB, Samoto T, Maruo T. Increased apoptosis in the syncytiotrophoblast in human term placentas complicated by either preeclampsia or intrauterine growth retardation. Am J Obstet Gynecol 2002;186(1):158–66.
[54] Sakuragi N, Matsuo H, Coukos G, Furth EE, Bronner MP, VanArsdale CM, et al. Differentiation-dependent expression of the BCL-2 proto-oncogene in the human trophoblast lineage. J Soc Gynecol Invest 1994;1(2):164–72.
[55] Nan J, Hu H, Sun Y, Zhu L, Wang Y, Zhong Z, et al. TNFR2 stimulation promotes mitochondrial fusion via Stat3- and NF-kB-dependent activation of OPA1 expression. Circ Res 2017;121(4):392–410.
[56] Youle RJ, van der Bliek AM. Mitochondrial fission, fusion, and stress. Science 2012;337(6098):1062.

[57] Chan DC. Mitochondrial fusion and fission in mammals. Annu Rev Cell Dev Biol 2006;22:79–99.

[58] Zhou X, Han TL, Chen H, Baker PN, Qi H, Zhang H. Impaired mitochondrial fusion, autophagy, biogenesis and dysregulated lipid metabolism is associated with preeclampsia. Exp Cell Res 2017;359(1):195–204.

[59] Chen H, Detmer SA, Ewald AJ, Griffin EE, Fraser SE, Chan DC. Mitofusins Mfn1 and Mfn2 coordinately regulate mitochondrial fusion and are essential for embryonic development. J Cell Biol 2003;160(2):189–200.

[60] Pang W, Zhang Y, Zhao N, Darwiche SS, Fu X, Xiang W. Low expression of Mfn2 is associated with mitochondrial damage and apoptosis in the placental villi of early unexplained miscarriage. Placenta 2013;34(7):613–8.

[61] Wasilewski M, Semenzato M, Rafelski SM, Robbins J, Bakardjiev AI, Scorrano L. Optic atrophy 1-dependent mitochondrial remodeling controls steroidogenesis in trophoblasts. Curr Biol 2012;22(13):1228–34.

[62] Marchi S, Patergnani S, Pinton P. The endoplasmic reticulum–mitochondria connection: one touch, multiple functions. Biochim Biophys Acta Bioenerg 2014;1837(4):461–9.

[63] Burton G, Yung H-W, Cindrova-Davies T, Charnock-Jones D. Placental endoplasmic reticulum stress and oxidative stress in the pathophysiology of unexplained intrauterine growth restriction and early onset preeclampsia. Placenta 2009;30:43–8.

[64] Yung HW, Atkinson D, Campion-Smith T, Olovsson M, Charnock-Jones DS, Burton GJ. Differential activation of placental unfolded protein response pathways implies heterogeneity in causation of early-and late-onset pre-eclampsia. J Pathol 2014;234(2):262–76.

[65] Gong J-S, Kim GJ. The role of autophagy in the placenta as a regulator of cell death. Clin Exp Reprod Med 2014;41(3):97–107.

[66] Chen B, Longtine MS, Nelson DM. Hypoxia induces autophagy in primary human trophoblasts. Endocrinology 2012;153(10):4946–54.

[67] Xiang AH, Peters RK, Trigo E, Kjos SL, Lee WP, Buchanan TA. Multiple metabolic defects during late pregnancy in women at high risk for type 2 diabetes. Diabetes 1999;48(4):848–54.

[68] Kirwan JP, Hauguel-De Mouzon S, Lepercq J, Challier J-C, Huston-Presley L, Friedman JE, et al. TNF-αis a predictor of insulin resistance in human pregnancy. Diabetes 2002;51(7):2207.

[69] Qu X, Yu H, Jia B, Yu X, Cui Q, Liu Z, et al. Association of downregulated HDAC 2 with the impaired mitochondrial function and cytokine secretion in the monocytes/macrophages from gestational diabetes mellitus patients. Cell Biol Int 2016;40(6):642–51.

[70] Chandler-Laney PC, Shepard DN, Schneider CR, Flagg LA, Granger WM, Mancuso MS, et al. Relatively low β-cell responsiveness contributes to the association of BMI with circulating glucose concentrations measured under free-living conditions among pregnant African American women. J Nutr 2016;146(5):994–1000.

[71] Catalano PM, Huston L, Amini SB, Kalhan SC. Longitudinal changes in glucose metabolism during pregnancy in obese women with normal glucose tolerance and gestational diabetes mellitus. Am J Obstet Gynecol 1999;180(4):903–16.

[72] Kulkarni RN, Wang ZL, Wang RM, Hurley JD, Smith DM, Ghatei MA, et al. Leptin rapidly suppresses insulin release from insulinoma cells, rat and human islets and, in vivo, in mice. J Clin Invest 1997;100(11):2729–36.

[73] Dekker Nitert M, Barrett HL, Denny KJ, McIntyre HD, Callaway LK, the B. Exercise in pregnancy does not alter gestational weight gain, MCP-1 or leptin in obese women. Aust N Z J Obstet Gynaecol 2015;55(1):27–33.

[74] Boyle KE, Newsom SA, Janssen RC, Lappas M, Friedman JE. Skeletal muscle MnSOD, mitochondrial complex II, and SIRT3 enzyme activities are decreased in maternal obesity during human pregnancy and gestational diabetes mellitus. J Clin Endocrinol Metabol 2013;98(10):E1601–9.
[75] Boyle KE, Hwang H, Janssen RC, DeVente JM, Barbour LA, Hernandez TL, et al. Gestational diabetes is characterized by reduced mitochondrial protein expression and altered calcium signaling proteins in skeletal muscle. PLoS One 2014;9(9). e106872.
[76] Barrett HL, Dekker Nitert M, Jones L, O'Rourke P, Lust K, Gatford KL, et al. Determinants of maternal triglycerides in women with gestational diabetes mellitus in the metformin in gestational diabetes (MiG) study. Diabetes Care 2013;36(7):1941–6.
[77] Jarvie E, Hauguel-de-Mouzon S, Nelson SM, Sattar N, Catalano PM, Freeman DJ. Lipotoxicity in obese pregnancy and its potential role in adverse pregnancy outcome and obesity in the offspring. Clin Sci (Lond) 2010;119(3):123–9.
[78] Boss O, Hagen T, Lowell BB. Uncoupling proteins 2 and 3: potential regulators of mitochondrial energy metabolism. Diabetes 2000;49(2):143.
[79] Barrett HL, Dekker Nitert M, McIntyre HD, Callaway LK. Normalizing metabolism in diabetic pregnancy: is it time to target lipids? Diabetes Care 2014;37(5):1484–93.
[80] White SL, Pasupathy D, Sattar N, Nelson SM, Lawlor DA, Briley AL, et al. Metabolic profiling of gestational diabetes in obese women during pregnancy. Diabetologia 2017;60(10):1903–12.
[81] Whitfield JB. Gamma glutamyltransferase. Crit Rev Clin Lab Sci 2001;38(4):263–355.
[82] Meng Q, Shao L, Luo X, Mu Y, Xu W, Gao C, et al. Ultrastructure of placenta of gravidas with gestational diabetes mellitus. Obstet Gynecol Int 2015;2015:9.
[83] Mele J, Muralimanoharan S, Maloyan A, Myatt L. Impaired mitochondrial function in human placenta with increased maternal adiposity. Am J Physiol Endocrinol Metab 2014;307(5):E419–25.
[84] Muralimanoharan S, Maloyan A, Myatt L. Mitochondrial function and glucose metabolism in the placenta with gestational diabetes mellitus: role of miR-143. Clin Sci 2016;130(11):931.
[85] Qiu C, Hevner K, Abetew D, Sedensky M, Morgan P, Enquobahrie DA, et al. Mitochondrial DNA copy number and oxidative DNA damage in placental tissues from gestational diabetes and control pregnancies: apilot study. Clin Lab 2013;59(0):655–60.
[86] Hastie R, Lappas M. The effect of pre-existing maternal obesity and diabetes on placental mitochondrial content and electron transport chain activity. Placenta 2014;35(9):673–83.
[87] Visiedo F, Bugatto F, Sánchez V, Cózar-Castellano I, Bartha JL, Perdomo G. High glucose levels reduce fatty acid oxidation and increase triglyceride accumulation in human placenta. Am J Physiol Endocrinol Metab 2013;305(2):E205–12.
[88] Zhang Y, Zhang Y, Ding GL, Liu XM, Ye J, Sheng JZ, et al. Regulation of hepatic pyruvate dehydrogenase phosphorylation in offspring glucose intolerance induced by intrauterine hyperglycemia. Oncotarget 2017;8(9):15205–12.
[89] Turdi S, Ge W, Hu N, Bradley KM, Wang X, Ren J. Interaction between maternal and postnatal high fat diet leads to a greater risk of myocardial dysfunction in offspring via enhanced lipotoxicity, IRS-1 serine phosphorylation and mitochondrial defects. J Mol Cell Cardiol 2013;55:117–29.
[90] Neufeld ND, Corbo L, Stoddard A, Klein AH, Tadokoro N. Oxygen consumption and guanosine diphosphate binding by fetal brown adipose tissue in diabetic pregnancy. Metabolism 1989;38(9):831–6.
[91] McPherson NO, Bell VG, Zander-Fox DL, Fullston T, Wu LL, Robker RL, et al. When two obese parents are worse than one! Impacts on embryo and fetal development. Am J Physiol Endocrinol Metab 2015;309(6):E568–81.
[92] Bournat JC, Brown CW. Mitochondrial dysfunction in obesity. Curr Opin Endocrinol Diabetes Obes 2010;17(5):446–52.

[93] Wang T, Si Y, Shirihai OS, Si H, Schultz V, Corkey RF, et al. Respiration in adipocytes is inhibited by reactive oxygen species. Obesity 2010;18(8):1493–502.
[94] Holland OJ, Cuffe JSM, Dekker Nitert M, Callaway L, Kwan Cheung KA, Radenkovic F, et al. Placental mitochondrial adaptations in preeclampsia associated with progression to term delivery. Cell Death Dis 2018;9(12):1150.
[95] Hung TH, Burton GJ. Hypoxia and reoxygenation: a possible mechanism for placental oxidative stress in preeclampsia. Taiwan J Obstet Gynecol 2006;45(3):189–200.
[96] Holland O, Dekker Nitert M, Gallo LA, Vejzovic M, Fisher JJ, Perkins AV. Review: placental mitochondrial function and structure in gestational disorders. Placenta 2016.
[97] McCarthy CM, Kenny LC. Mitochondrial [dys]function; culprit in pre-eclampsia? Clin Sci (Lond) 2016;130(14):1179–84.
[98] Shi Z, Long W, Zhao C, Guo X, Shen R, Ding H. Comparative proteomics analysis suggests that placental mitochondria are involved in the development of pre-eclampsia. PLoS One 2013;8(5). e64351.
[99] Wang Y, Walsh SW. Placental mitochondria as a source of oxidative stress in pre-eclampsia. Placenta 1998;19(8):581–6.
[100] Brownfoot FC, Hastie R, Hannan NJ, Cannon P, Tuohey L, Parry LJ, et al. Metformin as a prevention and treatment for preeclampsia: effects on soluble fms-like tyrosine kinase 1 and soluble endoglin secretion and endothelial dysfunction. Am J Obstet Gynecol 2016;214(3). 356.e1–e15.
[101] Vishnyakova PA, Volodina MA, Tarasova NV, Marey MV, Tsvirkun DV, Vavina OV, et al. Mitochondrial role in adaptive response to stress conditions in preeclampsia. Sci Rep 2016;6:32410.
[102] Kelley DE, He J, Menshikova EV, Ritov VB. Dysfunction of mitochondria in human skeletal muscle in type 2 diabetes. Diabetes 2002;51(10):2944–50.
[103] Widschwendter M, Schrocksnadel H, Mortl MG. Pre-eclampsia: a disorder of placental mitochondria? Mol Med Today 1998;4(7):286–91.
[104] Yan JY, Xu X. Relationships between concentrations of free fatty acid in serum and oxidative-damage levels in placental mitochondria and preeclampsia. Zhonghua Fu Chan Ke Za Zhi 2012;47(6):412–7.
[105] Vanderlelie J, Venardos K, Clifton VL, Gude NM, Clarke FM, Perkins AV. Increased biological oxidation and reduced anti-oxidant enzyme activity in pre-eclamptic placentae. Placenta 2005;26(1):53–8.
[106] Nezu M, Souma T, Yu L, Sekine H, Takahashi N, Wei AZ, et al. Nrf2 inactivation enhances placental angiogenesis in a preeclampsia mouse model and improves maternal and fetal outcomes. Sci Signal 2017;10(479).
[107] Pereira RD, De Long NE, Wang RC, Yazdi FT, Holloway AC, Raha S. Angiogenesis in the placenta: the role of reactive oxygen species signaling. BioMed Res Int 2015;2015:814543.
[108] Kweider N, Huppertz B, Kadyrov M, Rath W, Pufe T, Wruck CJ. A possible protective role of Nrf2 in preeclampsia. Ann Anatomy (Anatomischer Anzeiger) 2014;196(5):268–77.
[109] Holland OJ, Hickey AJR, Alvsaker A, Moran S, Hedges C, Chamley LW, et al. Changes in mitochondrial respiration in the human placenta over gestation. Placenta 2017;57:102–12.
[110] Burton GJ. Oxygen, the Janus gas; its effects on human placental development and function. J Anat 2009;215(1):27–35.
[111] Jauniaux E, Watson AL, Hempstock J, Bao YP, Skepper JN, Burton GJ. Onset of maternal arterial blood flow and placental oxidative stress. A possible factor in human early pregnancy failure. Am J Pathol 2000;157(6):2111–22.
[112] Kweider N, Huppertz B, Wruck CJ, Beckmann R, Rath W, Pufe T, et al. A role for Nrf2 in redox signalling of the invasive extravillous trophoblast in severe early onset IUGR associated with preeclampsia. PLoS One 2012;7(10). e47055.

[113] Florczyk U, Jazwa A, Maleszewska M, Mendel M, Szade K, Kozakowska M, et al. Nrf2 regulates angiogenesis: effect on endothelial cells, bone marrow-derived proangiogenic cells and hind limb ischemia. Antioxidants Redox Signal 2014;20(11):1693–708.
[114] Shibata E, Nanri H, Ejima K, Araki M, Fukuda J, Yoshimura K, et al. Enhancement of mitochondrial oxidative stress and up-regulation of antioxidant protein peroxiredoxin III/SP-22 in the mitochondria of human pre-eclamptic placentae. Placenta 2003;24(6):698–705.
[115] Rumbold A, Duley L, Crowther CA, Haslam RR. Antioxidants for preventing pre-eclampsia. Cochrane Database Syst Rev 2008;(1). Cd004227.
[116] Salles AM, Galvao TF, Silva MT, Motta LC, Pereira MG. Antioxidants for preventing preeclampsia: a systematic review. Sci World J 2012;2012:243476.
[117] Bartha JL, Visiedo F, Fernandez-Deudero A, Bugatto F, Perdomo G. Decreased mitochondrial fatty acid oxidation in placentas from women with preeclampsia. Placenta 2012;33(2):132–4.
[118] Rakheja D, Bennett MJ, Foster BM, Domiati-Saad R, Rogers BB. Evidence for fatty acid oxidation in human placenta, and the relationship of fatty acid oxidation enzyme activities with gestational age. Placenta 2002;23(5):447–50.
[119] Shekhawat PS, Matern D, Strauss AW. Fetal fatty acid oxidation disorders, their effect on maternal health and neonatal outcome: impact of expanded newborn screening on their diagnosis and management. Pediatr Res 2005;57(5 Pt 2):78r–86r.
[120] Challier JC, Basu S, Bintein T, Minium J, Hotmire K, Catalano PM, et al. Obesity in pregnancy stimulates macrophage accumulation and inflammation in the placenta. Placenta 2008;29(3):274–81.
[121] Lager S, Jansson N, Olsson AL, Wennergren M, Jansson T, Powell TL. Effect of IL-6 and TNF-alpha on fatty acid uptake in cultured human primary trophoblast cells. Placenta 2011;32(2):121–7.
[122] Lambertucci RH, Hirabara SM, SilveiraLdos R, Levada-Pires AC, Curi R, Pithon-Curi TC. Palmitate increases superoxide production through mitochondrial electron transport chain and NADPH oxidase activity in skeletal muscle cells. J Cell Physiol 2008;216(3):796–804.
[123] Myatt L, Maloyan A. Obesity and placental function. Semin Reprod Med 2016;34(1):42–9.
[124] Roberts VH, Smith J, McLea SA, Heizer AB, Richardson JL, Myatt L. Effect of increasing maternal body mass index on oxidative and nitrative stress in the human placenta. Placenta 2009;30(2):169–75.
[125] Padmini E, Lavanya S, Uthra V. Preeclamptic placental stress and over expression of mitochondrial HSP70. Clin Chem Lab Med 2009;47(9):1073–80.
[126] McCarthy C, Kenny LC. Therapeutically targeting mitochondrial redox signalling alleviates endothelial dysfunction in preeclampsia. Sci Rep 2016;6:32683.
[127] Shanklin DR, Sibai BM. Ultrastructural aspects of preeclampsia. II. Mitochondrial changes. Am J Obstet Gynecol 1990;163(3):943–53.
[128] Qiu C, Hevner K, Enquobahrie DA, Williams MA. A case-control study of maternal blood mitochondrial DNA copy number and preeclampsia risk. Int J Mol Epidemiol Genet 2012;3(3):237–44.
[129] Qiu C, Enquobahrie DA, Gelaye B, Hevner K, Williams MA. The association between leukocyte telomere length and mitochondrial DNA copy number in pregnant women: a pilot study. Clin Lab 2015;61(3–4):363–9.

PART 3

Genetic machinery and its function

CHAPTER 12

Gene–nutrient interaction: from fetal development to lifelong health

Andrea Maugeri, Martina Barchitta, Antonella Agodi
Department of Medical and Surgical Sciences and Advanced Technologies "GF Ingrassia", University of Catania, Catania, Italy

Contents

Introduction

Maternal nutritional status and diet may affect pregnancy outcomes through the alteration of maternal and fetal metabolism. The maternal supply of macronutrients and micronutrients plays a critical role in fetal growth and development because of their involvement in various biological functions such as enzymes activity, signal transduction, and transcription pathways [1]. Indeed, during the periconceptional and perinatal periods, the imbalance of macronutrients and micronutrients could potentially affect the fetus, by altering placental nutrient availability, tissue development, and functions. Although maternal nutrient supply is a major determinant of fetal growth and development, increasing evidence has led to the assertion that several genetic risk factors are associated to adverse neonatal outcomes. For example, polymorphisms in genes involved in the one-carbon metabolism are shown to modulate the normal metabolic functions, with adverse effects on maternal and fetal health. The study of the relationship between human

Molecular Nutrition
ISBN 978-0-12-813862-5
https://doi.org/10.1016/B978-0-12-813862-5.00012-8

genome, nutrition, and health, also known as Nutritional Genomics, is a rapidly developing discipline within nutrition. In this field, it becomes evident that single-nucleotide polymorphisms (SNPs) can create metabolic deficiencies, influencing dietary requirements for pregnant women [2]. Although the one-carbon metabolism is the most investigated, the role of genetic variants in fatty acids, proteins, and micronutrients metabolism has been assessed. Indeed, recent researches show that unhealthy maternal diet, imbalance of nutrients or supplements, as well as polymorphisms in both maternal and fetal genes, may influence fetal development, also resulting in low birth weight (LBW), small for gestational age babies, and intrauterine growth restriction (IUGR) [3–9,135–138].

There is also evidence that fetal and early-life nutrition may be of greater importance for lifelong health and chronic diseases in adults. Particularly, each stage of fetal development is influenced by maternal nutrient supply; several experimental models have confirmed that the timing of nutritional insults impacts differently on the risk of diseases that occur with aging, by programming postnatal physiological and metabolic states [10]. Genetic variants, such as polymorphisms of methylenetetrahydrofolate reductase (MTHFR) or apolipoprotein E variants, provide the predisposition to disease, but the etiology is characterized by the gene–environment or gene–nutrient interactions. For example, taking the C677T polymorphism of *MTHFR*, an adequate folate status reduces the risk of cardiovascular diseases and colorectal cancer that is associated to the TT genotype [11,12]. Furthermore, a decreased risk of cervical intraepithelial lesions in women homozygous for the MTHFR T allele, has been reported [134].

Epigenetics, the study of heritable and reversible molecular information outside of the DNA sequence, may explain how gene–environment interactions occur at the molecular level. The epigenetic factors, such as DNA methylation, histone modification, histone variants, long noncoding RNA (lncRNA), and microRNA (miRNA) regulation, represent potential mechanisms involved in disease heterogeneity and incomplete penetrance in genetic models [13]. Also lncRNAs are emerging as potentially important players in biological regulation. They are involved in physiology and disease, especially those relevant to endocrinology, reproduction, metabolism, immunology, neurobiology, muscle biology, and cancer [14]. As the placenta is the most exposed organ to environmental and nutritional insults, recent researches point to placental epigenetic profiles in fetal development. Indeed, increasing evidence from animal and human studies shows that DNA methylation [15–18], lncRNA [19,20], histone variants [21], microRNAs [22–24], and histone modifications [25,26] are involved in IUGR and other neonatal outcomes. In this context, maternal nutrient supply plays a critical role, by influencing the availability of macro- and micronutrients and mechanisms that regulate DNA stability [27]. Accordingly, the importance of maternal diet for epigenetic mechanisms that are involved in fetal growth and development has been confirmed [28–30].

Despite several researches having already been conducted in the field of gene–nutrient interaction during perinatal period, there are still significant gaps in our knowledge that require further investigations. Here we review current evidence and novel findings in relation to genetic variants in nutrient metabolism.

One-carbon metabolism

One-carbon metabolism is a crucial network of biochemical reactions for fetal growth and development, providing the transfer of methyl groups from one compound to another. The coenzymes necessary for several of the methyl transferase reactions include folate, vitamin B12, B6, and B2. Particularly, folate, methionine, and choline are important to maintain one-carbon flux, ensuring normal homocysteine conversion to methionine. Briefly, folate is metabolized to 5-methyltetrahydrofolate (5-methylTHF) in the intestine and/or liver. 5-MethylTHF is the primary folate constituent taken up by nonhepatic tissues, which then must be polyglutamated for cellular retention and 1-carbon cycle coenzyme function. Via the methionine synthase reaction, 5-methylTHF must be converted to tetrahydrofolate (THF), the most effective substrate for polyglutamate synthetase. When folic acid is consumed in fortified foods or supplements, it is metabolized primarily to 5-methylTHF during intestinal absorption and/or first pass in the liver, after which it behaves identically to natural dietary folate. Folic acid is normally first reduced to dihydrofolate by dihydrofolate reductase and subsequently to THF to enter the folate pool. Once the THF coenzyme is formed from either folic acid or dietary folate, it is first converted to 5,10-methyleneTHF by the vitamin B6–dependent enzyme serine hydroxymethyltransferase and subsequently irreversibly reduced to 5-methylTHF by 5,10-methylenetetrahydrofolate reductase (MTHFR). This reaction is important to maintain the flux of methyl groups for the remethylation of homocysteine (Hcy) to methionine via the vitamin B12–dependent methionine synthase reaction [31]. The alternative pathway for the methylation of Hcy to form methionine is catalyzed by betaine homocysteine methyltransferase [32], an enzyme whose activity has been associated to methionine concentration [33]. In this reaction, the methyl group donor is provided by the betaine, which is derived from dietary choline by the action of choline dehydrogenase. In fact, it is well established that supplemental oral betaine can reduce plasma homocysteine concentrations [34]. Therefore, nutrient deficiency [35,36], as well as SNPs in genes involved in these pathways, can result in the reduction of one-carbon groups availability and accumulation of homocysteine. High levels of homocysteine lead to the accumulation of SAH, an inhibitor of human DNA methyltransferase enzymes [37], which can cause DNA hypomethylation [38] and affect malignancy [39].

One-carbon metabolism and polymorphisms of the *MTHFR* gene

Accumulating evidence suggests that Hcy plays a crucial role in several developmental disorders [40]. In humans, polymorphisms in genes that encode enzymes involved in one-carbon metabolism, as well as folate and vitamin B6 and B12 deficiencies are the main factors that affect Hcy concentration. Among genetic variants, the SNPs of the *MTHFR* gene, which are commonly associated with hyperhomocysteinemia, became a research topic because of the role on the risk of adverse birth outcomes. During pregnancy, *MTHFR* polymorphisms not only are associated with increased levels of Hcy [41] but also are risk factors for neural tube defects (NTDs) [42,43], recurrent embryo loss [44], and first early pregnancy loss [41].

The best characterized *MTHFR* genetic polymorphism consists of a cytosine to thymine substitution at position 677 in exon 4 (*MTHFR* C677T), which results in an alanine to valine substitution in the catalytic domain of MTHFR [3]. This substitution leads to decreased enzyme activity, resulting in accumulation of plasma Hcy; in fact, homozygotes and heterozygotes have about a 70% and 35% reduced MTHFR activity in vitro, respectively. Carriers of T allele are about half the general population, and the frequency of the homozygous mutated genotype (677TT) ranges from 1% to 20% [45].

A second well-investigated polymorphism in the MTHFR gene is a 1298A > C transition, which results in an amino acid change from a glutamine to alanine in the regulatory region of the MTHFR enzyme

[46,47]. Although this variant has been reported to cause a reduction in MTHFR activity, its effect is considered to be less than that conferred by the 677C > T polymorphism [46,47], not significantly contributing to hyperhomocysteinemia.

The relationship between SNPs in *MTHFR* genes and nutrients involved in one-carbon metabolism is reciprocal. In fact, *MTHFR* mutated alleles reduce bioavailability of folate and vitamin B12 and increase Hcy concentration, as well as the combination between these polymorphisms and deficiency of folate and vitamin B12 inhibits the remethylation of Hcy to methionine [48].

Thus, the main effects of *MTHFR*-mutated alleles are to reduce bioavailability of folate and vitamin B12 and to increase homocysteine concentration. As folate- and vitamin B12–mediated one-carbon metabolism is crucial in cell proliferation and differentiation, the effects of these polymorphisms are especially detrimental during embryogenesis [46]. Accordingly, the above-mentioned polymorphisms have been associated to several developmental disorders, such as NTD [49,50], orofacial clefting [51], and Down syndrome [52]. For example, Wenstrom et al. report that the T allele of the 677C > T polymorphism increases the Hcy concentration in amniotic fluid, predisposing to NTDs of cervical–lumbar spine, lumbosacral spine, and occipital encephalocele [53].

As previously discussed, hyperhomocysteinemia is also a risk factor for recurrent embryo loss [42,44] and also for a first early embryo loss [41]. Moreover, previous studies showed an association between maternal *MTHFR* 677T allele and increased risk of recurrent spontaneous abortion [54,55]. However, as other authors reported no association between maternal T allele and nonrecurrent fetal loss [56–58], this evidence should be confirmed by future researches. A plausible explanation of this discrepancy could be attributed to differences in study design, ethnicity, and sample size.

Several studies evaluated the effect of neonatal *MTHFR* polymorphisms on adverse pregnancy outcomes, such as spontaneous abortion. A previous study by Isotalo et al. reported high prevalence of mutated *MTHFR* alleles in aborted embryos [59]. A similar study by Zetterberg et al. showed a positive association between the prevalence of one or more 677T and 1298C alleles and the risk of spontaneous abortion, indicating that the *MTHFR* polymorphisms may have a major impact on fetal survival [60].

Few studies analyzed the effect of *MTHFR* polymorphisms, folate, and vitamin B12 status on neonatal anthropometric measures. Among these,

Sukla et al. showed that the maternal *MTHFR* 677T allele and vitamin B12 and folate deficiencies were independently associated with the risk of LBW [61]. Moreover, among women carriers of allele 677T, a significant positive association was reported between maternal folate intake and birth weight [62]. In two Indian birth cohorts, maternal *MTHFR* 677TT genotype was associated to high plasma Hcy concentrations and LBW, independent of the offspring *MTHFR* genotype. However, adequate maternal folate status protects from the effect of maternal *MTHFR* 677TT genotype on birth weight [63].

Genetic variants and choline metabolism

During pregnancy, choline is considered an essential nutrient because previous studies reported that low choline concentration was associated with several adverse birth outcomes [64–66]. Several pathways are involved in choline metabolism, and genetic variants could influence how much choline is required from diet. Accordingly, there has been substantial interest about the effect of maternal and fetal genotype on choline requirements and metabolism. Particularly, SNPs in the folate pathway reduce the availability of methyltetrahydrofolate, which results in an increased use of choline as a methyl donor. Among these, polymorphisms in the gene methylenetetrahydrofolate dehydrogenase 1 (*MTHFD1*) were associated to choline deficiency [67]. Specifically, the A allele of *MTHFD1* G1958A polymorphism may affect homocysteine methylation when folate availability is low [67,68], increasing the risk of several congenital defects, such as NTD [69], Down's syndrome, cleft lip, and cleft palate [70]. These results were recently confirmed by several metaanalyses that have identified the associations between *MTHFD1* polymorphisms and birth defects [71–73].

In addition, the effects of polymorphisms in the *PEMT* gene, an enzyme required for de novo production of choline, have been well investigated. Particularly, two missense mutations (rs7946 and rs897453) in *PEMT* have been associated with increased homocysteine level [74], which results in neural tube defects [75]. A recent study measured choline and betaine levels in women with a current NTD-affected pregnancy. Although levels of choline and betaine did not differ between cases and controls, women, who had a current NTD-affected pregnancy, were significantly more likely to have the G allele of rs7946 polymorphism [70].

Improving our understanding of how maternal dietary requirements and genetics interact to affect fetal health has important public health implications. Identification of genetic variants affecting choline requirements could be used to refine our dietary recommendations in pregnancy.

Fatty acids metabolism and fetal development

The polyunsaturated fatty acids (PUFAs), important molecules for health and maintenance of metabolic functions, are closely related to numerous health outcomes like cardiovascular disease morbidity and mortality, metabolic syndrome, and psychiatric disorders [76,77]. It is well established that physiological effects of PUFA are considered to be primarily mediated by tissue concentrations of long-chain PUFAs (LC-PUFAs).

During pregnancy, the fetus relies entirely on the maternal supply of fatty acids in utero. Fatty acids pass through the placenta and their availability plays a crucial role in fetal growth and development [78]. During early childhood, LC-PUFAs are present in breast milk to accomplish their role in postnatal development [79,80]. Moreover, changes in the metabolic environment, due to insufficient or excessive maternal nutrient intake, can cause short- and long-term implications for cell structure and function [81]. Therefore, imbalances in fatty acid intake during fetal development cause structural and functional changes in metabolism [82]. An adequate supply of LC-PUFA arachidonic acid (AA) (20:4n-6) and docosahexaenoic acid (DHA) (22:6n-3) is critical for optimal brain development [83].

LC-PUFAs are synthesized from the precursor essential fatty acids, such as omega-6 (linoleic acid, LA) and omega-3 (alpha linolenic acid, ALA) fatty acids, or provided by diet. The synthesis from essential fatty acids involves biochemical reactions of elongation and desaturation, catalyzed by the enzymes delta-6-desaturases (D6D) and delta-5 desaturases (D5D). Particularly, LA is the precursor of AA, whereas ALA is the precursor of EPA (eicosapentaenoic acid) and DHA.

Both desaturases are membrane-bound enzymes, and they are thought to be the rate-limiting enzymes in the formation of LC-PUFA [84]. These enzymes are produced in several tissues; significant activity is found in the liver, adipose tissue, brain, heart, and lung, whereas a reduced activity has been reported in the placenta and pregnant uterus [85].

Because of the lack of desaturase activity in the utero and placenta, the fetus requires placental transfer of LC-PUFAs. Therefore, inadequate fatty acid intake and metabolism, during fetal development, could influence fatty acid levels in membrane phospholipids and stored triglycerides, disrupting the cellular environment and causing structural and functional modifications [82]. For example, it was reported that maternal low levels of n-3 fatty acids and high levels of omega-6 fatty acids were associated with LBW [86]. These results confirmed that inadequate maternal fatty acid intake is associated with defects in fetal growth and development.

Genetic variants in *FADS* gene cluster and fetal development

In humans, D5D and D6D are encoded by *FADS1* and *FADS2* genes, which are located head-to-head in a cluster on chromosome 11 (11q12-q13) [87]. Several *FADS1* and *FADS2* SNPs have been studied for their association with plasma fatty acids (cholesterol, LDL, HDL, triglycerides, etc.) [88–92]. Particularly, carriers of certain genotypes in the *FADS* gene cluster have consistently been shown to have higher biological status of PUFA precursors, LA and ALA, and lower status of LC-PUFA products, AA and EPA (20:5n-3), probably as a result of having lower expression of the functional enzymes [93–96]. Additional studies on cohorts of pregnant women confirmed the same results; maternal genetic variants in *FADS* cluster have been associated with lower concentrations of AA and EPA in breast milk and maternal and infant blood [97–99]. Although a previous study by Yeates et al. reported no significant association between maternal FADS genotype and fetal development, the authors found a trend of improved psychomotor development among newborns from women with the mutated allele of the rs3834458 polymorphism [100]. Genetic variants in the maternal FADS genotypes were associated to reduced *FADS1* and *FADS2* activity and lower cognitive development of infants, possibly owing to lower LC-PUFA status during critical stages of fetal development, suggesting an indirect association of the FADS genotype with neurodevelopment. Accordingly, results from the English mother–child ALSPAC cohort confirmed that children of mothers with the rs3834458 mutated allele performed better in tests of intelligence quotient [101].

Although previously mentioned studies agree on the robust association between *FADS* genotype and levels of several n-6 and n-3 fatty acids, the relationship with DHA levels is still under investigation. As DHA is necessary for the growth and maturation of infant's brain and retina, it is an important LC-PUFA during pregnancy and fetal development [102].

The relationship remains weak probably because of the "diluted" impact of genetic variation on DHA status [76]. In fact, only two previous studies reported an association between single *FADS* SNPs, DHA levels, and fetal development [99,103]. Particularly, Molto-Puigmarti et al. showed that, among carriers of the minor allele of the rs174556 polymorphism, newborns from mothers with higher DHA intake were heavier than those born to mothers with lower DHA intake [99]. However, DHA intake was not significantly associated with birthweight in carriers of the wild-type allele [104].

Early-life nutrition, genetic variants, and fetal programming

Several evidence suggest that the interaction between metabolism and genetic variability is complex, with several implications for nutrient requirements [105–107]. Of most interest, maternal nutritional factors have been related to health in later stages of life such as infancy and adulthood [108]. In the last 20 years, a growing body of evidence suggests that the intrauterine environment, including early nutrition, has a significant and lasting effect on the long-term health of the growing fetus and the development of chronic diseases in later life [109], such as cancer [110,111], diabetes [112,113], and nonalcoholic fatty liver disease [114,115]. This concept, known as fetal programming, implies that, during fetal development, permanent changes in molecular, cellular, and physiological mechanisms result from adverse intrauterine conditions. These changes may have long-term consequences, increasing the risk for developing adult life diseases [116]. Recent evidence suggests that IUGR could be associated with persistent changes in tissue structure and functionality, while a maternal obesogenic environment is most likely to be associated with metabolic reprogramming of glucose and lipid metabolism, increasing the long-term risk of metabolic syndrome, fatty liver, and insulin resistance [117]. Particularly, maternal feeding schedule has powerful effects on fetal physiology by influencing both maternal and fetal circadian rhythms [118]. In mammals, the circadian timing system is hierarchically coordinated by the suprachiasmatic nuclei of the hypothalamus, which controls peripheral organs such as the heart, lung, liver, kidney, pancreas, and uterus [119]. In these organs, circadian clock is regulated by transcriptional and translational feedback loops of key "clock genes." During pregnancy, the disruption of these rhythms leads to negative implications for long-life circadian, endocrine, and metabolic functions [120].

Although causal relationships have not been firmly established, a large number of studies provided novel insights into the epigenetic contributions to the mechanism of early-life predisposition to adult disease risk. The role of nutrients is clearly implicated in fetal programming [121], and the intake of several dietary factors (i.e., folate), as well as the effect of MTHFR polymorphisms, has been shown to affect the establishment of DNA methylation patterns in women of childbearing age [122,123]. The importance of one-carbon metabolism in fetal programming was reported through evidence indicating that maternal folate, vitamin B12, methionine, and choline levels were strongly associated to global and gene-specific methylation [124–129]. In addition, other groups reported that also LC-PUFA-induced DNA methylation changes in offsprings [130,131].

With regard to the effect of genetic variants in genes of nutrient metabolism, a study by Van Mil et al. reported a significant association between the maternal MTHFR C677T genotype and neonatal DNA methylation levels of fetal growth and neurodevelopmental genes. However, the researchers did not take into account the risk of adverse pregnancy outcomes [132]. To date, only the study by Chen et al. conducted on NTD-affected fetuses reported that MTHFR genotype contributes to global DNA hypomethylation, increasing the risk of NTDs [133].

In conclusion, although there is a substantial interest, lack of evidence already exists on gene–nutrient interaction and fetal health. Therefore, further researches are recommended to confirm the previously reported results and to investigate the relationship between genetic variants in genes of nutrient metabolisms, DNA methylation, fetal development, and health.

References

[1] McArdle HJ, Ashworth CJ. Micronutrients in fetal growth and development. Br Med Bull 1999;55:499–510.
[2] Stover PJ. Polymorphisms in 1-carbon metabolism, epigenetics and folate-related pathologies. J Nutrigenetics Nutrigenomics 2012;4:293–305.
[3] Wu G, Imhoff-Kunsch B, Girard AW. Biological mechanisms for nutritional regulation of maternal health and fetal development. Paediatr Perinat Epidemiol 2012;26:4–26.
[4] Alfaradhi MZ, Ozanne SE. Developmental programming in response to maternal overnutrition. Front Genet 2011;2.
[5] Berti C, et al. Micronutrients in pregnancy: current knowledge and unresolved questions. Clin Nutr 2011;30:689–701.

[6] Berti C, et al. Pregnancy and infants' outcome: nutritional and metabolic implications. Crit Rev Food Sci Nutr 2016;56:82–91.
[7] Yamada H, Sata F, Saijo Y, Kishi R, Minakami H. Genetic factors in fetal growth restriction and miscarriage. Semin Thromb Hemost 2005;31:334–45.
[8] Edwards DRV, et al. Polymorphisms in maternal and fetal genes encoding for proteins involved in extracellular matrix metabolism alter the risk for small-for-gestational-age. J Matern Fetal Neonatal Med 2011;24:362–80.
[9] Navarrete-Muñoz EM, et al. High doses of folic acid in the periconceptional period and risk of low weight for gestational age at birth in a population based cohort study. Eur J Nutr 2017;0:0.
[10] Langley-Evans SC. Nutrition in early life and the programming of adult disease: a review. J Hum Nutr Diet 2015;28:1–14.
[11] Homocysteine Studies Collaboration. Homocysteine and risk of ischemic heart disease and stroke: a meta-analysis. J Am Med Assoc 2002;288:2015–22.
[12] Kim J, et al. Dietary intake of folate and alcohol, MTHFR C677T polymorphism, and colorectal cancer risk in Korea. Am J Clin Nutr 2012;95:405–12.
[13] Jaenisch R, Bird A. Epigenetic regulation of gene expression: how the genome integrates intrinsic and environmental signals. Nat Genet 2003;33:245–54.
[14] Sun M, Kraus WL. From discovery to function: the expanding roles of long noncoding RNAs in physiology and disease. Endocr Rev 2015;36:25–64.
[15] Koukoura O, et al. Loss of imprinting and aberrant methylation of IGF2 in placentas from pregnancies complicated with fetal growth restriction. Int J Mol Med 2011;28:481–7.
[16] Koukoura O, et al. Hypomethylation along with increased H19 expression in placentas from pregnancies complicated with fetal growth restriction. Placenta 2011;32:51–7.
[17] Lambertini L, et al. Differential methylation of imprinted genes in growth-restricted placentas. Reprod Sci 2011;18:1111–7.
[18] Banister CE, et al. Infant growth restriction is associated with distinct patterns of DNA methylation in human placentas. Epigenetics 2011;6:920–7.
[19] McAninch D, Roberts CT, Bianco-Miotto T. Mechanistic insight into long noncoding RNAs and the placenta. Int J Mol Sci 2017;18.
[20] Bouckenheimer J, et al. Long non-coding RNAs in human early embryonic development and their potential in ART. Hum Reprod Update 2016;23:19–40.
[21] Kafer GR, Lehnert SA, Pantaleon M, Kaye PL, Moser RJ. Expression of genes coding for histone variants and histone-associated proteins in pluripotent stem cells and mouse preimplantation embryos. Gene Expr Patterns 2010;10:299–305.
[22] Mouillet JF, et al. The levels of hypoxia-regulated microRNAs in plasma of pregnant women with fetal growth restriction. Placenta 2010;31:781–4.
[23] Hromadnikova I, Kotlabova K, Doucha J, Dlouha K, Krofta L. Absolute and relative quantification of placenta-specific microRNAs in maternal circulation with placental insufficiency - related complications. J Mol Diagnostics 2012;14:160–7.
[24] Barchitta M, Maugeri A, Quattrocchi A, Agrifoglio O, Agodi A. The role of miRNAs as biomarkers for pregnancy outcomes: a comprehensive review. Int J Genomics 2017. https://doi.org/10.1155/2017/8067972.
[25] Pinney SE, Jaeckle Santos LJ, Han Y, Stoffers DA, Simmons RA. Exendin-4 increases histone acetylase activity and reverses epigenetic modifications that silence Pdx1 in the intrauterine growth retarded rat. Diabetologia 2011;54:2606–14.
[26] Sohi G, Marchand K, Revesz A, Arany E, Hardy DB. Maternal protein restriction elevates cholesterol in adult rat offspring due to repressive changes in histone modifications at the cholesterol 7alpha-hydroxylase promoter. Mol Endocrinol 2011;25:785–98.

[27] Sebert S, Sharkey D, Budge H, Symonds ME. The early programming of metabolic health: is epigenetic setting the missing link? Am J Clin Nutr 2011;94.
[28] Sundrani DP, Chavan Gautam PM, Mehendale SS, Joshi SR. Altered metabolism of maternal micronutrients and omega 3 fatty acids epigenetically regulate matrix metalloproteinases in preterm pregnancy: a novel hypothesis. Med Hypotheses 2011;77:878−83.
[29] Yan J, et al. Maternal choline intake modulates maternal and fetal biomarkers of choline metabolism in humans. Am J Clin Nutr 2012;95:1060−71.
[30] Chen JH, Martin-Gronert MS, Tarry-Adkins J, Ozanne SE. Maternal protein restriction affects postnatal growth and the expression of key proteins involved in lifespan regulation in mice. PloS One 2009;4.
[31] Weisberg IS, et al. The 1298A → C polymorphism in methylenetetrahydrofolate reductase (MTHFR): in vitro expression and association with homocysteine. Atherosclerosis 2001;156:409−15.
[32] Sunden SL, Renduchintala MS, Park EI, Miklasz SD, Garrow Ta. Betaine-homocysteine methyltransferase expression in porcine and human tissues and chromosomal localization of the human gene. Arch Biochem Biophys 1997;345:171−4.
[33] Holm PI, et al. Betaine as a determinant of postmethionine load total plasma homocysteine before and after B-vitamin supplementation. Arterioscler Thromb Vasc Biol 2004;24:301−7.
[34] Steenge GR, Verhoef P, Katan MB. Betaine supplementation lowers plasma homocysteine in healthy men and women. J Nutr 2003;133:1291−5.
[35] Shelnutt KP, et al. Folate status response to controlled folate intake is affected by the methylenetetrahydrofolate reductase 677C−>T polymorphism in young women. J Nutr 2003;133:4107−11.
[36] Jacques PF, et al. Determinants of plasma total homocysteine concentration in the Framingham Offspring cohort. Am J Clin Nutr 2001;73:613−21.
[37] Yi P, et al. Increase in plasma homocysteine associated with parallel increases in plasma S-adenosylhomocysteine and lymphocyte DNA hypomethylation. J Biol Chem 2000;275:29318−23.
[38] Liu J, Ward RL. Folate and one-carbon metabolism and its impact on aberrant DNA methylation in cancer. Adv Genet 2010;71.
[39] Nazki FH, Sameer AS, Ganaie BA. Folate: metabolism, genes, polymorphisms and the associated diseases. Gene 2014;533:11−20.
[40] Johnson WG. Teratogenic alleles and neurodevelopmental disorders. Bioessays 2003;25:464−77.
[41] Gris JC, et al. Antiphospholipid/antiprotein antibodies, hemostasis-related autoantibodies, and plasma homocysteine as risk factors for a first early pregnancy loss: a matched case-control study. Blood 2003;102:3504−13.
[42] Steegers-Theunissen RPM, et al. Maternal hyperhomocysteinemia: a risk factor for neural-tube defects? Metabolism 1994;43:1475−80.
[43] Mills JL, et al. Homocysteine metabolism in pregnancies complicated by neural-tube defects. Lancet 1995;345:149−51.
[44] Wouters MG, et al. Hyperhomocysteinemia: a risk factor in women with unexplained recurrent early pregnancy loss. Fertil Steril 1993;60:820−5.
[45] Botto LD, Yang Q5. 10-Methylenetetrahydrofolate reductase gene variants and congenital anomalies: a HuGE review. Am J Epidemiol 2000;151:862−77.
[46] van der Put NM, et al. A second common mutation in the methylenetetrahydrofolate reductase gene: an additional risk factor for neural-tube defects? Am J Hum Genet 1998;62:1044−51.

[47] Weisberg I, Tran P, Christensen B, Sibani S, Rozen R. A second genetic polymorphism in methylenetetrahydrofolate reductase (MTHFR) associated with decreased enzyme activity. Mol Genet Metabol 1998;64:169–72.
[48] Cortese C, Motti C. MTHFR gene polymorphism, homocysteine and cardiovascular disease. Publ Health Nutr 2001;4:493–7.
[49] van der Put NMJ, et al. Mutated methylenetetrahydrofolate reductase as a risk factor for spina bifida. Lancet 1995;346:1070–1.
[50] Whitehead a S, et al. A genetic defect in 5,10 methylenetetrahydrofolate reductase in neural tube defects. QJM 1995;88:763–6.
[51] Martinelli M, et al. C677T variant form at the MTHFR gene and CL/P: a risk factor for mothers? Am J Med Genet 2001;98:357–60.
[52] Scott JM, et al. MTRR and MTHFR polymorphism: link to Down syndrome? Am J Med Genet 2002;107:151–5.
[53] Wenstrom KD, et al. Amniotic fluid homocysteine levels, 5,10-methylenetetrahydrafolate reductase genotypes, and neural tube closure sites. Am J Med Genet 2000;90:6–11.
[54] Nelen WL, et al. Genetic risk factor for unexplained recurrent early pregnancy loss. Lancet 1996;350:861–9.
[55] Lissak A, et al. Polymorphism for mutation of cytosine to thymine at location 677 in the methylenetetrahydrofolate reductase gene is associated with recurrent early fetal loss. Am J Obstet Gynecol 1999;181:126–30.
[56] Murphy RP, et al. Prospective evaluation of the risk conferred by factor V Leiden and thermolabile methylenetetrahydrofolate reductase polymorphisms in pregnancy. Arterioscler Thromb Vasc Biol 2000;20:266–70.
[57] Alfirevic Z, et al. Postnatal screening for thrombophilia in women with severe pregnancy complications. Obstet Gynecol 2001;97:753–9.
[58] Gris JC, et al. Case-control study of the frequency of thrombophilic disorders in couples with late foetal loss and no thrombotic antecedent. Thromb Haemostasis 1999;81:891–9.
[59] Isotalo PA, Wells GA, Donnelly JG. Neonatal and fetal methylenetetrahydrofolate reductase genetic polymorphisms: an examination of C677T and A1298C mutations. Am J Hum Genet 2000;67:986–90.
[60] Zetterberg H, et al. Increased frequency of combined methylenetetrahydrofolate reductase C677T and A1298C mutated alleles in spontaneously aborted embryos. Eur J Hum Genet 2002;10:113–8.
[61] Sukla KK, Tiwari PK, Kumar A, Raman R. Low birthweight (LBW) and neonatal hyperbilirubinemia (NNH) in an Indian cohort: association of homocysteine, its metabolic pathway genes and micronutrients as risk factors. PloS One 2013;8.
[62] Kordas K, et al. Methylenetetrahydrofolate reductase (MTHFR) C677T, A1298C and G1793A genotypes, and the relationship between maternal folate intake, tibia lead and infant size at birth. Br J Nutr 2009;102:907–14.
[63] Yajnik CS, Deshmukh US. Fetal programming: maternal nutrition and role of one-carbon metabolism. Rev Endocr Metab Disord 2012;13:121–7.
[64] Shaw GM, et al. Choline and risk of neural tube defects in a folate-fortified population. Epidemiology 2009;20:714–9.
[65] Shaw GM, et al. Nested case-control study of one-carbon metabolites in mid-pregnancy and risks of cleft lip with and without cleft palate. Pediatr Res 2009;66:501–6.
[66] Zeisel SH. Choline: critical role during fetal development and dietary requirements in adults. Annu Rev Nutr 2006;26:229–50.

[67] Kohlmeier M, da Costa K-A, Fischer LM, Zeisel SH. Genetic variation of folate-mediated one-carbon transfer pathway predicts susceptibility to choline deficiency in humans. Proc Natl Acad Sci U S A 2005;102:16025–30.
[68] Ivanov A, Nash-Barboza S, Hinkis S, Caudill MA. Genetic variants in phosphatidylethanolamine N-methyltransferase and methylenetetrahydrofolate dehydrogenase influence biomarkers of choline metabolism when folate intake is restricted. J Am Diet Assoc 2009;109:313–8.
[69] Brody LC, et al. A polymorphism, R653Q, in the trifunctional enzyme methylenetetrahydrofolate dehydrogenase/methenyltetrahydrofolate cyclohydrolase/formyltetrahydrofolate synthetase is a maternal genetic risk factor for neural tube defects: report of the Birth Defects. Res. *Am. J. Hum. Genet.* 2002;71:1207–15.
[70] Mills JL, et al. Folate-related gene polymorphisms as risk factors for cleft lip and cleft palate. Birth Defects Res Part A - Clin Mol Teratol 2008;82:636–43.
[71] Victorino DB, De Godoy MF, Goloni-Bertollo EM, Pavarino ÉC. Genetic polymorphisms involved in folate metabolism and maternal risk for down syndrome: a meta-analysis. Dis Markers 2014;2014.
[72] Meng J, Han L, Zhuang B. Association between MTHFD1 polymorphisms and neural tube defect susceptibility. J Neurol Sci 2015;348:188–94.
[73] Zheng J, et al. MTHFD1 polymorphism as maternal risk for neural tube defects: a meta-analysis. Neurol Sci 2015;36:607–16.
[74] Yan J, Winter LB, Burns-Whitmore B, Vermeylen F, Caudill MA. Plasma choline metabolites associate with metabolic stress among young overweight men in a genotype-specific manner. Nutr Diabetes 2012;2:e49.
[75] Mills JL, et al. Maternal choline concentrations during pregnancy and choline-related genetic variants as risk factors for neural tube defects. Am J Clin Nutr 2014;100:1069–74.
[76] Lattka E, Illig T, Heinrich J, Koletzko B. Do FADS genotypes enhance our knowledge about fatty acid related phenotypes? Clin Nutr 2010;29:277–87.
[77] Lattka E, Illig T, Heinrich J, Koletzko B. FADS gene cluster polymorphisms: important modulators of fatty acid levels and their impact on atopic diseases. J Nutrigenetics Nutrigenomics 2009;2:119–28.
[78] Koletzko B, et al. The roles of long-chain polyunsaturated fatty acids in pregnancy, lactation and infancy: review of current knowledge and consensus recommendations. J Perinat Med 2008;36:5–14.
[79] Jensen RG. Lipids in human milk. Lipids 1999;34:1243–71.
[80] Innis SM. Essential fatty acids in growth and development. Prog Lipid Res 1991;30:39–103.
[81] Innis SM. Fatty acids and early human development. Early Hum Dev 2007;83:761–6.
[82] Innis SM. Metabolic programming of long-term outcomes due to fatty acid nutrition in early life. Matern Child Nutr 2011;7:112–23.
[83] Haggarty P. Fatty acid supply to the human fetus. Annu Rev Nutr 2010;30:237–55.
[84] Nakamura MT, Nara TY. Structure, function, and dietary regulation of delta6, delta5, and delta9 desaturases. Annu Rev Nutr 2004;24:345–76.
[85] Cho HP, Nakamura M, Clarke SD. Cloning, expression, and fatty acid regulation of the human delta-5 desaturase. J Biol Chem 1999;274:37335–9.
[86] Van Eijsden M, Hornstra G, Van der Wal MF, Vrijkotte TG, Bonsel GJ. Maternal n-3, n-6, and trans fatty acid profile early in pregnancy and term birth weight: a prospective cohort study. Am J Clin Nutr 2008;87:887–95.
[87] Marquardt A, Stöhr H, White K, Weber BH. cDNA cloning, genomic structure, and chromosomal localization of three members of the human fatty acid desaturase family. Genomics 2000;66:175–83.

[88] Malerba G, et al. SNPs of the FADS gene cluster are associated with polyunsaturated fatty acids in a cohort of patients with cardiovascular disease. Lipids 2008;43:289–99.
[89] Tanaka T, et al. Genome-wide association study of plasma polyunsaturated fatty acids in the InCHIANTI study. PLoS Genet 2009;5.
[90] Illig T, et al. A genome-wide perspective of genetic variation in human metabolism. Nat Genet 2010;42:137–41.
[91] Martinelli N, et al. FADS genotypes and desaturase activity estimated by the ratio of arachidonic acid to linoleic acid are associated with inflammation and coronary artery disease. Am J Clin Nutr 2008;88:941–9.
[92] Standl M, et al. FADS1 FADS2 gene cluster, PUFA intake and blood lipids in children: results from the GINIplus and LISAplus studies. PloS One 2012;7.
[93] Glaser C, Heinrich J, Koletzko B. Role of FADS1 and FADS2 polymorphisms in polyunsaturated fatty acid metabolism. Metab Clin Exp 2010;59:993–9.
[94] Howard TD, et al. DNA methylation in an enhancer region of the FADS cluster is associated with FADS activity in human liver. PloS One 2014;9.
[95] Lattka E, et al. Genetic variants in the FADS gene cluster are associated with arachidonic acid concentrations of human breast milk at 1.5 and 6 mo postpartum and influence the course of milk dodecanoic, tetracosenoic, and trans-9-octadecenoic acid concentrations over the. Am J Clin Nutr 2011;93:382–91.
[96] Reardon HT, et al. Insertion-deletions in a FADS2 intron 1 conserved regulatory locus control expression of fatty acid desaturases 1 and 2 and modulate response to simvastatin. Prostagl Leukot Essent Fat Acids 2012;87:25–33.
[97] Koletzko B, Lattka E, Zeilinger S, Illig T, Steer C. Genetic variants of the fatty acid desaturase gene cluster predict amounts of red blood cell docosahexaenoic and other polyunsaturated fatty acids in pregnant women: findings from the Avon Longitudinal Study of Parents and Children. Am J Clin Nutr 2011;93:211–9.
[98] Lattka E, et al. Umbilical cord PUFA are determined by maternal and child fatty acid desaturase (FADS) genetic variants in the Avon Longitudinal Study of Parents and Children (ALSPAC). Br J Nutr 2013;109:1196–210.
[99] Moltó-Puigmartí C, et al. FADS1 FADS2 gene variants modify the association between fish intake and the docosahexaenoic acid proportions in human milk. Am J Clin Nutr 2010;91:1368–76.
[100] Yeates AJ, et al. Genetic variation in FADS genes is associated with maternal long-chain PUFA status but not with cognitive development of infants in a high fish-eating observational study. Prostagl Leukot Essent Fat Acids 2015;102–103:13–20.
[101] Steer CD, Lattka E, Koletzko B, Golding J, Hibbeln JR. Maternal fatty acids in pregnancy, FADS polymorphisms, and child intelligence quotient at 8 y of age1-3. Am J Clin Nutr 2013;98:1575–82.
[102] Larque E, Demmelmair H, Koletzko B. Perinatal supply and metabolism of long-chain polyunsaturated fatty acids: importance for the early development of the nervous system. Ann N Y Acad Sci 2002;967:299–310.
[103] Xie L, Innis SM. Genetic variants of the FADS1 FADS2 gene cluster Are associated with altered (n-6) and (n-3) essential fatty acids in plasma and erythrocyte phospholipids in women during pregnancy and in breast milk during lactation 1,2. J Nutr 2008;138:2222–8.
[104] Molto-Puigmarti C, et al. Maternal but not fetal FADS gene variants modify the association between maternal long-chain PUFA intake in pregnancy and birth weight. J Nutr 2014;144:1430–7.
[105] Agodi A, et al. Increase in the prevalence of the MTHFR 677 TT polymorphism in women born since 1959: potential implications for folate requirements. Eur J Clin Nutr 2011;65:1302–8.

[106] Agodi A, et al. Dietary folate intake and blood biomarkers reveal high-risk groups in a mediterranean population of healthy women of childbearing potential. Ann Nutr Metab 2013;63:179–85.
[107] Barchitta M, Quattrocchi A, Adornetto V, Marchese AE, Agodi A. Tumor necrosis factor-alpha 308 G >A polymorphism, adherence toMediterranean diet, and risk of overweight/obesity in young women. BioMed Res Int 2014;2014.
[108] Harding J. The nutritional basis of the fetal origins of adult disease. Int J Epidemiol 2001;30:15–23.
[109] Seki Y, Williams L, Vuguin PM, Charron MJ. Minireview: epigenetic programming of diabetes and obesity: animal models. Endocrinology 2012;153:1031–8.
[110] Dessypris N, et al. Association of maternal and index child's diet with subsequent leukemia risk: a systematic review and meta analysis. Cancer Epidemiology 2017;47:64–75.
[111] Nguyen NM, et al. Maternal intake of high n-6 polyunsaturated fatty acid diet during pregnancy causes transgenerational increase in mammary cancer risk in mice. Breast Cancer Res 2017;19.
[112] Huang Y, et al. Maternal high folic acid supplement promotes glucose intolerance and insulin resistance in male mouse offspring fed a high-fat diet. Int J Mol Sci 2014;15:6298–313.
[113] Dunn GA, Bale TL. Maternal high-fat diet promotes body length increases and insulin insensitivity in second-generation mice. Endocrinology 2009;150:4999–5009.
[114] Mouralidarane A, et al. Maternal obesity programs offspring non-alcoholic fatty liver disease through disruption of 24-h rhythms in mice. Int J Obes 2015;39:1339–48.
[115] Soeda J, et al. Hepatic rhythmicity of endoplasmic reticulum stress is disrupted in perinatal and adult mice models of high-fat diet-induced obesity. Int J Food Sci Nutr 2017;68:455–66.
[116] Warner MJ, Ozanne SE. Mechanisms involved in the developmental programming of adulthood disease. Biochem J 2010;427:333–47.
[117] Sookoian S, Gianotti TF, Burgueño AL, Pirola CJ. Fetal metabolic programming and epigenetic modifications: a systems biology approach. Pediatr Res 2013;73:531–42.
[118] Ohta H, et al. Maternal feeding controls fetal biological clock. PloS One 2008;3.
[119] Hastings M, O'Neill JS, Maywood ES. Circadian clocks: regulators of endocrine and metabolic rhythms. J Endocrinol 2007;195:187–98.
[120] Varcoe TJ, Gatford KL, Kennaway DJ. Maternal circadian rhythms and the programming of adult health and disease. Am J Physiol - Regul Integr Comp Physiol 2017. https://doi.org/10.1152/ajpregu.00248.2017. ajpregu.00248.2017.
[121] Mcmillen IC. Developmental origins of the metabolic syndrome: prediction, plasticity, and programming. Physiol Rev 2005;85:571–633.
[122] Agodi A, et al. Low fruit consumption and folate deficiency are associated with LINE-1 hypomethylation in women of a cancer-free population. Genes Nutr 2015;10(5):480.
[123] Agodi A, Quattrocchi A, Maugeri A, Barchitta M. The link between MTHFR C677T polymorphism, folate metabolism and global DNA methylation: a literature review. In: Methylenetetrahydrofolate reductase (MTHFR) in health and disease; 2015. p. 71–81.
[124] Sinclair KD, et al. DNA methylation, insulin resistance, and blood pressure in offspring determined by maternal periconceptional B vitamin and methionine status. Proc Natl Acad Sci Unit States Am 2007;104:19351–6.
[125] Lillycrop KA, Phillips ES, Jackson AA, Hanson MA, Burdge GC. Dietary protein restriction of pregnant rats induces and folic acid supplementation prevents epigenetic modification of hepatic gene expression in the offspring. J Nutr 2005;135:1382–6.

[126] Cooper WN, et al. DNA methylation profiling at imprinted loci after periconceptional micronutrient supplementation in humans: results of a pilot randomized controlled trials. World Rev Nutr Diet 2014;109:2—3.
[127] Fryer AA, et al. LINE-1 DNA methylation is inversely correlated with cord plasma homocysteine in man: a preliminary study. Epigenetics 2009;4:394—8.
[128] Mehedint MG, Craciunescu C, Zeisel SH. Maternal dietary choline deficiency alters angiogenesis in fetal mouse hippocampus. Proc Natl Acad Sci U S A 2010;107:12834—9.
[129] Niculescu MD, Craciunescu CN, Zeisel SH. Dietary choline deficiency alters global and gene-specific DNA methylation in the developing hippocampus of mouse fetal brains. Faseb J 2006;20:43—9.
[130] Hoile SP, et al. Supplementation with N-3 long-chain polyunsaturated fatty acids or olive oil in men and women with renal disease induces differential changes in the DNA methylation of FADS2 and ELOVL5 in peripheral blood mononuclear cells. PloS One 2014;9:e109896.
[131] Lee HS, et al. Modulation of DNA methylation states and infant immune system by dietary supplementation with v-3 PUFA during pregnancy in an intervention study. Am J Clin Nutr 2013;98:480—7.
[132] Van Mil NH, et al. Determinants of maternal pregnancy one-carbon metabolism and newborn human DNA methylation profiles. Reproduction 2014;148:581—92.
[133] Chen X, et al. Global DNA hypomethylation is associated with NTD-affected pregnancy: a case-control study. Birth Defects Res Part A - Clin Mol Teratol 2010;88:575—81.
[134] Agodi A, et al. Distribution of p53, GST, and MTHFR polymorphisms and risk of cervical intraepithelial lesions in sicily. Int J Gynecol Cancer 2010;20(1):141—6.
[135] Barchitta M, Maugeri, et al. Dietary folate intake and folic acid supplements among pregnant women from Southern Italy: Evidence from the "Mamma & Bambino" cohort. Int J Environ Res Public Health 2020;17(2):638.
[136] Barchitta, et al. Single nucleotide polymorphisms in vitamin D receptor gene affect birth weight and the risk of preterm birth: results from the "Mamma & Bambino" cohort and a meta-analysis. Nutrients 2018;10(9):1172.
[137] Maugeri A, Barchitta M, Blanco I, Agodi A. Effects of vitamin D supplementation during pregnancy on birth size: a systematic review and meta-analysis of randomized controlled trials. Nutrients 2019;11(2):442.
[138] Maugeri, et al. Maternal dietary patterns are associated with pre-pregnancy body mass index and gestational weight gain: results from the "Mamma & Bambino" cohort. Nutrients 2019;11(6):1308. https://doi.org/10.3390/nu11061308. Published 2019 Jun 10.

CHAPTER 13

Pregnancy loss and polymorphisms in folic acid genes

Fabio Coppedè
Department of Translational Research and of New Surgical and Medical Technologies, Section of Medical Genetics, University of Pisa, Pisa, Italy

Contents

Introduction

Folate is the general term for vitamin B9, a water-soluble compound which is naturally found in green leafy vegetables, beans, cereals, liver, egg yolks, some citric fruits, kiwis, and strawberries [1]. Dietary folates are essential for normal cell growth and replication, since they work as donors and acceptors of one-carbon units during the synthesis of nucleic acids, amino acids, and *S*-adenosylmethionine (SAM), the main intracellular methylating agent (Fig. 13.1). Therefore, a folate restriction results in aberrant cell growth, leads to hyperhomocysteinemia (Hhcy), impairs DNA methylation, and increases the rate of point mutations, chromosome damage, and aneuploidy [1]. DNA methylation is an epigenetic mechanism consisting of the

Molecular Nutrition
ISBN 978-0-12-813862-5
https://doi.org/10.1016/B978-0-12-813862-5.00013-X

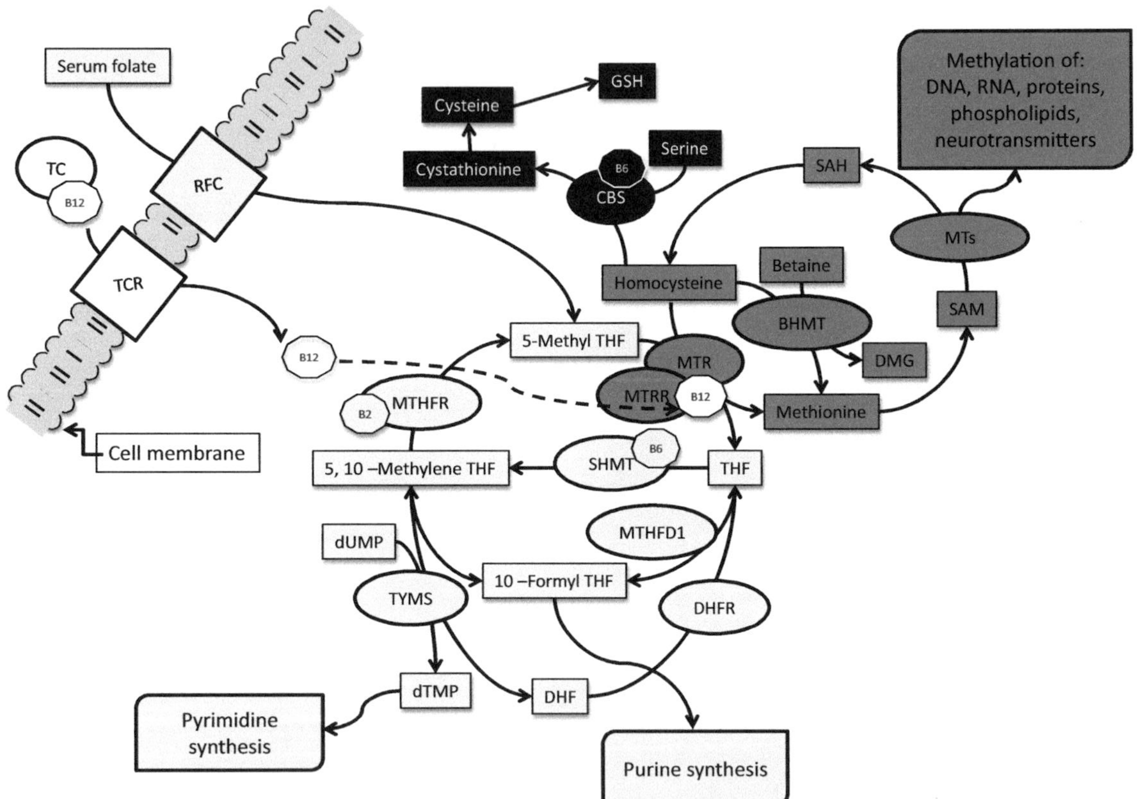

Figure 13.1 ***Overview of the folate metabolic pathway.*** The "DNA synthesis" pathway is shown in light gray and the "homocysteine remethylation" pathway in dark grey. The black color is used for the "transsulfuration" pathway, while cobalamin metabolism is shown in white (see the text for details). Enzymes: *BHMT*, betaine-homocysteine methyltransferase; *CBS*, cystathionine β-synthase; *DHFR*,

dihydrofolate reductase; *MTHFD1*, methylenetetrahydrofolate dehydrogenase; *MTHFR*, methylenetetrahydrofolate reductase; *MTR*, methionine synthase; *MTRR*, methionine synthase reductase; *MTs*, methyltransferases; *RFC1*, reduced folate carrier; *SHMT*, serine hydroxymethyltransferase; *TC*, transcobalamin; *TCR*, transcobalamin receptor; *TYMS*, thymidylate synthase. Metabolites: *DHF*, dihydrofolate; *dTMP*, deoxythymidine monophosphate; *dUMP*, deoxyuridine monophosphate; *GSH*, glutathione; *THF*, tetrahydrofolate; *SAH, S*-adenosyl homocysteine; *SAM, S*-adenosylmethionine. Cofactors: *B2*, vitamin *B2; B6*, vitamin *B6; B12*, vitamin *B12* or cobalamin. *(Adapted from Coppedè F. The genetics of folate metabolism and maternal risk of birth of a child with Down syndrome and associated congenital heart defects. Front Genet 2015;6:223.)*

addition of a methyl group to the DNA, mainly to cytosine in a CpG dinucleotide context, mediated by enzymes called DNA methyltransferases and allowing a cell-specific regulation of gene expression levels. Particularly, DNA methylation induces chromatin condensation and gene silencing and represents a physiological mechanism required for embryonic development, cell differentiation, X-chromosome inactivation, genomic imprinting, repression of repetitive elements, and maintenance of the cellular identity [2]. Owing to the functions of folate in DNA synthesis, DNA methylation, and cell division, the need for this vitamin increases during pregnancy to support enlargement of the uterus, and development of the placenta and fetus [3]. For these reasons numerous studies have investigated the associations between polymorphisms of genes involved in folate metabolism and risk of human aneuploidy, trisomy 21, spontaneous abortion, and recurrent pregnancy loss (RPL) [4,5]. RPL is a highly heterogeneous condition defined as two or more successive clinical pregnancy losses before 20 weeks of gestation and affects 1%–2% of fertile women worldwide [5]. RPL could be due to chromosome abnormalities in the parents, uterine alterations, infections, and endocrinological and autoimmune diseases; nevertheless, approximately 50% of RPL cases remain unexplained and are called idiopathic [5]. Several investigators reported increased homocysteine (hcy) levels as a risk factor for RPL, and common polymorphisms in folate-related genes have been investigated for their contribution to Hhcy, aneuploidy, and RPL [6,7]. This chapter provides an update of studies investigating genes involved in folate/hcy metabolism as risk factors for RPL. Some of these polymorphisms have been extensively investigated, with dozens of available case–control studies, and in such cases this chapter will critically discuss their most recent systematic reviews and meta-analyses in order to provide a general overview of their contribution to RPL in different ethnic groups, rather than a boring discussion of each single study. Other polymorphisms have been less frequently investigated, some of them in only one or a few case–control studies, so that general considerations cannot yet be drawn. For these polymorphisms, the limits of the available literature will be critically discussed. The frequency of certain of the described polymorphisms varies among different populations and this might help explaining ethnic or regional effects in the magnitude of the associated RPL risk, but the most important factor to take into account when assessing their potential contribution to RPL risk is the gene-nutrient interaction. Indeed, a proper dietary intake of foods rich in folate, or a proper supplementation with folic acid during pregnancy, can mask or minimize the effect of certain polymorphisms, such as the *MTHFR* 677C>T one. By contrast, the effect of this polymorphism is exacerbated in poor countries, without governmental programs of food fortification with folic acid, or characterized by a scarce availability of high quality foods for the general population [4,8].

Folate metabolism: an overview

Fig. 13.1 provides a general overview of the complex folate metabolic pathway [4], which is summarized below. Before discussing folate metabolism, it is also worth to clarify that the term folate is used for the naturally occurring vitamin found in foods, while the term folic acid refers to the synthetic form of vitamin B9 that is found in fortified foods or as dietary supplements. According to the recommendations of the World Health Organization, all women, from the moment they begin trying to conceive until 12 weeks of gestation, should take a folic acid supplement (400 μg folic acid daily) in order to prevent birth defects or congenital malformations such as neural tube defects, and for this reason several countries have introduced mandatory folic acid fortification of flour, while in other countries a daily intake of 400 μg of folic acid is recommended to women when planning a pregnancy [9]. After absorption in the intestinal lumen, dietary folates are reduced and methylated into the liver to form 5-methyltetrahydrofolate (5-MTHF), which is the main circulating form taken up by the cells through folate carriers or receptors, such as the ubiquitously expressed carrier (solute carrier family 19 member 1: SLC19A1), commonly known as reduced folate carrier (RFC1). Inside the cells, 5-MTHF functions as a methyl donor for hcy remethylation in a reaction catalyzed by the methionine synthase/methionine synthase reductase complex (MTR/MTRR) that requires cobalamin (vitamin B12) as a cofactor to produce methionine and tetrahydrofolate (THF). Once generated, methionine can be converted to SAM, the main intracellular methylating agent (Fig. 13.1). Hcy can also enter the transsulfuration pathway and be condensed with serine to form cystathionine in a reaction catalyzed by cystathionine β-synthase (CBS), which requires vitamin B6 as a cofactor. Cystathionine is then hydrolyzed to cysteine, the precursor of the antioxidant compound glutathione (GSH). Folate metabolism is also essential for the synthesis of nucleic acid precursors, and THF, resulting from the MTR/MTRR activity, can be converted to 5,10-methyleneTHF by serine hydroxymethyltransferase (SHMT). Depending on cellular demands, 5,10-methyleneTHF can be used for thymidylate synthesis, for purine synthesis, or for the production of 5-methylTHF, required for hcy remethylation (Fig. 13.1). Particularly, 5,10-methyleneTHF can be reduced to 5-methylTHF by methylenetetrahydrofolate reductase (MTHFR), a vitamin B2 (riboflavin)-dependent enzyme, which is of great importance to shift folate derivatives toward hcy remethylation or DNA synthesis reactions [4]. Many of the enzymes coding for folate-related genes are polymorphic and have been investigated as risk factors for RPL. Each of them will be discussed in details in the following sections.

Genetic polymorphisms in folic acid genes and pregnancy loss

MTHFR polymorphisms

Common polymorphisms of the *MTHFR* gene are by far the most studied as risk factors for pregnancy loss among those in folate-related genes. A functional polymorphism in the *MTHFR* gene, namely 677C>T (rs1801133), results in alanine to valine substitution at position 222 in the MTHFR protein [10,11]. MTHFR works as a dimer which is stabilized by physiological levels of folates, and the mutant TT enzyme is less stable and prone to dissociate into monomers at 37°C, particularly under conditions of reduced folate bioavailability [12,13]. As a consequence, the mutant TT enzyme has a resultant mean activity, which is 40%–50% lower than the wild-type CC one [10], resulting in increased circulating hcy levels [13–15]. Since 1999, the *MTHFR* 677C>T polymorphism has been associated with maternal risk for the birth of a child with Down syndrome (DS), resulting from maternal chromosome 21 malsegregation, and particularly in women subjected to nutritional and/or environmental factors leading to reduced folate bioavailability [16–18].

Numerous studies have investigated the association between the *MTHFR* 677C>T polymorphism and the risk of spontaneous abortion, yielding controversial results, but comprehensive systematic reviews and meta-analyses of those papers are available, all suggesting a potential contribution of the *MTHFR* 677T allele as a risk factor for RPL [6,19–21]. Particularly, in 2013, Cao et al. performed a meta-analysis of 46 published studies addressing the contribution of the *MTHFR* 677C>T polymorphism as a risk factor for unexplained RPL, including a total of 3559 RPL cases and 5097 healthy controls, and observing an overall significant increased risk for the 677T allele [odds ratio (OR) = 1.34; 95% confidence interval (CI) = 1.13–1.58]. A further stratification into ethnic groups confirmed association in East Asian and mixed populations, but not in Caucasians [19]. More recently, 16 articles involving 1420 RPL cases and 1408 controls from China were included in a meta-analysis that revealed a significant increased risk for RPL in carriers of the 677T allele (OR = 1.83; 95% CI = 1.64–2.05) [20]. A similar meta-analysis was performed in the same year, and included 29 Asian studies for a total of 3725 cases and 4105 controls [21]. Again the study revealed a significant association of the *MTHFR* 677T allele with risk of RPL (OR = 1.35; 95% CI = 1.09–1.68) [21]. Another systematic analysis of the literature included a total of 57 articles, and particularly 6078 maternal cases and 9441 female controls, 395 fetal cases and 404 controls, as well as 718 paternal cases and 403 male controls [6]. In the maternal group, the *MTHFR* 677C>T polymorphism showed a significant pooled odds ratio for the homozygous comparison (TT vs. CC: OR = 2.28, 95% CI = 1.70–3.07), and in the paternal group for the heterozygous comparison (CT vs. CC: OR = 1.97, 95% CI = 1.45–2.68). Subgroup stratification for ethnicity in the maternal group revealed association in both Asians (TT vs. CC: OR = 2.78, 95% CI = 1.99–3.89) and Caucasians (TT vs. CC: OR = 1.92, 95% CI = 1.24–2.96) [6]. Taken collectively, systematic analyses of the studies performed so far have provided substantial evidence that the *MTHFR* 677C>T polymorphism is likely a maternal risk factor for RPL in Asian populations, while data in Caucasians are still controversial. However, the frequency of the *MTHFR* 677T allele varies extensively in different countries, according to ethnic and regional differences. For example, it has been reported to range from 1% in eastern India to 17% in northern India [22], and from 25% in southern China to 53% in northern China [23]. It also ranges from 25% to almost 50% according to the different Chinese ethnic groups [23]. Allele frequencies higher than 30% have been often reported for most Caucasian populations, but again regional differences are observed [43]. Despite that these differences might account for a different magnitude in the risk for RPL, the gene–nutrient interaction seems to represent the most important factor. Indeed, a recent meta-analysis that stratified RPL cases according to the development level of the country revealed a significant association of the *MTHFR* 677C>T polymorphism with RPL risk in developing countries (OR = 1.36, 95% CI = 1.22–1.51), but not in developed ones (OR = 0.87, 95% CI = 0.68–1.11), suggesting that folic acid fortification programs, a better living environment, and different dietary regimens can make the difference [24]. In order to understand the gene—environment interaction, it is of fundamental importance to remember that the MTHFR enzyme works as a dimer that is stabilized by physiological levels of folates, and that *MTHFR* 677TT individuals are particularly subjected to dimer destabilization under conditions of reduced folate bioavailability [12].

Another common *MTHFR* polymorphism, the 1298A>C one (rs1801131), results in a glutamate to alanine substitution at codon 429 and is in linkage disequilibrium with the *MTHFR* 677C>T one. Particularly, the *MTHFR* 677T-1298C haplotype is rare, and the double homozygous *MTHFR* 677TT-1298CC genotype leads to MTHFR protein instability and inactivity, often resulting in prenatal death [12]. In 2013, eight relevant studies were available addressing the contribution of the *MTHFR* 1298A>C polymorphism and risk for unexplained RPL, for a total of 1163 RPL cases and 1061 healthy controls; their meta-analysis revealed no association between this polymorphism and RPL risk [19]. Similar negative findings were obtained in a recent meta-analysis of Asian studies, which included a total of 453 RPL cases and 376 controls [20]. Another meta-analysis, that included 16 studies with 2924 maternal cases and 4759 female controls revealed a significant association with maternal RPL risk (CC vs. AA: OR = 1.65; 95% CI = 1.14—2.38), and the C allele was found more frequently also in fetal RPL cases [6]. However, stratification into ethnic groups revealed association only in Caucasian mothers, but not in Asians [6]. More recently, no significant relationship was found between *MTHFR* 1298A>C and RPL (OR = 1.04; 95% CI = 0.93—1.18), even after stratification of the literature into studies performed in developed or developing countries [24]. Collectively, concerning the association between the *MTHFR* 1298A>C polymorphism and RPL risk, results are still largely controversial [6,24]. Additional studies are therefore required to further address this issue. However, we must remember that the *MTHFR* 1298A>C polymorphism is in strong linkage with the *MTHFT* 677C>T one, and that the haplotype containing both mutations (677T-1298C) is very rare in living humans as it leads to a severe enzyme instability, so that genotypes with four 677TT/1298CC or three mutations (677TT/1298AC and 677CT/1298CC) are extremely rare [12]. For all these reasons, assessing the contribution of only *MTHFR* 1298A>C to RPL risk, without investigating for *MTHFR* 677C>T and folate bioavailability, does not really make sense.

MTR and *MTRR* polymorphisms

MTR and MTRR are essential for hcy remethylation to methionine. Particularly, MTR transfers a methyl group from folate cofactors to hcy forming methionine, the precursor of the intracellular methylating agent SAM. Vitamin B12 is a cofactor in this reaction and MTRR is required for the maintenance of MTR in its active state (Fig. 13.1). Two common polymorphisms in these genes, namely *MTR* 2756A>G (rs1805087), leading to Asp919Gly substitution, and *MTRR* 66A>G (rs1801394), resulting in an Ile22Met amino acidic change, have been largely investigated for their contribution to circulating hcy levels and aneuploidy [4]. Large cohort studies in mothers of DS individuals as well as literature meta-analyses revealed that the *MTR* 2756A>G polymorphism is not a maternal risk factor for chromosome 21 malsegregation [18,25], while the *MTRR* 66A>G one was linked to increased maternal risk for trisomy 21 in Caucasian women [26]. Only a few studies have addressed the contribution of these polymorphisms to RPL risk. The analysis of a cohort of 353 RPL patients and 226 control subjects from South Korea reported association of the *MTR* 2756G allele with reduced RPL risk (OR = 0.59; 95% CI = 0.42–0.85) [44], and similar results were observed in a cohort of 125 RPL cases from China (OR = 0.51; 95% CI = 0.27–0.95) [27]. However, no association of the *MTR* 2756A>G polymorphism with RPL risk was observed in 89 women with a history of idiopathic recurrent miscarriage and 150 control women from Brazil [28]. No association of the *MTRR* 66A>G polymorphism with RPL risk was observed in the two previously described Asian studies [27,44], and similar results were obtained by Guo and coworkers in a cohort of 200 Chinese Han couples with unexplained spontaneous recurrent abortion and 76 control couples [29]. However, another case–control study conducted in 118 patients with unexplained recurrent spontaneous abortion and 174 healthy women of Chinese Han origin showed an increased frequency of the *MTRR* 66G allele in the case group [30]. Collectively, concerning both *MTR* and *MTRR* polymorphisms and RPL risk results are still conflicting and the available studies are limited in sample size; furthermore, except for one single study [28], data have been collected almost exclusively in Asian populations, and literature meta-analyses are missing due to the scarce number of available case–control studies. Information on the nutritional status of the mother at peri-conception is a limiting factor in most of these small case–control studies because, as previously discussed for *MTHFR* polymorphisms, dietary restrictions of B-group vitamins or enzymatic cofactors could potentiate the effect of any given polymorphism of this pathway. Alcohol intake should be also evaluated, because it is known to impair MTR activity and the hcy to methionine conversion [4]. Therefore, only future studies empowered in sample size and completed by a food-intake evaluation will clarify whether or not these polymorphisms should be taken into account in the maternal risk for RPL.

RFC1 (SLC19A1) polymorphisms

The ubiquitously expressed reduced folate carrier is the major transport system in mammalian cells and tissues for folate cofactors, and a common *RFC1* 80A>G polymorphism (rs1051266), resulting in Arg27His replacement, was suggested to impair folate uptake [31]. Subsequent studies have linked this polymorphism to the maternal risk of chromosome 21 malsegregation [18,32], making it a good candidate for aneuploidy predisposition and pregnancy loss. Therefore, at least four different case–control studies have addressed the contribution of rs1051266 to RPL risk, but none of them observed a statistically significant difference in allele or genotype distributions between RPL cases and controls [27,33–35]. However, two of these studies reported association between haplotypes generated by three different *RFC1* polymorphisms, namely −43T>C (rs1131596), 80G>A and 696C>T (rs12659), and RPL risk [33,35]. In addition, the two other studies observed that combined genotypes including *MTHFR* 677C>T, *MTHFR* 1298A>C, *RFC1* 80A>G, and *RFC1* 696C>T polymorphisms [34], or *MTHFR* 677C>T, *MTHFR* 1298A>C, *MTR* 2756G>A, and *RFC1* 80A>G polymorphisms [27], respectively, were linked to RPL risk. Despite that these studies are limited in sample size, a possible contribution of *RFC1* polymorphisms or haplotypes to the risk of pregnancy loss cannot be factored out, and further studies are required to clarify this issue.

Transcobalamin (*TCN2*) polymorphisms

Vitamin B12, or cobalamin, is an important cofactor for hcy remethylation in the reaction catalyzed by MTR, and vitamin B12 deficiency can lead to Hhcy thus increasing the risk for RPL [36]. In the circulation, transcobalamin (TC) is the transport protein of vitamin B12, required for its cellular uptake mediated by specific membrane receptors (TCRs) (Fig. 13.1). A common *TCN2* 776C>G polymorphism, resulting in Arg232Pro replacement, has been associated with RPL risk in early studies [37,38], but most recent ones including larger case–control cohorts have failed to find a statistically significant difference in the distribution of this polymorphism between case mothers and control mothers [36,39]. The most recent study in this field, however, revealed association of another *TCN2* polymorphism, namely *TCN2* 67A>G leading to Ile23Val substitution, and RPL risk [36]. The study included 378 RPL cases and 208 controls from South Korea, and revealed an increased frequency of the *TCN2* 67G allele in the case group (OR = 3.30; 95% CI = 1.38–7.92) [36]. However, the frequency of this polymorphism was lower than 5% in both case and control cohort [36], suggesting that additional studies empowered in sample size are required to clarify the contribution of *TCN2* polymorphisms in the risk of spontaneous abortion.

Methylenetetrahydrofolate dehydrogenase (*MTHFD1*) polymorphisms

MTHFD1 is a trifunctional enzyme that mediates the interconversion of folate cofactors for either nucleic acid synthesis or hcy remethylation (Fig. 13.1). The *MTHFD1* 1958G>A polymorphism (rs2236225), leading to Arg653Gln substitution, reduces enzyme stability and activity and was suggested as a risk factor for pregnancy loss [39]. The analysis of 125 Irish women who had at least one unexplained spontaneous abortion or intrauterine fetal death and 625 control women with no history of prior pregnancy loss revealed an association between the *MTHFD1* 1958G>A polymorphism and the maternal risk of having an unexplained second trimester pregnancy loss. Particularly, homozygous *MTHFD1* 1958AA women had a 1.64-fold (OR 1.64; 95%CI = 1.05–2.57) increased risk of having an unexplained second trimester loss compared to those with 1958AG or 1958GG genotypes [39]. However, two subsequent studies have failed to find association between this polymorphism and RPL risk. Particularly, Crisan and coworkers [40] investigated 131 women from Romania with a history of at least two consecutive spontaneous abortions, and failed to find *MTHFD1* allele differences with respect to a matched number of controls. Similarly, a study performed in a cohort of 353 RPL cases and 226 control subjects from South Korea revealed no *MTHFD1* 1958G>A allele or genotype differences between cases and controls [3]. Similar conflicting results were obtained when addressing the contribution of the *MTHFD1* 1958G>A polymorphism as a maternal risk factor for chromosome 21 aneuploidy [4]. Therefore, additional studies are required to clarify if this polymorphism really contributes to chromosome malsegregation, human abortion, and RPL risk.

Other polymorphisms in folate-related genes

Other polymorphisms in genes participating in folate metabolism have been investigated even less extensively than the previous ones, and in most of the cases data have been collected in a single case–control study, so that our understanding of their potential contribution to RPL risk is still in its infancy, and only future investigation could clarify this issue. For example, cystathionine β-synthase (CBS) is a hemoprotein that catalyzes the condensation of hcy and serine to form cystathionine in the transsulfuration pathway (Fig. 13.1), and a common *CBS* polymorphism consists of the insertion of 68-bp within exon8 (*CBS* 844ins68), resulting in the duplication of a splice site at the intron7/exon8 junction of the gene.[28] investigated this polymorphism in 89 Brazilian women with a history of idiopathic recurrent miscarriage and 150 controls and found that there were no significant differences in allele or genotype distributions between case and control women. However, the frequency of the 844ins68 allele in the *CBS* gene was higher among women with a history of loss during the third trimester of pregnancy, suggesting that additional studies are required to clarify this issue [28].

Thymidylate synthase (TYMS) converts deoxyuridine monophosphate (dUMP) and 5,10-methyleneTHF to deoxythymidine monophosphate (dTMP) and dihydrofolate (DHF) in the de novo synthesis of pyrimidines (Fig. 13.1). A 6-bp deletion (1494ins/del) polymorphism in the 3′-UTR (rs34489327) of the *TYMS* gene, that affects mRNA stability into the cytoplasm [41], was investigated in a cohort of 353 RPL patients and 226 control subjects in South Korea, but no difference was observed in the distribution of both allele and genotype frequencies between groups [3]. However, the authors suggested that combinations of this polymorphism with the *MTR* 2756A>G one could increase RPL risk [3]. To the best of the author knowledge, no other group has investigated this gene combination with respect to RPL risk, so that also these findings are pending replication.

Discussion

Table 13.1 provides a summary of the main outcomes of studies addressing the potential contribution of polymorphisms in folate-related genes as risk

Table 13.1 Polymorphisms of folate-related genes and risk of recurrent pregnancy loss.

Gene	Polymorphism	Results	References
MTHFR	677C>T	Several recent meta-analyses support a contribution to RPL risk in different ethnic groups, particularly in Asians and developing countries	[6,19−21,24]
MTHFR	1298A>C	Conflicting results from association studies and meta-analyses	[6,19,20]
MTR	2756A>G	Associated with reduced RPL risk in two Asian studies, but not in Brazil. No data are available from other populations	[27,28,44]
MTRR	66A>G	Only one out of four different case−control studies reported an increased frequency of this polymorphism in women with RPL. All the studies were performed in Asian women	[27,29,30,44]
RFC1 (SLC19A1)	80A>G	Four different case−control studies failed to find association with RPL risk	[27,33−35]
RFC1 (SLC19A1)	−43T>C/ 80A>G/ 696C>T	Two independent studies suggest that haplotypes generated by these three polymorphisms could affect RPL risk. Additional studies are required to confirm these findings and clarify ethnic and gene−nutrient interactions	[33,35]
TCN2	776C>G	Conflicting results in genetic association studies. Data are still limited to perform a meta-analysis	[36−39]
TCN2	67A>G	Associated with RPL risk in a recent Asian study. Replication is pending	[36]
MTHFD1	1958G>A	Conflicting results in genetic association studies. Data are	[3,39,40]

Continued

Table 13.1 Polymorphisms of folate-related genes and risk of recurrent pregnancy loss.—cont'd

Gene	Polymorphism	Results	References
		still limited to perform a meta-analysis	
CBS	844ins68	A single study in Brazilian women reported an increased frequency among women with a history of loss during the third trimester of pregnancy. The sample size of this study was very low and replication is pending	[28]

factors for pregnancy loss. Overall, only for *MTHFR* polymorphisms there are enough studies available to perform meta-analyses and reach some conclusions. Indeed, according to the available literature, the *MTHFR* 677T allele can be considered as a maternal risk factor for RPL, particularly in Asians and in developing countries. Data in Caucasians are still controversial, but the available literature suggests that the magnitude of the risk is higher in Asians than in Caucasians, and this difference is more likely resulting from gene—nutrient interactions than from differences in the frequency of the polymorphism among different populations [24]. Indeed, the most recent meta-analysis revealed that the *MTHFR* 677C>T polymorphism is associated to RPL risk only in developing countries, but not in developed ones, and that the magnitude of the association is moderate [24]. Addressing this issue is however difficult because of a large heterogeneity among the available studies. Data on food intake are often missing from the different case—control cohorts, so that gene—nutrient interaction cannot be adequately assessed in the meta-analyses [6,19—21,24]. For what is concerning the *MTHFR* 1298A>C polymorphism data are still uncertain warranting some further investigation. Noteworthy, *MTHFR* 677C>T and 1298A>C polymorphisms are in linkage disequilibrium, so that it is likely that their combinations (haplotypes) could account for RPL risk, as suggested by some investigators [12,34]. Because of the still conflicting nature of the findings, most of the professional organizations in western countries, including the American College of Medical Genetics, do not recommend testing for *MTHFR* 677C>T or 1298A>C polymorphisms in the evaluation for RPL [42].

Several investigators have suggested that haplotypes generated by different *RFC1* polymorphisms could increase RPL risk [33–35], but data come from relatively small case–control studies, so that further investigation is required to better address this issue. For all the other investigated polymorphisms, evidence of an association with RPL risk is limited to one or two case–control studies, results are conflicting among different investigators, or replication is missing, so that none of them is clearly emerging as a potential RPL risk factor. Reasons for the discordant results obtained so far are likely due to the small sample size of case–control cohorts, often limited to 100–200 individuals each. In addition, ethnic differences in the distribution of the studied polymorphisms coupled to different dietary habits and folate bioavailability at peri-conception could have contributed to the observed discordant findings. However, a proper evaluation of the ethnic or regional effects to the magnitude of RPL risk is not an easy task for most of these polymorphisms, because the available data are limited to very few studies, mainly from Asian countries. Studies in European Caucasians or mixed American populations are often missing or limited to a single study, and this might be due to the fact that programs of mandatory folic acid fortifications of foods or a better socioeconomic status allowing accessibility to folic acid supplements, coupled to the conflicting nature of the findings concerning the association of *MTHFR* 677C>T and RPL risk in Caucasians [6,19,24], have reduced the interest in the investigation of polymorphisms of this pathway. On the other hand, data from several of the poorest regions of the world, such as central and southern Africa, are missing. Even more difficult is to evaluate gene–nutrient interactions or the correlation between a certain polymorphism and the prevalence of RPL in a given population, because most of the studies from the available literature are retrospective, and often lack a proper nutritional and socioeconomic evaluation at peri-conception.

Some authors have also suggested that combinations of polymorphisms in folate-related genes, rather than each single one, could increase RPL risk. Within this context, we already discussed the potential contribution of both *MTHFR* and *RFC1* haplotypes, but authors have suggested also other interactions, such as between *TYMS* and *MTR* [3], or even more complex ones involving three/four different genes [45]. Unfortunately, each single study has included different polymorphisms in the analysis, so that data are difficult to confirm. Furthermore, the small sample size of the available studies drastically reduces the statistical power to address those interactions. Given the complexity of the folate metabolic pathway (Fig. 13.1), it is likely that combinations of polymorphisms of folate-related genes could interact in increasing RPL risk, but only future prospective studies empowered in sample size, and containing a proper evaluation of the nutritional status, could clarify this issue.

Conclusions

Accumulating evince suggests a possible contribution for the *MTHFR* 677C>T polymorphism as a risk factor for pregnancy loss, especially in developing countries. It is therefore likely that also *MTHFR* haplotypes, involving combinations of its major polymorphisms, could represent RPL risk factors, but gene–nutrient interactions should be taken into account when addressing this issue. There is also evidence that other polymorphisms in folate-related genes, their haplotypes, as well as combinations of different polymorphisms, might represent maternal risk factors for pregnancy loss. Studies are, however, limited in sample size, often conflicting, and restricted to few populations, so that additional investigation is required to clarify the complex contribution of the genetics of folate metabolism to RPL risk. The nutritional status of the studied populations should be properly evaluated, in order to reveal the most important gene–nutrient interactions.

References

[1] Fenech M. Folate (vitamin B9) and vitamin B12 and their function in the maintenance of nuclear and mitochondrial genome integrity. Mutat Res 2012;733(1–2):21–33.
[2] Martín-Subero JI. How epigenomics brings phenotype into being. Pediatr Endocrinol Rev 2011;9(Suppl. 1):506–10.
[3] Kim JH, Jeon YJ, Lee BE, Kang H, Shin JE, Choi DH, Lee WS, Kim NK. Association of methionine synthase and thymidylate synthase genetic polymorphisms with idiopathic recurrent pregnancy loss. Fertil Steril 2013;99:1674–80.
[4] Coppedè F. The genetics of folate metabolism and maternal risk of birth of a child with Down syndrome and associated congenital heart defects. Front Genet 2015;6:223.
[5] Arias-Sosa LA, Acosta ID, Lucena-Quevedo E, Moreno-Ortiz H, Esteban-Pérez C, Forero-Castro M. Genetic and epigenetic variations associated with idiopathic recurrent pregnancy loss. J Assist Reprod Genet 2018. https://doi.org/10.1007/s10815-017-1108-y [Epub ahead of print].
[6] Yang Y, Luo Y, Yuan J, Tang Y, Xiong L, Xu M, Rao X, Liu H. Association between maternal, fetal and paternal MTHFR gene C677T and A1298C polymorphisms and risk of recurrent pregnancy loss: a comprehensive evaluation. Arch Gynecol Obstet 2016;293(6):1197–211.
[7] Serapinas D, Boreikaite E, Bartkeviciute A, Bandzeviciene R, Silkunas M, Bartkeviciene D. The importance of folate, vitamins B6 and B12 for the lowering of homocysteine concentrations for patients with recurrent pregnancy loss and MTHFR mutations. ReprodToxicol 2017;72:159–63.

[8] Friso S, Choi SW. Gene-nutrient interactions in one-carbon metabolism. Curr Drug Metabol 2005;6(1):37−46.
[9] World Health Organization. Guideline: optimal serum and red blood cell folate concentrations in women of reproductive age for prevention of neural tube defects. Geneva: World Health Organization; 2015.
[10] Rozen R. Genetic predisposition to hyperhomocysteinemia: deficiency of methylenetetrahydrofolate reductase (MTHFR). Thromb Haemostasis 1997;78:523−6.
[11] Yamada K, Zhoutao C, Rima R, Mathews RG. Effects of common polymorphisms on the properties of recombinant human methylenetetrahydrofolate reductase. Proc Natl Acad Sci USA 2001;98:14853−8.
[12] Martínez-Frías ML. The biochemical structure and function of methylenetetrahydrofolate reductase provide the rationale to interpret the epidemiological results on the risk for infants with Down syndrome. Am J Med Genet A 2008;146A:1477−82.
[13] Nishio K, Goto Y, Kondo T, Ito S, Ishida Y, Kawai S, Naito M, Wakai K, Hamajima N. Serum folate and methylenetetrahydrofolate reductase (MTHFR) C677T polymorphism adjusted for folate intake. J Epidemiol 2008;18:125−31.
[14] Devlin AM, Clarke R, Birks J, Evans JG, Halsted CH. Interactions among polymorphisms in folate-metabolizing genes and serum total homocysteine concentrations in a healthy elderly population. Am J Clin Nutr 2006;83:708−13.
[15] Coppedè F, Tannorella P, Pezzini I, Migheli F, Ricci G, Ienco EC, Piaceri I, Polini A, Nacmias B, Monzani F, Sorbi S, Siciliano G, Migliore L. Folate, homocysteine, vitamin B12, and polymorphisms of genes participating in one-carbon metabolism in late-onset Alzheimer's disease patients and healthy controls. Antioxidants Redox Signal 2012;17:195−204.
[16] James SJ, Pogribna M, Pogribny IP, Melnyk S, Hine RJ, Gibson JB, Yi P, Tafoya DL, Swenson DH, Wilson VL, Gaylor DW. Abnormal folate metabolism and mutation in the methylenetetrahydrofolate reductase gene may be maternal risk factors for Down syndrome. Am J Clin Nutr 1999;70:495−501.
[17] Coppedè F, Colognato R, Bonelli A, Astrea G, Bargagna S, Siciliano G, Migliore L. Polymorphisms in folate and homocysteine metabolizing genes and chromosome damage in mothers of Down syndrome children. Am J Med Genet A 2007;143A:2006−15.
[18] Yang M, Gong T, Lin X, Qi L, Guo Y, Cao Z, Shen M, Du Y. Maternal gene polymorphisms involved in folate metabolism and the risk of having a Down syndrome offspring: a meta-analysis. Mutagenesis 2013;28:661−71.
[19] Cao Y, Xu J, Zhang Z, Huang X, Zhang A, Wang J, Zheng Q, Fu L, Du J. Association study between methylenetetrahydrofolate reductase polymorphisms and unexplained recurrent pregnancy loss: a meta-analysis. Gene 2013;514:105−11.
[20] Chen H, Yang X, Lu M. Methylenetetrahydrofolate reductase gene polymorphisms and recurrent pregnancy loss in China: a systematic review and meta-analysis. Arch Gynecol Obstet 2016;293:283−90.
[21] Rai V. Methylenetetrahydrofolate reductase C677T polymorphism and recurrent pregnancy loss risk in Asian population: ameta-analysis. Indian J Clin Biochem 2016;31(4):402−13.
[22] Saraswathy KN, Asghar M, Samtani R, Murry B, Mondal PR, Ghosh PK, Sachdeva MP. Spectrum of MTHFR gene SNPs C677T and A1298C: a study among 23 population groups of India. Mol Biol Rep 2012;39(4):5025−31.
[23] Wang X, Fu J, Li Q, Zeng D. Geographical and ethnic distributions of the MTHFR C677T, A1298C and MTRR A66G gene polymorphisms in Chinese populations: ameta-analysis. PLoS One 2016;11(4):e0152414.

[24] Zhang Y, He X, Xiong X, Chuan J, Zhong L, Chen G, Yu D. The association between maternal methylenetetrahydrofolate reductase C677T and A1298C polymorphism and birth defects and adverse pregnancy outcomes. Prenat Diagn 2019;39(1):3–9.
[25] Coppedè F, Bosco P, Lorenzoni V, Migheli F, Barone C, Antonucci I, Stuppia L, Romano C, Migliore L. The *MTR* 2756A>G polymorphism and maternal risk of birth of a child with Down syndrome: a case-control study and a meta-analysis. Mol Biol Rep 2013;40:6913–25.
[26] Coppedè F, Bosco P, Lorenzoni V, Denaro M, Anello G, Antonucci I, Barone C, Stuppia L, Romano C, Migliore L. The MTRR 66A>G polymorphism and maternal risk of birth of a child with Down syndrome in Caucasian women: a case-control study and a meta-analysis. Mol Biol Rep 2014;41:5571–83.
[27] Luo L, Chen Y, Wang L, Zhuo G, Qiu C, Tu Q, Mei J, Zhang W, Qian X, Wang X. Polymorphisms of genes involved in the folate metabolic pathway impact the occurrence of unexplained recurrent pregnancy loss. Reprod Sci 2015;22:845–51.
[28] Boas WV, Gonçalves RO, Costa OL, Goncalves MS. Metabolism and gene polymorphisms of the folate pathway in Brazilian women with history of recurrent abortion. Rev Bras Ginecol Obstet 2015;37:71–6.
[29] Guo QN, Liao SX, Kang B, Zhang JX, Wang RL, Ding XB, Zhang WH. Association of methionine synthase reductase gene polymorphism with unexplained recurrent spontaneous abortion. Zhonghua Fu Chan Ke Za Zhi 2012;47:742–6.
[30] Zhu L. Polymorphisms in the methylene tetrahydrofolate reductase and methionine synthase reductase genes and their correlation with unexplained recurrent spontaneous abortion susceptibility. Genet Mol Res 2015;14:8500–8.
[31] Chango A, Emery-Fillon N, de Courcy GP, Lambert D, Pfister M, Rosenblatt DS, Nicolas JP. A polymorphism (80G>A) in the reduced folate carrier gene and its associations with folate status and homocysteinemia. Mol Genet Metabol 2000;70:310–5.
[32] Coppedè F, Marini G, Bargagna S, Stuppia L, Minichilli F, Fontana I, Colognato R, Astrea G, Palka G, Migliore L. Folate gene polymorphisms and the risk of Down syndrome pregnancies in young Italian women. Am J Med Genet A 2006;140:1083–91.
[33] Rah H, Choi YS, Jeon YJ, Choi Y, Cha SH, Choi DH, Ko JJ, Shim SH, Kim NK. Solute Carrier Family 19, member 1 (SLC19A1) polymorphisms (-43T>C, 80G>A, and 696C>T), and haplotypes in idiopathic recurrent spontaneous abortion in a Korean population. Reprod Sci 2012;19(5):513–9.
[34] Cao Y, Zhang Z, Zheng Y, Yuan W, Wang J, Liang H, Chen J, Du J, Shen Y. The association of idiopathic recurrent early pregnancy loss with polymorphisms in folic acid metabolism-related genes. Genes Nutr 2014;9:402.
[35] Mohtaram S, Sheikhha MH, Honarvar N, Sazegari A, Maraghechi N, Feizollahi Z, Ghasemi N. An association study of the SLC19A1 gene polymorphisms/haplotypes with idiopathic recurrent pregnancy loss in an Iranian population. Genet Test Mol Biomarkers 2016;20(5):235–40.
[36] Kim HS, Lee BE, Jeon YJ, Rah H, Lee WS, Shin JE, Choi DH, Kim NK. Transcobalamin II (TCN2 67A>G and TCN2 776C>G) and transcobalamin II receptor (TCblR 1104C>T) polymorphisms in Korean patients with idiopathic recurrent spontaneous abortion. Am J Reprod Immunol 2014;72(3):337–46.
[37] Zetterberg H, Regland B, Palmér M, Rymo L, Zafiropoulos A, Arvanitis DA, Spandidos DA, Blennow K. The transcobalamin codon 259 polymorphism influences the risk of human spontaneous abortion. Hum Reprod 2002;17:3033–6.
[38] Zetterberg H, Zafiropoulos A, Spandidos DA, Rymo L, Blennow K. Gene-gene interaction between fetal MTHFR 677C>T and transcobalamin 776C>G polymorphisms in human spontaneous abortion. Hum Reprod 2003;18:1948–50.

[39] Parle-McDermott A, Pangilinan F, Mills JL, Signore CC, Molloy AM, Cotter A, Conley M, Cox C, Kirke PN, Scott JM, Brody LC. A polymorphism in the MTHFD1 gene increases a mother's risk of having an unexplained second trimester pregnancy loss. Mol Hum Reprod 2005;11:477–80.
[40] Crisan TO, Trifa A, Farcas M, Militaru M, Netea M, Pop I, Popp R. The MTHFD1 c.1958 G>A polymorphism and recurrent spontaneous abortions. J Matern Fetal Neonatal Med 2011;24(1):189–92.
[41] Ulrich CM, Bigler J, Bostick R, Fosdick L, Potter JD. Thymidylate synthase promoter polymorphism, interaction with folate intake, and risk of colorectal adenomas. Cancer Res 2002;62:3361–4.
[42] Levin BL, Varga E. MTHFR: addressing genetic counseling dilemmas using evidence-based literature. J Genet Counsel 2016;25(5):901–11.
[43] Nefic H, Mackic-Djurovic M, Eminovic I. The frequency of the 677CT and 1298AC polymorphisms in the methylenetetrahydrofolate reductase (MTHFR) gene in the population. Med Arch 2018;72(3):164–9. https://doi.org/10.5455/medarh.2018.72.164-169.
[44] Kim JH, Jeon YJ, Lee BE, Kang H, Shin JE, Choi DH, Lee WS, Kim NK. Association of methionine synthase and thymidylate synthase genetic polymorphisms with idiopathic recurrent pregnancy loss. Fertil Steril 2013;99(6):1674–80. https://doi.org/10.1016/j.fertnstert.2013.01.108.
[45] Luo L, Chen Y, Wang L, Zhuo G, Qiu C, Tu Q, Mei J, Zhang W, Qian X, Wang X. polymorphisms of genes involved in the folate metabolic pathway impact the occurrence of unexplained recurrent pregnancy loss. Reprod Sci 2015;22(7):845–51. https://doi.org/10.1177/1933719114565033.

CHAPTER 14

Perinatal lipid nutrition

Alicia I. Leikin-Frenkel[1,2]
[1]The Sackler Faculty of Medicine Ramat Aviv and Bert Strassburger Lipid Center, Sheba, Tel Hashomer Ramat Gan, Israel; [2]The Bert Strassburger Lipid Center, Sheba, Tel Hashomer, Tel Aviv University, Tel Aviv, Israel

Contents

Molecular Nutrition
ISBN 978-0-12-813862-5
https://doi.org/10.1016/B978-0-12-813862-5.00014-1

Nutrition during the perinatal period has long-term implications for neonates. Molecular and cellular events initiated during this period have the potential to generate lifelong phenotypic changes to infants. Experimental evidence in animals has demonstrated that essential fatty acid (EFA) deficiency during early brain development has deleterious and permanent effects. Disnutrition, either by a high caloric load or by deficiency of essential nutrients, is associated with an increased risk of baby and adult-onset diseases. Therefore, an understanding of the properties and relevance of lipids during this period is important.

Lipids

Lipids are utilized by mammals for multiple functions including energy, structure, metabolic regulation, and temperature insulation. Most needed lipids can be novo synthetized, except for linoleic (LA omega-6) and alpha-linolenic (ALA omega-3), fatty acids which must be compulsory incorporated with the diet and are therefore called EFAs [1].

Lipid classes

Fatty acids

Their structure contains a carboxyl group that enables their esterification to biological alcohols to form complex lipids. The carbon chain, typically between 4 and 24 carbons long, may be saturated or unsaturated depending on the presence of double bonds, in either a cis or trans geometric isomerism, which significantly affects the molecule's configuration. Most naturally occurring fatty acids are of cis configuration [2]. Double bonds introduce flexibility to the fatty acid chains, playing an important role in the structure and function of cell membranes.

Glycerolipids

These compounds present one to the three hydroxyl groups of the alcohol glycerol, of carbohydrate origin, esterified usually by different fatty acids.

Triglycerides

The three hydroxyl groups of glycerol are esterified with three fatty acids. They provide compact energy storage and are found in the fat of animal tissues and oil of vegetable seeds. They are majoritarian dietary lipid contribution for humans and animals. They are important as a source of energy for immediate utilization by the body or as reserve in adipose tissue. The hydrolysis of the ester bonds of glycerides with the release of glycerol and fatty acids from adipose tissue is the initial steps in fat metabolism [3].

Glycerophospholipids

One hydroxyl group of glycerol is bound to a phosphate group to give phosphatidic acid to which different polar groups can bind to produce the molecules called phospholipids. They are key components of the lipid bilayer of cell membranes [2] as well as main players in metabolism and cell signaling [4]. Main glycerophospholipids found in biological membranes are phosphatidylcholine, phosphatidylethanolamine, and phosphatidylserine. In addition to be primary cellular membranes components phosphatidylinositols and phosphatidic acid are precursors of membrane-derived second messengers [5] in signaling. Plasmalogens are also important molecules of this group in which beside the ester bond exists a vinyl bond [6].

Sphingolipids

The sphingoid backbone bases their structure on the alcohol sphingol. They include ceramides, phosphosphingolipids, glycosphingolipids, and other compounds, with sphingomyelins (ceramide phosphocholines) being the major phosphosphingolipid of mammals [7].

Sterols

Based on a tetracyclic structure, they are important components of membrane lipids, along with the glycerophospholipids and sphingomyelins [8,9]. Their derived steroids have different biological roles as hormones, whereas cholesterol, quantitatively the major sterol, is oxidized in the liver to produce bile acids, salts, and their conjugates derivatives [10,11].

Regulatory functions

Lipid signaling is a vital part of the cell signaling mechanism. It may occur via activation of G protein–coupled or nuclear receptors. Among lipid categories identified as signaling molecules and cellular messengers [12,13], sphingosine-1-phosphate is involved in regulating calcium mobilization, cell growth, and apoptosis; diacylglycerol (DAG) and the phosphatidylinositol phosphates (PIPs) are involved in calcium-mediated activation of protein kinase C, prostaglandins are involved in inflammation and immunity, steroid hormones such as estrogen, testosterone, and cortisol, modulate a host of functions such as reproduction, metabolism, and blood pressure and oxysterols such as 25-hydroxy-cholesterol are liver X receptor agonists [14]. Besides, phosphatidylserine lipids signal for the phagocytosis of apoptotic cells [15].

Lipid metabolism

Humans are able to synthesize all lipids required for bodily functions except EFA and liposoluble vitamins. The metabolic processes are also responsible for the stimulated transformation of membrane lipids in biologically active regulatory molecules like that of eicosanoids, resolvins, lipoxines, etc. [16].

Synthesis

Humans convert the unused excess of an oversupply of dietary carbohydrate to triglycerides. The acetyl molecule produced by degradation of carbohydrates is the starting point for fatty acids. The newly synthesized fatty acids produce triglycerides by esterification to glycerol [17] that are stored in adipose tissue. Their hydrophobic nature allows the accumulation of several molecules in the smaller possible volume away from the hydrophilic environment in the adipocyte, or fat cell. The continuous synthesis and breakdown of triglycerides in animals is controlled, mainly, by the activation of hormone-sensitive enzyme lipase [18]. The complete oxidation of fatty acids provides twice the calories, about 9 kcal/g compared with 4 kcal/g for the breakdown of carbohydrates and proteins.

The synthesis of unsaturated fatty acids involves the introduction of double bonds into the fatty acyl chain by enzymatic desaturation. Thus, SCD-1 or Δ9 desaturase introduce the first double bond in saturated fatty acids (SFAs) transforming them into monounsaturated fatty acids (MUFA). Essential Linoleic (omega-6) and alpha-linolenic acids (omega-3) are the starting point in polyunsaturated fatty acid metabolism. Thus, Arachidonic acid or ARA is the product of Linoleic acid desaturation by Δ5 desaturase or FADS1 and elongation. Eicosapentenoic (EPA) and Docosahexenoic (DHA) are products of ALA elongation and desaturation by or Δ6 desaturase FADS2 [19]. Cholesterol, Triglyceride, and Phospholipid synthesis take place in the endoplasmic reticulum by individual metabolic pathway [20].

Degradation

Fatty acids released from complex lipids are broken down in the mitochondria or in peroxisomes generating acetyl-CoA by beta oxidation. For the most part, fatty acids are oxidized liberating acetyl-CoA molecules that ultimately produce ATP, CO_2, and H_2O.Therefore, fat is a source of energy when there is little or no glucose available [21,22].

Lipid nutrition

Nutritional lipids can be of animal or vegetal origin, which determines their differential fatty acids array. Besides their importance as energy suppliers, vegetable triglycerides carry essential and polyunsaturated fatty acids, whereas animal triglycerides carry mainly saturated and monounsaturated fatty acids as well as cholesterol. Therefore, the origin of nutritional lipid supply will determine the quality of fatty acids incorporated by mammals with the diet and determine their molecular effects on health [23].

Quality

Fatty acids

Humans and other mammals have a dietary requirement for EFAs, LA and ALA, because they cannot synthesize them from simple precursors in the diet. Safflower, sunflower, and corn oils are rich in LA, whereas the green leaves of plants and selected seeds, nuts, and legumes (in particular flax, rapeseed, walnut, and soy) are rich in ALA [24]. Fish oils are particularly rich in the longer-chain omega-3 fatty acids eicosapentaenoic acid (EPA) and docosahexaenoic acid (DHA) that are not essential since they that can be also produced by mammals from ALA [25,26]. Some studies have shown positive health benefits associated with consumption of DHA and EPA omega-3 fatty acids on infant development, cancer, cardiovascular diseases, and various mental illnesses [27]. Conversely, trans fats present in partially hydrogenated vegetable oils are a recognized risk factor for cardiovascular disease [28].

Studies on fatty acid's requirements performed in developed countries are generally in use as a model for worldwide nutritional regulations with disregard for regional nutritional habits and the existence of individual fatty acids enzyme isoforms. Therefore, research should be pursued considering those facts before the establishment of dietary guidance for the population in general and pregnant women in particular [29].

Liposoluble vitamins

Nutritional intervention strategy may be advisable to improve the quality of life of patients, once the actual deficiency is recognized. Thus, vitamins like A, D, E, K, and carotenoids are an important part of the human nutrition [30,31].

Quantity

Nutritional lipids, incorporated mainly as triglycerides, provide twice the amount of calories, per weigh, than sugars and proteins. The connection between percentage of calories from fat and risk of cancer, heart disease, or weight gain has nevertheless not yet been proved [32].

Perinatal lipid nutrition

Maternal nutrition during pregnancy lactation can induce significant changes in body composition and physiology and can have long-term effects on the offspring. During the course of mammalian development, fatty acids are transferred to the fetus through the placenta [33] and their composition depends, to a great extent, on the maternal diet [34]. In this context not only quantitative but also qualitative deficiency, like that of EFAs, play a primary role in growth and development and it imbalances in EFA intake during pregnancy and lactation may result in permanent changes that affect appetite control, neuroendocrine function, and energy metabolism in the fetus, thus influencing the metabolic programming [35,36].

Placental metabolism

The human placenta is responsible for the adequate supply of nutrients essential for proper embryonic and fetal development such as glucose, amino acids, and lipids. The processes involved in the placental transport of these nutrients are complex and tightly regulated and involve many transporters, receptors, and regulators [37]. Maternal plasma lipoproteins do not cross the placental barrier directly. Also, placental lipase activities increase and lipoprotein lipase (LPL) activity decrease drastically during the last trimester of pregnancy, resulting in depleted triacylglycerol storage [38]. The released triacylglycerol is substrate for the placental lipase activity that releases free fatty acids for fetal transport [39]. The placental LPL hydrolyzes triacylglycerol from posthepatic low density lipoproteins and very low density lipoproteins (VLDLs) but not from chylomicrons [40–42].These activities have consequences on the regulation of quality and quantity of fatty acids delivered to the fetus [43]. Endothelial lipase (EL) and LPL [44] seem to be the only lipases expressed in the first trimester in trophoblasts, cells responsible for the embryo's nutrition. At term, only EL is expressed in trophoblasts and endothelial cells. In total placental tissue EL expression prevails in first trimester and at term [45]. There is an increased breakdown of fat depots during the last trimester of pregnancy due to increased lipolytic activity in adipose tissue. EL expression in endothelial cells and LPL in smooth muscle cells surrounding blood vessels may account for major lipase activity. Lipoprotein receptors have been detected both on placental macrophages and syncytiotrophoblasts, the interface between maternal blood and embryonic extracellular fluid, where the passive exchange of material between the mother and the embryo occurs [38,40]. It is assumed that these receptors are involved in fatty acid uptake by the placenta [46,47].

Fatty acids transport

The regulation of different lipases expressed in placenta and their roles in fatty acid transport across the human placenta [48] is far from understood and much work is still required. Free fatty acids in the maternal circulation are the major source of fatty acids for transport across the placenta [43] since triglycerides are not transported intact [49]. Fatty acids either free or derived from lipoproteins by LPL and EL are transported into the placenta by multiple fatty acid transporters: plasma membrane fatty acid binding protein (FABPpm) [50], fatty acid binding protein 1-5 (FABP1-5), fatty acid translocase (FAT)/CD36, and fatty acid transport protein 1–4 and 6 (FATP1–4,6) [51]. Fatty acids are then either metabolized in the placenta for energy production or storage in lipid droplets or transported to the fetal circulation by passive diffusion or carried by FAT/CD36 or FATP1–4, 6. Placenta seems to express all the enzymes necessary for mitochondrial fatty acid oxidation [52]. Fatty acids are used as a major metabolic fuel by human placentas at all gestational ages and defects within the production of energy may jeopardize the growth, differentiation, and functionality of the placenta, with detrimental consequences on fetal growth and development [53].

In trophoblasts, saturated and monounsaturated fatty acids may be esterified as triglycerides and enter lipid droplets for storage. Polyunsaturated fatty acids like DHA, in turn, would be directed transferred toward the fetus without esterification. Although FA transporters seem to lack specificity [53], this step is critical to define how maternal FA quality impacts the fetal FA accretion and future well-designed competitive studies between different fatty acids would deepen the understanding of this important process. The exact mechanism of how fatty acids are transferred across the plasma membrane needs to be disclosed [52]. Long-chain polyunsaturated fatty acids can enter cells by passive diffusion through and from the placenta to the fetus. However, plasma membrane transport and binding proteins such as fatty acid translocase [54] (FAT/CD36), plasma membrane fatty acid binding protein (FABPpm), fatty acid transport protein family (FATP1–6), and intracellular FABPs may also contribute to mother–fetus flow [55]. The direction and magnitude of fatty acid flux is mainly dictated by the relative abundance of available binding sites in binding proteins in human placenta. They may be essential to facilitate the preferential transport of maternal plasma fatty acids in order to meet the requirements of the growing fetus. These fatty acid transport/binding proteins and placental functions are regulated by different hormones [56] and FA-activated transcription factors (PPARs, LXR, RXR, and SREBP-1) [54,57]. Their involvement is critical in the expression of genes responsible for fatty acids uptake, placental trophoblast differentiation, and hCG production. These receptors are, therefore, potential regulators of placental lipid transfer and homeostasis [58].

Fatty acid uptake by placental trophoblast cells

The underlying mechanisms responsible for the selective uptake and concentration of FA in fetal tissues are not fully understood. Moreover, in vitro and in placental perfusion system competitive studies seem to indicate a preferential uptake of omega-3 fatty acids versus omega-6 fatty acids at similar concentrations [59]. However, not all fatty acids have been studied and, more importantly, not competitive studies testing variable concentrations of different EFAs have been performed [60]. Further work is required to understand the implication of supplementation of different FA during pregnancy which may increase general fatty acid uptake by the placenta and its impact on feto-placental growth and development [60].

FATs and fatty acid transporter proteins (FATP) are located on both sides of the bipolar placental trophoblasts. Their lack of specificity allows bidirectional transport of all FFAs, from the mother to the fetus and vice versa. Placenta-specific plasma membrane fatty acid–binding protein (p-FABPpm) sequesters maternal plasma DHA/ARA to the placenta for critical supply to fetal brain development in utero. Cytoplasmic fatty acid–binding proteins (FABPs) are responsible for trans-cytoplasmic movement of FA or to the fetal circulation via placental basal membranes. Each one of these steps suggest a regulation by the fatty acid molecular species and their competition, leading to design a perinatal molecular nutrition aimed to the best health outcomes for the offspring [51].

Maternal lipid metabolism

Maternal needs

Lipid metabolism during pregnancy must fulfill both maternal requirements for lipid stores and energy reserves for lactation and as lipid substrates required by the fetus. Although the mechanisms are still poorly understood, it seems that during the first part of pregnancy intracellular accumulation of triglycerides is the product of low lipolytic activity together with high synthesis [61,62]. Studies show that these pathways are stimulated by insulin and enhanced insulin responsiveness in early pregnancy in women and in rats as the driving force for the net fat depot accumulation at this stage [63].

Lipid use

Conversely, during the last third of gestation high plasma levels of placental hormones with lipolytic effects (i.e., human placental lactogen) augmented production of catecholamines secondary to maternal insulin–resistant condition present at this stage seem to produce net lipolysis of maternal depots, with consequent increments in plasma-free FA and glycerol levels [64,65]. Part of the lipolytic products released from maternal adipose tissue is reesterified for the synthesis of triglycerides in the maternal liver, transferred to VLDL particles and released into the circulation. The fatty acids oxidation releases energy and induces ketone body synthesis, whereas glycerol may be used for gluconeogenesis [66]. Ketone bodies, that are efficiently transferred in the placenta [67], may be used by the fetus as oxidative fuels as well as substrates for brain lipid synthesis. The insulin-resistant condition present in late pregnancy controls these metabolic changes [68].

Lipid transfer

Lipoproteins cross the placenta mediated by receptors, lipase activities, and fatty acid binding proteins that allow for the efficient transfer of maternal

FA to the fetus [37]. The cholesterol moiety of lipoproteins can be taken up by the cholesterol receptors, metabolized in the placenta or can be exported to the fetal circulation by the ATP-binding cassette transporters A1 (ABCA1) and G1 (ABCG1) [69]. Cholesterol synthesis is also an important source of fetal cholesterol. The human placenta, in addition to its roles as a nutrient transfer and endocrine organ, functions as a selective barrier to protect the fetus against the harmful effects of exogenous and endogenous toxins. Members of the ATP-binding cassette (ABC) family of transport proteins limit the entry of xenobiotics into the fetal circulation via vectorial efflux from the placenta to the maternal circulation. Several members of the ABC family, including proteins from the ABCA, ABCB, ABCC, and ABCG subfamilies, have been shown to be functional in the placenta with clinically significant roles in xenobiotic efflux. Several studies in primary human trophoblast cells and animal models have demonstrated decreased expression and activity of placental ABC transporters in cases of inflammatory, oxidative, or metabolic stress. Several clinical studies in pregnancies complicated by inflammatory conditions such as preeclampsia and gestational diabetes support these findings, although the clinical relevance requires further studies to determine of the relationships between placental ABC transporter expression and activity, and placental function in stressed pregnancies. Such studies are necessary and important to fully understand the consequences of pregnancy disorders on placental function and viability in order to optimize pregnancy care and maximize fetal growth and health [70].

Major changes take place during pregnancy in lipid metabolism [37]. These are mainly controlled by the insulin resistance seen during the third trimester. Maternal adipose tissue and hyperlipidemia contribute to the metabolic adaptations that benefit fetal growth, particularly under conditions of dietary shortage [71].

Nuclear transcription factors and prostaglandins

Fatty acid—activated transcription factors (PPARs, LXR, RXR, and SREBP-1) regulate fatty acid transport/binding proteins and placental functions. Maternal dietary fatty acids therefore may regulate their own placental transport as well as placental function via several fatty acid—activated transcriptions. PPARs may play essential roles in placental development and function [72,73]. PPARc and PPARd are essential for multiple physiological functions of the trophoblastic and amniotic parts, leading to major involvement of PPARs in the pathophysiology of gestational diseases [74]. Trophoblastic lipid uptake and accumulation are also regulated in part PPARc ligands leading to increased uptake and accumulation of fatty acids in human placenta [80,89]. PPARs also regulate a number of placental fatty acid and lipid metabolism [75]. The dietary origin of maternal fatty acids may affect their placental transport as well as placental biological processes [76]. The maternal blood may also be a source of PPAR ligands for the human placenta [77,78].

During pregnancy, placenta is the major source of prostaglandins (PGs) generated from dietary fatty acids within intrauterine tissues. PUFAs supply the precursors for prostaglandin (PG) synthesis and PGs in turn influence many aspects of reproduction. Although prostaglandin (PG) levels are the lowest in early pregnancy and their increase jeopardizes the process, production by intrauterine tissues plays also a key part in the control of pregnancy and parturition [79,80]. Thus, the output of bioactive PGs from placenta is controlled by both their synthesis and metabolism within placenta. The enzymes necessary to convert prostaglandins are correlated to PPARc in placenta [81] [82]. Prostaglandins (PGs) are produced by a variety of utero-placental tissues during pregnancy and are released into the fetal fluid sacs and both the uterine and umbilical circulations [83]. The availability of glucose and FFA to the gravid uterus therefore has an important role in controlling utero-placental PG production and metabolism in late gestation. Data suggest that high omega-6 dietary fatty acids reduce the endometrial capacity to produce PGs and may therefore have implications for the control of luteolysis and other PG-mediated events, at least in cows [84].

The major source of PGE2, in ovine pregnancy, is the placenta, with secretion occurring bidirectionally into fetal and maternal circulations. The placental output of PGE2 appears to increase when demand on placental function is increased, suggesting that the normally observed increase in its concentration toward term is driven by the growing demands of the fetus [85].

Molecular nutrition

In the context of molecular nutrition, it should be emphasized that the main lipids of high concern are EFA, essential fatty acids of critical importance in fetal growth and development [86], precursors of eicosanoids, constituents of the membrane lipids that maintain cellular and organelle integrity, and important intracellular mediators of gene expression [87]. Because of these fundamental roles of EFA, the maternal, fetal, and neonatal EFA status is an important determinant of health and disease in infancy and later life [88,89]. The EFA metabolic products increase in the fetus is rapid during growth, and it a deficit of a specific component which would be in detriment of brain development [90].

The dietary EFAs, linoleic acid and alpha-linolenic acid, are important for infant growth and development. EFA as starting point and their long-chain metabolites long-chain polyunsaturated fatty acids (LC-PUFAs) also play important roles in reproduction. There is currently no evidence that the absolute amounts of EFA provided by any cultural dietary pattern are neither adequate nor inadequate to meet the needs for growth of the placenta, the fetus, or the infant [91]. Both blood and tissue levels of PUFA are influenced not only by diet but to a large extent also by genetic heritability [92]. Delta-5 (D5D) and Delta-6 desaturases (D6D), encoded, respectively, by FADS1 and FADS2 genes, are the rate-limiting enzymes for PUFA conversion and are recognized as main determinants of PUFA levels [29]. Alterations of D5D/D6D activity have been associated with several diseases, from metabolic derangements to neuropsychiatric illnesses, from type 2 diabetes [93] to cardiovascular disease [34], and inflammation [94,95]. Similar results have been found by investigations on FADS1/FADS2 genotypes. Recent genome-wide association studies showed that FADS1/FADS2 genetic locus, beyond being the main determinant of PUFA, was strongly associated with plasma lipids and glucose metabolism [96]. Other analyses suggested potential link between FADS1/FADS2 polymorphisms and cognitive development [97,98], immunological illnesses [99], and cardiovascular disease [100,101]. Lessons from both animal models and rare disorders in humans further emphasized the key role of desaturases in health and disease, like obesity and diabetes [102,103]. Remarkably, some of the above-mentioned associations appear to be influenced by the environmental context/PUFA dietary intake, in particular the relative prevalence of omega-3 and omega-6 PUFA [104].

However, the roles of EFAs and the mechanisms by which they impact the long-term health of the offspring are far from being elucidated [8]. The importance of the FA composition in the diet has been spotted both in adults and in maternal diets during pregnancy [10,36]. DHA is regarded as an important dietary ingredient required in early placentation, feto-placental growth, and development to the maintenance of general health. An optimal level of DHA sources, either from maritime or terrestrial origin, is especially important for pregnant mothers to ensure adequate feto-placental growth and supply for fetal brain structure and function [78,89,105]. Essential fatty acids impact on fetal brain development is an area that deserves further research.

Early life

Embryo

FA levels in the embryo and newborn babies are directly associated with maternal FA levels and composition; therefore, the maternal intake of FAs is fundamental for fetal growth, development, and health [106]. It has been shown that breastfeeding exposes babies to the maternal genetic FADS variations through their effects on milk quality and quantity of fatty acids that, in turn, affect the proper visual and cognitive development of newborn children. Consequently, the influence of FADS2 polymorphisms in the mother is of uttermost importance for the array of FAs transferred from mother to child during uterine development and breastfeeding. This knowledge reinforces the importance of a nutritional adjustment during the critical perinatal period [107].

Regulatory mechanisms

It has been suggested that longer chain length and higher number of double bonds in omega-3 FA family confer unique properties as related to the modulation of enzymes associated with signaling pathways/incorporation of EPA and DHA into membrane phospholipids and direct effects on gene expression, among others [108].

Epigenetics

Environmental factors such as diet during fetal development can induce long-term modifications in the fetus genes. Human epidemiological data and animal studies at embryonic day 7.25 corroborate the impact of diet in the perinatal period and its lasting effect on gene expression and metabolism [65,109,110]. Epigenetic mechanisms in animals include DNA methylation, histone modifications, and noncoding RNAs. They alter DNA accessibility and chromatin structure, thereby regulating patterns of gene expression. These processes are crucial to normal development and differentiation of distinct cell lineages in the adult organism. In DNA methylation, methyl groups are added to the DNA molecule, changing the activity of a DNA segment without changing the sequence. When located in a gene promoter, DNA methylation typically acts to repress gene transcription. Histone acetylation and deacetylation are the processes by which the lysine residues within the N-terminal tail are acetylated and deacetylated. Histone acetylation and deacetylation are essential parts of gene regulation. MicroRNA is a small noncoding RNA molecule able to produce RNA silencing and posttranscriptional located in a gene promoter, DNA methylation typically acts to repress gene transcription. Histone acetylation and deacetylation are the processes by which the lysine residues within the N-terminal tail are acetylated and deacetylated. Histone acetylation and deacetylation are essential parts of gene regulation. MicroRNA is a small noncoding RNA molecule able to produce RNA silencing and post-transcriptional regulation of gene expression. The question, how do FAs influence the establishment of an epigenotype [111], regulate genome activity and gene expression leading to proteins that affect fetal programming and organ physiology with lifelong consequences [112]. A positive correlation between FA and FADS2 promoter methylation in maternal and offspring livers was described with modified expression of DNA methyltransferases in early pregnancy [113]. Possible epigenetic modifications should be further detected to account for implications of the observed changes, in terms of postnatal growth and predisposition for disease and the extrapolation to humans.

Maternal obesity

The factors predisposing to obesity may become established in the womb. Maternal overnutrition, in particular when it leads to obesity and diabetes, perpetuates an intergenerational cycle of obesity through its effects on placental function and fetal metabolism. Thus, metabolic changes associated with maternal obesity affect placental nutrient handling. Altered placental nutrient handling may induce proadipogenic changes in the fetus, in particular increased fetal insulin. Understanding the effects of maternal obesity on the placenta will aid the development of effective interventions to optimize pregnancy outcomes. Obesity during pregnancy has an impact on the health of both mothers and developing babies who have, consequently, a greater risk of developing obesity and cardiovascular disease in later life [114–117]. Maternal hyperlipidemia contributes to placental lipid droplet accumulation, perinatal mortality, and aberrant FA profiles that may influence the health of the developing offspring [118]. Obese women, on average, give birth to babies with high fat mass [119].

Placental lipid metabolism alters fetal lipid delivery and maybe neonatal adiposity, yet how it is affected by maternal obesity is poorly understood [120]. Impaired placental function of obese women may alter the supply long-chain fatty acids (FAs) to the fetus [121]. Placentas of obese women are characterized by lipid accumulation, inflammation [122], and oxidative stress [123]. Long-chain FA uptake is generally decreased in placentas of obese women. FA beta oxidation is also decreased due to reduced mitochondrial function. Enzymes mRNA and protein levels, related to FA esterification PPARg, acetyl-CoA carboxylase, stearoyl-CoA desaturase 1, and diacylglycerol O-acyltransferase-1, are overexpressed resulting in increased FA esters. Altogether, these changes in placental lipid metabolism may affect the transfer of maternal lipids to the fetus and, consequently, growth, fat accretion, and development [62]. Obesity, in general, may account for the lipid accumulation in the placenta by either an increased FA hydrolysis or by changes of the intracellular lipid compartmentalization [124,125].

Maternal high fat diet seems to programs liver fatty acid metabolism in rodent's offspring [126]. In offspring exposed in utero to a maternal diet high in fat (HF), adult offspring at 6 months of age had significantly higher body weights, greater adiposity, and increased triacylglycerol (TAG) levels as compared to controls. Decreased plasma and liver palmitic acid desaturation indices were decreased in HF newborns, but increased in the adult offspring, whereas liver SCD-1 expression was increased in the HF adult offspring. These data show that the maternal HF diet during pregnancy and lactation increases offspring liver SCD-1 protein abundance and alters the liver palmitic to palmitoleic desaturase pathway [127].

Pregravid obesity significantly modifies the expression of placental genes related to transport and storage of neutral lipids. It has been proposed that the upregulation of CGI-58, a master regulator of triglycerides hydrolysis, contributes to the turnover of intracellular lipids in placenta of obese women and is tightly regulated by metabolic factors of the mother [125]. Growing evidence in the literature suggests that maternal prepregnancy obesity appeared to be at a greater risk of developing adverse pregnancy outcomes related to metabolic disease in mother and child [39,128]. Maternal obesity has been found associated with increased content in placental TGs despite similar circulating maternal TG in lean and obese groups. Placental pathways for lipid storage and mobilization PLIN2, ATGL, and CGI-58 showed a strong positive correlation with maternal pregravid obesity [125].

Adipose triglyceride lipase (ATGL) hydrolyzes FA from TG stores. In the adipose tissue, ATGL is responsible for maintaining basal lipolytic activity and can be activated by its master regulator CGI-58. Beside its role as coactivator of TG hydrolysis, the proposed lysophosphatidic acid acyltransferase activity of CGI-58 may generate lipid mediators involved in insulin signaling and thereby obesity, role currently under debate. However, the concomitant increase in placental TG content and CGI-58 expression in placentas of obese women suggests a regulatory role for CGI-58 in placental lipid turnover, which might be under influence of elevated insulin levels in the obese mother. The important information is worth further research.

Conclusion

Perinatal lipid nutrition is of paramount importance for both mother and fetus. Moreover, the influence of molecular lipid species like EFAs shows the potential to impact genes in the programming of the offspring health later in life. Therefore, quality beyond quantity of lipids is important, which enhances the relevance of nutrigenetic approaches when designing maternal perinatal nutritional guidance. Dietary lipid molecules affect the placental development from the very beginning. The placenta has its own independent lipid metabolism and the complex synchronization between fatty acids uptake, transport, and delivery determines how much benefit or damage the fetus will receive. On one side, fatty acid nutrients affect the nuclear factors that regulate the synthesis of uptake, transport, and delivery proteins. On the other, the quantity and quality of the transferred fatty acids will determine the anatomical, physiological, and possibly epigenetic development of the fetus. Qualitative lipid malnutrition in the form of excess or deficits will affect fetal—offspring health. Qualitative lipid molecular malnutrition in the form of proportionally high levels of saturated fatty acids or lack of balance between the EFA in the form of high omega-6 LA and low omega-3 levels will undoubtedly impact the mother's own lipid metabolism and placental function. Moreover, that unbalance will determine the fetus fate of health or disease.

Problems of high priority for research are (1) mother/fetus requirements for specific fatty acids, particularly the EFAs and long-chain polyunsaturated fatty acids (LC-PUFA); (2) influence of dietary lipids on the mechanisms for their transfer across the placenta; (3) and fatty acid metabolism in the maternal liver during pregnancy. Competition between EFAs omega-6 and omega-3 should be studied.

Studies from developed countries have been in use as model for dietary fat intake recommendation during pregnancy and lactation. However, the different existing regional dietary habits should be considered when lying down those recommendations. Once the importance of EFA in maternal diet during pregnancy and lactation is understood, efforts should be invested to control the proportions of EFA due to their competition for the same enzymes and their different isoforms.

The importance of fatty acids as possible epigenetic agents has begun to be recognized and a thorough nutrigenetic approach in research is necessary in order to better understand developmental fetal programming.

Maternal obesity, as a disease, has direct negative influence on the fetal development and health. Nowadays, obesity becomes one of the most important, modifiable risk factors for the development of preeclampsia. Emerging evidence suggests that dysregulation of maternal and placental lipid metabolism is involved in the pathogenesis of the condition.

Altogether, the impact of nutritional FAs on whole body and brain development and their long-term influence on the offspring's susceptibility to diseases remains a research subject of outermost relevance for developed and underdeveloped countries as one.

References

[1] Spector AA, Kim HY. Discovery of essential fatty acids. J Lipid Res 2015;56(1):11–21.

[2] Singer SJ, Nicolson GL. The fluid mosaic model of the structure of cell membranes. Science 1972;175(4023):720–31.

[3] Natarajan SK, et al. Structure, function and metabolism of hepatic and adipose tissue lipid droplets: implications in alcoholic liver disease. Curr Mol Pharmacol 2017;10(3):237–48.

[4] Brindley DN, et al. Lipid phosphate phosphatases regulate signal transduction through glycerolipids and sphingolipids. Biochim Biophys Acta 2002;1582(1–3):33–44.

[5] Hartl WH, Wolfe RR. The phospholipid/arachidonic acid second messenger system: its possible role in physiology and pathophysiology of metabolism. J Parenter Enter Nutr 1990;14(4):416–27.

[6] Koivuniemi A. The biophysical properties of plasmalogens originating from their unique molecular architecture. FEBS Lett 2017;591(18):2700–13.

[7] Iqbal J, et al. Sphingolipids and lipoproteins in health and metabolic disorders. Trends Endocrinol Metabol 2017;28(7):506–18.

[8] Kim JH, et al. The effect of sterol structure upon clathrin-mediated and clathrin-independent endocytosis. J Cell Sci 2017;130(16):2682–95.

[9] Moser H. [Biochemical, histological and clinical findings in a four-year-old female carrier of benign X-linked muscular dystrophy (Becker type)]. Humangenetik 1971;11(4):328–35.

[10] Paththinige CS, Sirisena ND, Dissanayake V. Genetic determinants of inherited susceptibility to hypercholesterolemia - a comprehensive literature review. Lipids Health Dis 2017;16(1):103.

[11] Goldstein HS, et al. Psychological differentiation and specificity of response. J Nerv Ment Dis 1970;151(2):97–103.

[12] De Craene JO, et al. Phosphoinositides, major actors in membrane trafficking and lipid signaling pathways. Int J Mol Sci 2017;18(3).

[13] Nickol HJ. Xerostomia as accident sequela. Arch Klin Exp Ohren- Nasen- Kehl-kopfheilkd 1969;194(2):621–5.

[14] Willy PJ, et al. LXR, a nuclear receptor that defines a distinct retinoid response pathway. Genes Dev 1995;9(9):1033–45.

[15] Marino G, Kroemer G. Mechanisms of apoptotic phosphatidylserine exposure. Cell Res 2013;23(11):1247–8.
[16] Bistrian BR. Clinical aspects of essential fatty acid metabolism: jonathan Rhoads Lecture. J Parenter Enter Nutr 2003;27(3):168–75.
[17] Postic C, Girard J. Contribution of de novo fatty acid synthesis to hepatic steatosis and insulin resistance: lessons from genetically engineered mice. J Clin Invest 2008;118(3):829–38.
[18] Duncan RE, et al. Regulation of lipolysis in adipocytes. Annu Rev Nutr 2007;27:79–101.
[19] Lee H, Park WJ. Unsaturated fatty acids, desaturases, and human health. J Med Food 2014;17(2):189–97.
[20] Suzuki M. Regulation of lipid metabolism via a connection between the endoplasmic reticulum and lipid droplets. Anat Sci Int 2017;92(1):50–4.
[21] Rambold AS, Cohen S, Lippincott-Schwartz J. Fatty acid trafficking in starved cells: regulation by lipid droplet lipolysis, autophagy, and mitochondrial fusion dynamics. Dev Cell 2015;32(6):678–92.
[22] Sarma PS, Gazdar AF. Recent progress in studies of mouse type-C viruses. Curr Top Microbiol Immunol 1974;68:1–28.
[23] Mourot J, Camara M, Fevrier C. [Effects of dietary fats of vegetable and animal origin on lipid synthesis in pigs]. C R Acad Sci III 1995;318(9):965–70.
[24] Simopoulos AP, Leaf A, Salem Jr N. Essentiality of and recommended dietary intakes for omega-6 and omega-3 fatty acids. Ann Nutr Metab 1999;43(2):127–30.
[25] Blondeau N, et al. Alpha-linolenic acid: an omega-3 fatty acid with neuroprotective properties-ready for use in the stroke clinic? BioMed Res Int 2015:519830. 2015.
[26] Simopoulos AP. The importance of the omega-6/omega-3 fatty acid ratio in cardiovascular disease and other chronic diseases. Exp Biol Med 2008;233(6):674–88.
[27] Calder PC, Yaqoob P. Omega-3 polyunsaturated fatty acids and human health outcomes. Biofactors 2009;35(3):266–72.
[28] Mozaffarian D, Aro A, Willett WC. Health effects of trans-fatty acids: experimental and observational evidence. Eur J Clin Nutr 2009;63(Suppl. 2):S5–21.
[29] Simopoulos AP. Genetic variants in the metabolism of omega-6 and omega-3 fatty acids: their role in the determination of nutritional requirements and chronic disease risk. Exp Biol Med 2010;235(7):785–95.
[30] Catani MV, et al. Essential dietary bioactive lipids in neuroinflammatory diseases. Antioxidants Redox Signal 2018;29(1):37–60.
[31] Asson-Batres MA, Rochette-Egly C. The nutritional importance of liposoluble compounds, such as vitamin A. Foreword. Subcell Biochem 2014;70:v–vi.
[32] Longo VD, Fontana L. Calorie restriction and cancer prevention: metabolic and molecular mechanisms. Trends Pharmacol Sci 2010;31(2):89–98.
[33] Innis SM. Essential fatty acid transfer and fetal development. Placenta 2005;26(Suppl. A):S70–5.
[34] Barker DJ. The fetal origins of coronary heart disease. Acta Paediatr Suppl 1997;422:78–82.
[35] Kabaran S, Besler HT. Do fatty acids affect fetal programming? J Health Popul Nutr 2015;33:14.
[36] Leikin-Frenkel AI. Is there A Role for alpha-linolenic acid in the fetal programming of health? J Clin Med 2016;5(4).
[37] Dube E, Desparois G, Lafond J. Placental lipid transport. Methods Mol Biol 2018;1710:305–16.
[38] Herrera E. Lipid metabolism in pregnancy and its consequences in the fetus and newborn. Endocrine 2002;19(1):43–55.

[39] Dube E, et al. Modulation of fatty acid transport and metabolism by maternal obesity in the human full-term placenta. Biol Reprod 2012;87(1):14. 1-11.
[40] Herrera E, Ortega-Senovilla H. Lipid metabolism during pregnancy and its implications for fetal growth. Curr Pharmaceut Biotechnol 2014;15(1):24−31.
[41] Alvarez JJ, et al. Longitudinal study on lipoprotein profile, high density lipoprotein subclass, and postheparin lipases during gestation in women. J Lipid Res 1996;37(2):299−308.
[42] Iglesias A, et al. Changes in cholesteryl ester transfer protein activity during normal gestation and postpartum. Clin Biochem 1994;27(1):63−8.
[43] Lewis RM, Wadsack C, Desoye G. Placental fatty acid transfer. Curr Opin Clin Nutr Metab Care 2018;21(2):78−82.
[44] Gauster M, et al. Dysregulation of placental endothelial lipase and lipoprotein lipase in intrauterine growth-restricted pregnancies. J Clin Endocrinol Metab 2007;92(6):2256−63.
[45] Lindegaard ML, et al. Endothelial and lipoprotein lipases in human and mouse placenta. J Lipid Res 2005;46(11):2339−46.
[46] Harmon CM, McGonigal S, Larkin JC. Impairment of trophoblast survival and differentiation by LXR ligands is prevented by cholesterol but not ABCA1 silencing. Placenta 2018;69:50−6.
[47] Lewis RM, Childs CE, Calder PC. New perspectives on placental fatty acid transfer. Prostaglandins Leukot Essent Fatty Acids 2018;138:24−9.
[48] Dutta-Roy AK. Transport mechanisms for long-chain polyunsaturated fatty acids in the human placenta. Am J Clin Nutr 2000;71(1 Suppl. l):315S−22S.
[49] Gil-Sanchez A, Koletzko B, Larque E. Current understanding of placental fatty acid transport. Curr Opin Clin Nutr Metab Care 2012;15(3):265−72.
[50] Makkar A, et al. Fatty acid binding protein-4 is expressed in the mouse placental labyrinth, yet is dispensable for placental triglyceride accumulation and fetal growth. Placenta 2014;35(10):802−7.
[51] Scifres CM, et al. Fatty acid binding protein 4 regulates intracellular lipid accumulation in human trophoblasts. J Clin Endocrinol Metab 2011;96(7):E1083−91.
[52] Shekhawat PS, Matern D, Strauss AW. Fetal fatty acid oxidation disorders, their effect on maternal health and neonatal outcome: impact of expanded newborn screening on their diagnosis and management. Pediatr Res 2005;57(5 Pt 2):78R−86R.
[53] Gil-Sanchez A, et al. Mechanisms involved in the selective transfer of long chain polyunsaturated Fatty acids to the fetus. Front Genet 2011;2:57.
[54] Glatz JF, Luiken JJ. From fat to FAT (CD36/SR-B2): understanding the regulation of cellular fatty acid uptake. Biochimie 2017;136:21−6.
[55] Wang P, et al. Fatty acid-binding protein 4 in endometrial epithelium is involved in embryonic implantation. Cell Physiol Biochem 2017;41(2):501−9.
[56] Ruiz-Palacios M, et al. Insulin treatment may alter fatty acid carriers in placentas from gestational diabetes subjects. Int J Mol Sci 2017;18(6).
[57] Nikolova V, et al. Changes in LXR signaling influence early-pregnancy lipogenesis and protect against dysregulated fetoplacental lipid homeostasis. Am J Physiol Endocrinol Metab 2017;313(4):E463−72.
[58] Duttaroy AK. Fetal growth and development: roles of fatty acid transport proteins and nuclear transcription factors in human placenta. Indian J Exp Biol 2004;42(8):747−57.
[59] Haggarty P, et al. Long-chain polyunsaturated fatty acid transport across the perfused human placenta. Placenta 1997;18(8):635−42.
[60] Islam A, et al. Fatty acid binding protein 3 is involved in n-3 and n-6 PUFA transport in mouse trophoblasts. J Nutr 2014;144(10):1509−16.

[61] Magnusson-Olsson AL, et al. Effect of maternal triglycerides and free fatty acids on placental LPL in cultured primary trophoblast cells and in a case of maternal LPL deficiency. Am J Physiol Endocrinol Metab 2007;293(1):E24–30.
[62] Barbour LA, Hernandez TL. Maternal lipids and fetal overgrowth: making fat from fat. Clin Therapeut 2018;40(10):1638–47.
[63] Ramos MP, et al. Fat accumulation in the rat during early pregnancy is modulated by enhanced insulin responsiveness. Am J Physiol Endocrinol Metab 2003;285(2):E318–28.
[64] Herrera E, Amusquivar E. Lipid metabolism in the fetus and the newborn. Diabetes Metab Res Rev 2000;16(3):202–10.
[65] Herrera E, Ortega-Senovilla H. Implications of lipids in neonatal body weight and fat mass in gestational diabetic mothers and non-diabetic controls. Curr Diabetes Rep 2018;18(2):7.
[66] Butte NF. Carbohydrate and lipid metabolism in pregnancy: normal compared with gestational diabetes mellitus. Am J Clin Nutr 2000;71(5 Suppl. l):1256S–61S.
[67] Herrera E, et al. Relationship between maternal and fetal fuels and placental glucose transfer in rats with maternal diabetes of varying severity. Diabetes 1985;34 (Suppl. 2):42–6.
[68] Herrera E. Metabolic adaptations in pregnancy and their implications for the availability of substrates to the fetus. Eur J Clin Nutr 2000;54(Suppl. 1):S47–51.
[69] Zhang R, et al. Modulation of cholesterol transport by maternal hypercholesterolemia in human full-term placenta. PloS One 2017;12(2):e0171934.
[70] Aye IL, Keelan JA. Placental ABC transporters, cellular toxicity and stress in pregnancy. Chem Biol Interact 2013;203(2):456–66.
[71] Lopez-Soldado I, Ortega-Senovilla H, Herrera E. Maternal adipose tissue becomes a source of fatty acids for the fetus in fasted pregnant rats given diets with different fatty acid compositions. Eur J Nutr 2018;57(8):2963–74.
[72] Fournier T, et al. Involvement of PPARgamma in human trophoblast invasion. Placenta 2007;28(Suppl. A):S76–81.
[73] Lendvai A, et al. The peroxisome proliferator-activated receptors under epigenetic control in placental metabolism and fetal development. Am J Physiol Endocrinol Metab 2016;310(10):E797–810.
[74] Capparuccia L, et al. PPARgamma expression in normal human placenta, hydatidiform mole and choriocarcinoma. Mol Hum Reprod 2002;8(6):574–9.
[75] Bildirici I, et al. The lipid droplet-associated protein adipophilin is expressed in human trophoblasts and is regulated by peroxisomal proliferator-activated receptor-gamma/ retinoid X receptor. J Clin Endocrinol Metab 2003;88(12):6056–62.
[76] Meher AP, Joshi AA, Joshi SR. Maternal micronutrients, omega-3 fatty acids, and placental PPARgamma expression. Appl Physiol Nutr Metabol 2014;39(7):793–800.
[77] Capobianco E, et al. Effects of natural ligands of PPARgamma on lipid metabolism in placental tissues from healthy and diabetic rats. Mol Hum Reprod 2008;14(8):491–9.
[78] Wadhwani N, Patil V, Joshi S. Maternal long chain polyunsaturated fatty acid status and pregnancy complications. Prostaglandins Leukot Essent Fatty Acids 2018;136:143–52.
[79] Gao L, et al. Differential regulation of prostaglandin production mediated by corticotropin-releasing hormone receptor type 1 and type 2 in cultured human placental trophoblasts. Endocrinology 2008;149(6):2866–76.
[80] Gibb W. The role of prostaglandins in human parturition. Ann Med 1998;30(3):235–41.
[81] Bogacka I, et al. In vitro effect of peroxisome proliferator activated receptor (PPAR) ligands on prostaglandin E2 synthesis and secretion by porcine endometrium during the estrous cycle and early pregnancy. J Physiol Pharmacol 2013;64(1):47–54.
[82] Challis JR, et al. Prostaglandins and mechanisms of preterm birth. Reproduction 2002;124(1):1–17.

[83] Fowden AL, Ralph MM, Silver M. Nutritional regulation of uteroplacental prostaglandin production and metabolism in pregnant ewes and mares during late gestation. Exp Clin Endocrinol 1994;102(3):212–21.
[84] Cheng Z, et al. Effect of dietary polyunsaturated fatty acids on uterine prostaglandin synthesis in the cow. J Endocrinol 2001;171(3):463–73.
[85] Young IR, Thorburn GD. Prostaglandin E2, fetal maturation and ovine parturition. Aust N Z J Obstet Gynaecol 1994;34(3):342–6.
[86] Truong H, et al. Does genetic variation in the Delta6-desaturase promoter modify the association between alpha-linolenic acid and the prevalence of metabolic syndrome? Am J Clin Nutr 2009;89(3):920–5.
[87] Mennitti LV, et al. Type of fatty acids in maternal diets during pregnancy and/or lactation and metabolic consequences of the offspring. J Nutr Biochem 2015;26(2):99–111.
[88] Swanson D, Block R, Mousa SA. Omega-3 fatty acids EPA and DHA: health benefits throughout life. Adv Nutr 2012;3(1):1–7.
[89] Akerele OA, Cheema SK. A diet enriched in longer chain omega-3 fatty acids reduced placental inflammatory cytokines and improved fetal sustainability of C57BL/6 mice. Prostaglandins Leukot Essent Fatty Acids 2018;137:43–51.
[90] Burdge GC, et al. Effect of reduced dietary protein intake on hepatic and plasma essential fatty acid concentrations in the adult female rat: effect of pregnancy and consequences for accumulation of arachidonic and docosahexaenoic acids in fetal liver and brain. Br J Nutr 2002;88(4):379–87.
[91] Lauritzen L, Carlson SE. Maternal fatty acid status during pregnancy and lactation and relation to newborn and infant status. Matern Child Nutr 2011;7(Suppl. 2):41–58.
[92] Hornstra G. Essential fatty acids in mothers and their neonates. Am J Clin Nutr 2000;71(5 Suppl. l):1262S–9S.
[93] Kroger J, Schulze MB. Recent insights into the relation of Delta5 desaturase and Delta6 desaturase activity to the development of type 2 diabetes. Curr Opin Lipidol 2012;23(1):4–10.
[94] Labrousse VF, et al. Dietary omega-3 deficiency exacerbates inflammation and reveals spatial memory deficits in mice exposed to lipopolysaccharide during gestation. Brain Behav Immun 2018;73:427–40.
[95] Peng J, et al. Maternal eicosapentaenoic acid feeding promotes placental angiogenesis through a Sirtuin-1 independent inflammatory pathway. Biochim Biophys Acta Mol Cell Biol Lipids 2018;1864(2):147–57.
[96] Tosi F, et al. Delta-5 and delta-6 desaturases: crucial enzymes in polyunsaturated fatty acid-related pathways with pleiotropic influences in health and disease. Adv Exp Med Biol 2014;824:61–81.
[97] Morales E, et al. Genetic variants of the FADS gene cluster and ELOVL gene family, colostrums LC-PUFA levels, breastfeeding, and child cognition. PloS One 2011;6(2):e17181.
[98] Brookes KJ, et al. Association of fatty acid desaturase genes with attention-deficit/hyperactivity disorder. Biol Psychiatr 2006;60(10):1053–61.
[99] Standl M, et al. FADS gene variants modulate the effect of dietary fatty acid intake on allergic diseases in children. Clin Exp Allergy 2011;41(12):1757–66.
[100] Martinelli N, et al. FADS genotypes and desaturase activity estimated by the ratio of arachidonic acid to linoleic acid are associated with inflammation and coronary artery disease. Am J Clin Nutr 2008;88(4):941–9.
[101] Malerba G, et al. SNPs of the FADS gene cluster are associated with polyunsaturated fatty acids in a cohort of patients with cardiovascular disease. Lipids 2008;43(4):289–99.

[102] Kelsall CJ, et al. Vascular dysfunction induced in offspring by maternal dietary fat involves altered arterial polyunsaturated fatty acid biosynthesis. PloS One 2012;7(4):e34492.
[103] Brayner B, et al. FADS polymorphism, omega-3 fatty acids and diabetes risk: asystematic review. Nutrients 2018;10(6).
[104] Chilton FH, et al. Precision nutrition and omega-3 polyunsaturated fatty acids: acase for personalized supplementation approaches for the prevention and management of human diseases. Nutrients 2017;9(11).
[105] Leveille P, Rouxel C, Plourde M. Diabetic pregnancy, maternal and fetal docosahexaenoic acid: a review of existing evidence. J Matern Fetal Neonatal Med 2018;31(10):1358–63.
[106] Gimpfl M, et al. Modification of the fatty acid composition of an obesogenic diet improves the maternal and placental metabolic environment in obese pregnant mice. Biochim Biophys Acta (BBA) - Mol Basis Dis 2017;1863(6):1605–14.
[107] Church MW, et al. Abnormal neurological responses in young adult offspring caused by excess omega-3 fatty acid (fish oil) consumption by the mother during pregnancy and lactation. Neurotoxicol Teratol 2009;31(1):26–33.
[108] Young PA, et al. Long-chain acyl-CoA synthetase 1 interacts with key proteins that activate and direct fatty acids into niche hepatic pathways. J Biol Chem 2018;293(43):16724–40.
[109] Kaur P, et al. The epigenome as a potential mediator of cancer and disease prevention in prenatal development. Nutr Rev 2013;71(7):441–57.
[110] Yang KF, et al. Maternal high-fat diet programs Wnt genes through histone modification in the liver of neonatal rats. J Mol Endocrinol 2012;49(2):107–14.
[111] Burdge GC, Lillycrop KA. Fatty acids and epigenetics. Curr Opin Clin Nutr Metab Care 2014;17(2):156–61.
[112] Ramaiyan B, Talahalli RR. Dietary unsaturated fatty acids modulate maternal dyslipidemia-induced DNA methylation and histone acetylation in placenta and fetal liver in rats. Lipids 2018;53(6):581–8.
[113] He Z, et al. FADS1-FADS2 genetic polymorphisms are associated with fatty acid metabolism through changes in DNA methylation and gene expression. Clin Epigenet 2018;10(1):113.
[114] Reynolds RM, et al. Maternal obesity during pregnancy and premature mortality from cardiovascular event in adult offspring: follow-up of 1 323 275 person years. BMJ 2013;347:f4539.
[115] Cameron CM, et al. Maternal pregravid body mass index and child hospital admissions in the first 5 years of life: results from an Australian birth cohort. Int J Obes 2014;38(10):1268–74.
[116] Osmond C, Barker DJ. Fetal, infant, and childhood growth are predictors of coronary heart disease, diabetes, and hypertension in adult men and women. Environ Health Perspect 2000;108(Suppl. 3):545–53.
[117] Kuhle S, et al. Maternal pre-pregnancy obesity and health care utilization and costs in the offspring. Int J Obes 2019;43:735–43.
[118] Muhlhausler BS, et al. Pregnancy, obesity and insulin resistance: maternal overnutrition and the target windows of fetal development. Horm Mol Biol Clin Invest 2013;15(1):25–36.
[119] Sewell MF, et al. Increased neonatal fat mass, not lean body mass, is associated with maternal obesity. Am J Obstet Gynecol 2006;195(4):1100–3.
[120] Modi N, et al. The influence of maternal body mass index on infant adiposity and hepatic lipid content. Pediatr Res 2011;70(3):287–91.
[121] Segura MT, et al. Maternal BMI and gestational diabetes alter placental lipid transporters and fatty acid composition. Placenta 2017;57:144–51.

[122] R B, Tr R. Dietary n-3 but not n-6 fatty acids down-regulate maternal dyslipidemia induced inflammation: a three-generation study in rats. Prostaglandins Leukot Essent Fatty Acids 2018;135:83–91.
[123] Hoch D, et al. Diabesity-associated oxidative and inflammatory stress signalling in the early human placenta. Mol Aspect Med 2019;66:21–30.
[124] Calabuig-Navarro V, et al. Effect of maternal obesity on placental lipid metabolism. Endocrinology 2017;158(8):2543–55.
[125] Hirschmugl B, et al. Maternal obesity modulates intracellular lipid turnover in the human term placenta. Int J Obes 2017;41(2):317–3tl23.
[126] Shomonov-Wagner L, Raz A, Leikin-Frenkel A. Alpha linolenic acid in maternal diet halts the lipid disarray due to saturated fatty acids in the liver of mice offspring at weaning. Lipids Health Dis 2015;14:14.
[127] Seet EL, et al. Maternal high-fat-diet programs rat offspring liver fatty acid metabolism. Lipids 2015;50(6):565–73.
[128] Gazquez A, et al. Placental lipid droplet composition: effect of a lifestyle intervention (UPBEAT) in obese pregnant women. Biochim Biophys Acta Mol Cell Biol Lipids 2018;1863(9):998–1005.

CHAPTER 15

Vitamin D as a modifier of genomic function and phenotypic expression during pregnancy*

Bruce W. Hollis, Carol L. Wagner
Pediatrics Medical University of South Carolina, Charleston, SC, United States

Contents

Introduction

In 1986, David Barker noted a connection between small infant size and risk of heart disease later in adult life [1]. The theory that certain adult-onset diseases might have their roots in nutritional insults sustained in the perinatal period has since become known as "the Barker hypothesis." The idea

* Funded in part by NIH/NICHD R01 HD043921, U01HL091528 from NHLBI, NIH/NCATS UL1RR029882, and the Thrasher Research Fund.

Molecular Nutrition
ISBN 978-0-12-813862-5
https://doi.org/10.1016/B978-0-12-813862-5.00015-3

that early-life influences can have important downstream consequences is attractive and is supported by such known instances as perinatal thyroid function, which is absolutely essential for early-life brain development and maturation. In this example, iodine deficiency and its consequences certainly qualify as an instance of the Barker hypothesis in operation. A critical feature of diseases occurring by way of the Barker hypothesis is the nutritional irreversibility of the disorders that result. Beyond certain critical points in development, full nutrient repletion is not able to correct or reverse the earlier inadequacy.

Another nutrient deficiency during the perinatal period resulting in a catastrophic event is folic acid deficiency resulting in spina bifida [2]. In the 1960s, Hibbard and Smithells established a register of malformed babies born in Liverpool, England [3]. This register enabled him to identify families who had babies with the specific defect of spina bifida establishing a link between the condition and a poor diet. Smithells went on to define the lack of folic acid in the early perinatal period as the cause of spinal bifida [4], a truly remarkable association.

During this early period, only the phenotypic result could be observed as a consequence of any given nutritional deficiency. Presently, we have the capabilities of not only observing the phenotype but also the genetic changes contributing to any given phenotype. The purpose of this review is to shed light on the potential of dietary vitamin D during the prenatal and perinatal periods as a contributor to maternal/infant afflictions, and thus its role in instituting examples of the Barker hypothesis at both the genetic and phenotypic levels. These afflictions include but are not limited to auto-immune disorders, complications of pregnancy, immune function, and respiratory disease. We will not be discussing vitamin D metabolism in this text as that information is readily available elsewhere [5,6].

Defining a "normal" circulating 25(OH)D concentration in humans

Defining a "normal" circulating level of 25(OH)D, the prehormone to the active hormone 1,25(OH)$_2$D, in humans is not an easy task. For instance, the most recent Institute of Medicine (IOM) concludes that a circulating concentration of 20 ng/mL is adequate to meet human physiological requirements [7]. Conversely, the Endocrine Society concludes that a concentration of 30 ng/mL 25(OH)D is what is needed [8]. The IOM recommendation was based solely on skeletal integrity stating that extra-skeletal functions had not been proven [7]. The Endocrine Society used not only skeletal studies but other afflictions such as cancer, immune function, and pregnancy complications [8]. What recommendation does one adhere to that not only includes circulating concentrations of 25(OH)D but also the amount of dietary vitamin D to be consumed on a daily basis?

To properly define "normal" circulating 25(OH)D status in humans, it makes sense to measure 25(OH)D concentrations in "healthy subjects" who are sunbathers, fieldworkers that are sun-exposed and indigenous people living and functioning in environments to which they are native. Why is this important? When ultraviolet light B in the range of ~290–320 nm hits the skin, specifically the epidermis, a chemical reaction occurs such that epidermal 7-dehydrocholesterol is converted to precholecalciferol or pre-vitamin D_3, and with an additional thermal conversion that takes place in the skin, the previtamin D_3 is converted to vitamin D_3 (cholecalciferol), the parent compound of vitamin D.

Humans did not evolve in today's sun-shy culture so "normal," with respect to circulating 25(OH)D concentrations, should not be defined by the current average or medium population concentrations. We would not even be having this controversy if a landmark study by Haddad and Chyu had been interpreted correctly [5]. This study assessed the circulating concentration of 25(OH)D in "normal individuals" and lifeguards where the lifeguards had circulating 25(OH)D concentrations 2.5 times higher than the "normal" subjects. If Haddad and Chyu had set "normal" as a 25(OH)D concentration based on the sun-exposed lifeguards and not the sun-shy "normal" subjects, the current controversy would not exist. Why was this not done? The biggest reason likely is attributed to the dietary recommendation of the era, which was approximately 400 IU/d vitamin D. To reach a circulating concentration of 60 ng/mL, which is the concentration of individuals with full access to sunlight living in a sun-rich environment and was the concentration achieved by the sun-exposed lifeguards [5], a dietary intake of 4000–6000 IU/d is required [6]; this was unacceptable to regulators since they had set the requirement at 400 IU/d [7]. Thus, normal physiology and science was ignored. Since that time, we have made significant advances on this front, although many regulators still cling to the outdated recommendations [7].

A final important question is: how much vitamin D do I need to take to achieve any given desired circulating 25(OH)D concentration? The 400 IU/d dose that is recommended by the IOM for older children and adults also is recommended for breastfeeding neonates a few days after birth [7,9]. When taking a dietary supplement of vitamin D containing 400 IU, on a per kilogram basis, the reference newborn infant weighing 3 kg receives ~133 IU/kg and the reference 60 kg pregnant woman receives 6.7 IU/kg. Based on pharmacokinetics, unless the pregnant woman has access to sunlight exposure, her circulating 25(OH)D concentration, serving as the indicator of her vitamin D status, will be around 15–25 ng/mL, whereas the newborn infant on 400 IU/day will have achieved circulating 25(OH) D concentrations in the mid-40s [10,11]. One thing is for sure—the amount listed by the IOM will not get you there [6]. Beyond that, the same amount of vitamin D taken orally will result in a wide variety of circulating 25(OH) concentrations among individuals [6]. Thus, the only way to know for sure is to have a circulating 25(OH)D concentration measured. Just to be clear, a daily intake of 10,000 IU/d vitamin D is deemed to be safe [8].

Vitamin D deficiency during pregnancy: animal models and human studies

Neurodevelopment

Animal model studies are required to give us guidance and insight into any given human disease. In the case of vitamin D and pregnancy, studies have been undertaken since the early 1980s and focused primarily on vitamin D deficiency and skeletal integrity because at the time it was thought to be the sole function of vitamin D [12]. As the role of vitamin D on bodily systems other than skeletal unfolded, the role of vitamin D during pregnancy expanded. The first extraskeletal studies focused on vitamin D deficiency during pregnancy and brain development. Vitamin D is a potent neurosteroid which mediates numerous actions in the brain. Localization studies have shown the presence of vitamin D activating enzyme CYP27B1 and catabolic enzyme CYP24A1 in neural cells of the cerebral cortex and cerebellar Purkinje cells, suggesting that vitamin D can be activated and/or degraded locally in the brain [13]. Early on, Eyles et al. [14] performed the first studies on this topic using rats. These investigators demonstrated that rats born to vitamin D-deficient mothers had profound alterations in the brain at birth. The cortex was longer but not wider, the lateral ventricles were enlarged, the cortex was proportionally thinner, and there was more cell proliferation throughout the brain. Further, there were reductions in brain content of nerve growth factor and glial cell line–derived neurotrophic factor and reduced expression of $p75^{NTR}$, the low-affinity neurotrophic receptor [14]. Further studies by this group demonstrated vitamin D deficiency in utero resulted in embryos and pups having significantly less apoptotic cells and more mitotic cells [15]. Targeted gene arrays specific for apoptosis and cell cycle genes confirmed a transcriptomic deregulation in the vitamin D-deficient group [16]. This study also demonstrated that vitamin D deficiency during pregnancy reduced fetal crown—rump length and head size [16]. Moreover, lateral ventricle volume was reduced in deficient fetuses. Expression of neurotrophic genes brain-derived neurotrophic factor and transforming growth factor-beta 1 was altered. Brain expression of forkhead box protein, a gene important in human speech and language, was altered. Further, Foxp2 immunoreactive cells in the developing cortex were reduced due to vitamin D deficiency. Brain tyrosine hydroxylase gene expression was reduced as was its localization in the substantia nigra [16]. Needless to say, these are profound brain changes involved in neurodevelopment. How these changes could relate to human neurodevelopment and brain function has significant implications.

The association between vitamin D and autism spectrum disorders (ASDs) was first proposed by Dr. John Cannell [17]. ASD includes autistic disorder, Asperger's syndrome, Rett's syndrome, childhood disintegrative disorder, and pervasive development disorders. Epidemiological studies have suggested a potential role for vitamin D deficiency in the development of ASD [18]. Vuillermot et al. [19] have recently presented a murine model of autism and demonstrated that vitamin D treatment during pregnancy attenuates and/or prevents neurodevelopment disorders following maternal inflammation during pregnancy. This study investigated whether some of the phenotypes present in offspring could be alleviated following maternal treatment with the active hormonal form of vitamin D called calcitriol or $1,25(OH)_2D$. The study demonstrated that prenatal administration of $1,25(OH)_2D$ abolished all behavioral defects in polyriboinosinic polyribocytidylic acid (poly[I:C])-treated juvenile mice with autism. However, this result could not be attributed to antiinflammatory mechanisms [19]. Other recent studies involving rodents have demonstrated maternal vitamin D deficiency results in the offspring expressing spatial learning deficiencies [20] as well as reproductive dysfunction in female mice offspring through adverse effects in the neuroendocrine axis [21].

Placental function

The IOM have estimated the annual costs for the burden of morbidity disability and mortality associated with preterm birth in the United States to be at least $26 billion [22], much of which is attributed to placental dysfunction leading to preeclampsia. Observational studies have linked vitamin D deficiency with preeclampsia in humans [23]. To date, there is no preventive or treatment measure for this condition. Preeclampsia, typically characterized by maternal hypertension, proteinuria, and a variation of other signs and symptoms, is the leading cause of premature delivery. Preeclampsia complicates up to 10% of all pregnancies, 3% severely with potential life-threatening consequences [24]. Again, causes and treatments remain unknown.

Liu et al. [25] hypothesized that low vitamin D status in pregnant mice could lead to symptoms of preeclampsia. The study used female BL6 mice raised on vitamin D-sufficient or vitamin D-deficient diets and then mated with vitamin D-sufficient BL6 males. The resulting pregnant mice were either allowed to deliver and monitored for blood pressure (BP) or euthanized prior to delivery for analysis of serum, placental/kidney tissues, and fetuses. Vitamin D-deficient pregnant mice exhibited both elevated systolic and arterial pressure. This elevation continued through pregnancy until 7 days postpartum but returned to baseline at 14 days postpartum. Maternal kidney analysis showed increased expression of mRNA for renin and the angiotensin II receptor due to deficiency. Histological analysis of deficient placentas showed decreased vascular diameter within the labyrinth region. Resupplementation of vitamin D post conception partially reversed the effects of vitamin D deficiency. Overall, these data provide evidence that low vitamin D status may predispose pregnant women to dysregulated placental development and elevated BP.

The findings of Liu et al. [25] were supported by a recent study by our group involving healthy pregnant women enrolled in a vitamin D supplementation trial. Specifically, a focused analysis of placental mRNA expression related to angiogenesis, pregnancy maintenance, and vitamin D metabolism was conducted in placentas from 43 subjects enrolled in a randomized controlled trial supplementing 400 IU or 4400 IU of vitamin D_3 (cholecalciferol, the parent compound) per day during pregnancy [26]. Placental mRNA was isolated from biopsies within 1 hour of delivery, followed by quantitative PCR. We classified pregnant women with circulating concentrations of <100 nmoles vitamin D/L as deficient and those with ≥100 nmoles vitamin D/L as sufficient, the threshold previously shown by our group where conversion of 25(OH)D to $1,25(OH)_2D$ is optimized [10]. We found that soluble FMS-like tyrosine kinase 1 (sFlt-1) and vascular endothelial growth factor (VEGF) gene expression was significantly downregulated in women with circulating 25(OH)D $\geq$ 100 ng/mL compared to those with a concentration <100 ng/mL. This was the first report of a significant association between maternal vitamin D status and the expression of sFlt-1 and VEGF at the mRNA level. Achieving maternal circulating 25(OH) D $\geq$ 100 nmoles/L suggests that the impact of maternal vitamin D_3 supplementation on gene transcription in the placenta may be through the downregulation of antiangiogenic factors that may contribute to vascular pregnancy complications.

Incomplete human extra-villous trophoblast invasion of the decidua and maternal spiral arteries is characteristic of preeclampsia [27]. It is hypothesized that dysregulated vitamin D action in utero of placental tissues disrupts extra-villous invasion leading to malplacentation [28]. Chan et al. [28] demonstrated that vitamin D significantly increased extra-villous trophoblast invasion. This was accomplished by increased promatrix metalloproteinases. These data support a role for vitamin D in extra-villous trophoblast invasion and preeclampsia. Further studies by this group have shown that vitamin D is an important component of antiinflammatory immune responses during pregnancy, with the placenta and fetal sex playing pivotal roles in this process [29]. Finally, consistent with the work of Schulz et al., [26] vitamin D supplementation prevents placental ischemia—induced endothelial dysfunction by downregulating placental soluble FMS-like tyrosine kinase 1 leading to preeclampsia [30].

Lung maturation and function

Vitamin D deficiency is recognized worldwide and there are data indicating that circulating concentrations have decreased over time, coincident with the rise in autoimmunity and asthma [31,32]. Vitamin D also has effects on the developing lung that are upregulated in early lung development; and these same genes (for example, matrix metallopeptidase9; NF-k light polypeptide gene enhancer in B cells inhibitor; epidermal growth factor receptor; E1A binding protein p300) are linked to the later development of asthma [33]. Zosky et al., using a relevant BALB/c mouse model of vitamin D deficiency, studied somatic growth, lung function, and lung structure at 2 weeks of age [34]. It was determined that volume dependence of lung mechanics was altered by vitamin D deficiency, suggesting altered tissue structure. It was determined that the primary histological difference between vitamin D-deficient and replete groups was primarily explained by differences in lung volume, thus providing evidence linking vitamin D deficiency and lung development. The same group subsequently published the effects of in utero vitamin D deficiency on airway smooth muscle mass and function [33]. Their data demonstrated that gene pathways involved in embryonic organ development, pattern formation, branching morphogenesis, wingless/Int, and inflammation were differently expressed in vitamin D-deficient mice. Genes differentially expressed include hubs matrix metallopeptidase 9, NF-k light polypeptide gene enhancer in B cells inhibitor, an epidermal growth factor receptor, and E1A binding protein p300 [33]. *In utero*, vitamin D deficiency was sufficient to increase airway smooth muscle mass and baseline airway resistance and alter lung function [34]. Collectively, these data suggest that in utero vitamin D deficiency can alter lung structure and function and increase inflammation, contributing to symptoms such as asthma.

A more recent animal study investigated if vitamin D supplementation could block pulmonary structural and functional changes in a rat model of perinatal vitamin D deficiency [35]. This study found that only a high dose of vitamin D corrected the increase in tracheal contractility. In addition to altering alveolar epithelial–mesenchymal signaling, perinatal vitamin D deficiency also altered airway contractility, providing insights into asthma pathogenesis in perinatally vitamin D-deficient offspring [35]. Thus, significant animal model data suggest a strong link between perinatal vitamin D deficiency and the development of respiratory abnormalities such as asthma in offspring.

Other diseases

Autoimmune diseases, including rheumatoid, multiple sclerosis (MS), Crohn's disease, and celiac disease, result from an aberrant activation of the immune system whereby the immune response is directed against harmless self-antigens. The immunomodulatory effects of vitamin D provide opportunities to enhance the treatment of autoimmune diseases [36].

MS ethology has been an active field with respect to vitamin D [37]. In experimental animals, Experimental Autoimmune Encephalomyelitis (EAE) is used as a model for MS [38]. Fernandes de Abreu et al. [39] demonstrated that adult mice from mothers exposed to vitamin D deficiency during pregnancy developed a less severe and delayed EAE when compared to controls. Fernandes de Abreu et al. [40] subsequently showed that maternal vitamin D deficiency induces inverted transgenerational effects on the immune system of offspring, with the first generation being less sensitive. EAE symptoms in the second generation are equally increased if it is either the first generation mother or father who has been vitamin D-deprived during embryogenesis [40]. It is possible that vitamin D could inhibit the production of autocrine IL-6 and IL-21 in 2D2 T cells, which, in turn, could reduce their TL 17 differentiation, thus impacting autoimmune reaction [41].

Vitamin D deficiency during pregnancy: human studies

Observational studies

Again, this chapter will not discuss the role of vitamin D and skeletal function during pregnancy since this has been discussed endlessly in the past, and truth be told, minimal supplemental vitamin D is required to meet these needs [42]. Certainly, these needs would be met and exceeded by recommendations we make here with respect to nonskeletal functions of vitamin D.

Beyond skeletal issues, what would these other issues be with respect to vitamin D in pregnancy? To discover what these might be, we rely on associative or observational studies, and in the past 15 years many of these studies have been performed. Of high interest is the association of dietary vitamin D_3 intake in pregnant women and preeclampsia [43]. Olsen and Secher [43] point out that in the early 1940s, studies were performed giving pregnant women halibut liver oil, a rich source of vitamin D_3, with decreases in preterm birth and preeclampsia observed, which the authors attributed to marine n-3 fatty acids, with no mention of vitamin D and its potential effect [43]. But why would they, since that connection would make no sense to them at the time? As we moved through the recent decades, it became clear that vitamin D's actions in the human body could exist well beyond skeletal events, and thus people started looking at the link between vitamin D and other disease states and conditions [44–59]. Early observational studies uncovered strong relationships between maternal circulating levels of 25(OH)D and preeclampsia [23,53–55], altered placental vascular pathology [56], cesarean section [57], glucose tolerance [58], adverse birth outcomes due to race [59], brain function [52], and respiratory function [45]. More recent studies have pointed to maternal vitamin D deficiency as a risk factor for abnormal fetal growth patterns, adverse birth outcomes, reproductive failure [60–64], and further strengthened vitamin D's role as a contributing agent for preeclampsia [65,66]. Also, a recent metaanalysis of observational studies has confirmed the fact that maternal vitamin D deficiency increases the risk of preterm birth [67].

While public policy cannot be set for supplementation practices based on observational studies, this information is invaluable at pointing research in the direction that could yield public policy changes in vitamin D consumption. These next steps are interventional studies or better yet, randomized clinical trials (RCTs). One has to exhibit caution, however, even with RCTs, whose results can be problematic when analyzed on an intent-to-treat basis and when there is high nonadherence to protocol (as is often the case), thereby diluting the potential good or harm of a given treatment at higher doses. Also, unlike a pharmaceutical, everyone has a given amount of circulating 25(OH)D, which certainly confounds any such trial. As such, a biomarker of a drug or in this case "vitamin" or preprohormone is better served. For these reasons, analyses of effect of vitamin D therapies using 25(OH)D concentration are a far better indicator of true effect.

Randomized clinical trials

Enthusiasm for evidence-based medicine (EBM) has resulted in the extension of its methods to the evaluation of nutrient effects. Heaney [68] pointed out that EBM, as applied in the evaluation of drugs, is poorly suited to the study of nutrients. In a drug trial, the placebo group should be totally devoid of the compound in question; not so for a nutrient like vitamin D. To perform a true RCT for vitamin D, one would have to make sure all subjects were vitamin D-deficient at the study onset. For the duration of the study, all subjects would have to remain indoors to avoid any sun exposure. Then and only then could a true RCT be performed for any given function of vitamin D. Of course, what we have suggested here is unethical and is never going to take place. How then does one proceed? Heaney [68] has provided excellent guidance in this regard. He proposed five rules for individual clinical studies of nutrient effects. These rules are as follows: (1) basal nutrient status must be measured, used as an inclusion criterion for entry into the study, and recorded in the report of the trial; (2) the intervention must be large enough to change nutrient status and must be quantified by suitable analysis; (3) the change in nutrient status produced in those enrolled in the report of the trial must be measured and reported; (4) the hypothesis to be tested must be that a change in nutrient status produces the sought-after effect; and (5) conutrient status must be optimized in order to ensure that the nutrient is the only nutrition-related, limiting factor in the response. We would add one additional rule to this group, that being: the nutrient in question has to follow an appropriate dosing schedule matching the physiologic system being investigated [69]. Needless to say, while almost all vitamin D RCTs to this point would fail based on these criteria, evaluation of existing evidence with respect to pregnancy will become the basis for optimizing dietary and clinical recommendations.

Vitamin D supplementation trials involving pregnant women have been performed since 1980 [70]. These early studies were small; did not look at meaningful endpoints (such as accurate bone mineral density measurements [such methods did not exist at that time], or the role of vitamin D on the incidence of such disease states as preeclampsia [23,53–55], asthma [45,71–74], preterm birth [67,75–77], and autoimmune dysfunction [78–82]; and/or supplemented with nominal doses of vitamin D (0–400 IU/day) [70]. As a result, no meaningful information or public policy changes occurred because of them.

In 2001, our group conceived a large RCT investigating the supplementation of vitamin D to a pregnant population. Our study was radical in design in that we proposed supplementing pregnant women less than 16 weeks of gestation with up to 4000 IU/d vitamin D_3 until delivery in a double-blind fashion. The goal of the study was to see how much vitamin D was required to raise circulating maternal 25(OH)D concentrations to at least 32 ng/mL by the end of gestation. Using mathematical calculations from previous studies [6,83], we calculated how much vitamin D_3 we would need to provide to achieve this endpoint. We selected the 32 ng/mL concentration of circulating 25(OH)D based on the suppression of secondary hyperparathyroidism [84]. At the initiation of these RCTs, our endpoints were safety of the dosing, attained circulating level of maternal 25(OH)D, growth parameters of the infant, and bone–mineral density of the mother and infant. As for the other factors mentioned in the previous section on vitamin D relationships based on observational studies, those associations had not been made at study initiation, and as a result we had no idea to even look for them, and certainly not to propose them as endpoints. As such, these endpoints were analyzed as *post hoc* analyses.

The results of these RCTs have been presented and published over the last few years [10,85–94]. The main finding of these studies was that a 4000 IU/d dose of vitamin D_3 safely elevates circulating 25(OH)D to a concentration that, regardless of race, fully normalizes vitamin D metabolism, and calcium homeostasis in the pregnant women. Using repeated measures, the concentration of 25(OH)D that fully normalized $1,25(OH)_2D$ in our study cohort was determined on each subject and plotted to determine the point at which first order kinetics went to zero order [10]. This point at which the 25(OH)D concentration was 40 ng/mL, the production of $1,25(OH)_2D$ became substrate independent [10]. Further, elevated dosing was safe with not a single adverse event observed attributable to vitamin D supplementation [10,85–94].

When our studies were completed in 2009–10, we were aware of the observational data suggesting favorable efforts of vitamin D on pregnancy outcomes beyond calcium homeostasis. Therefore, other collected data on our patients were subsequently analyzed. We demonstrated increased vitamin D supplementation decreased complications of pregnancy and C-section births [75,86]. Further, RCT data and analysis by our group and others have clearly demonstrated that higher doses of vitamin D during pregnancy improve birth outcome data [75,76,88].

RCT studies beyond our own have recently demonstrated vitamin D to greatly decrease complications of birth and gestational diabetes [58,88,89,91], aeroallergen sensitization [90], and markers of regulatory immunity [92]. The most informative of these RCT studies was performed by Sablok et al.[88]. These investigators took a vitamin D-deficient population of pregnant women, with circulating 25(OH)D concentrations of <10 ng/mL and supplemented the treatment arm with substantial amounts of vitamin D starting at 20 weeks of gestation. The control group received placebo and thus remained profoundly vitamin D-deficient throughout pregnancy. Vitamin D treatment in these women with 100% adherence to protocol resulted in a substantial decline in the complications of pregnancy. A study of this type could never be performed in most of the western countries as it would be deemed unethical. Be that as it may, it demonstrated the massive effect of vitamin D supplementation on the complications of pregnancy.

Vitamin D-induced genomic alterations during pregnancy

If one looks at our original pregnancy study from an intent-to-treat perspective, the results are muddled most likely due to nonadherence [10]; however, taking adherence into account by using circulating 25(OH)D concentrations as a variable, the true effect on vitamin D supplementation

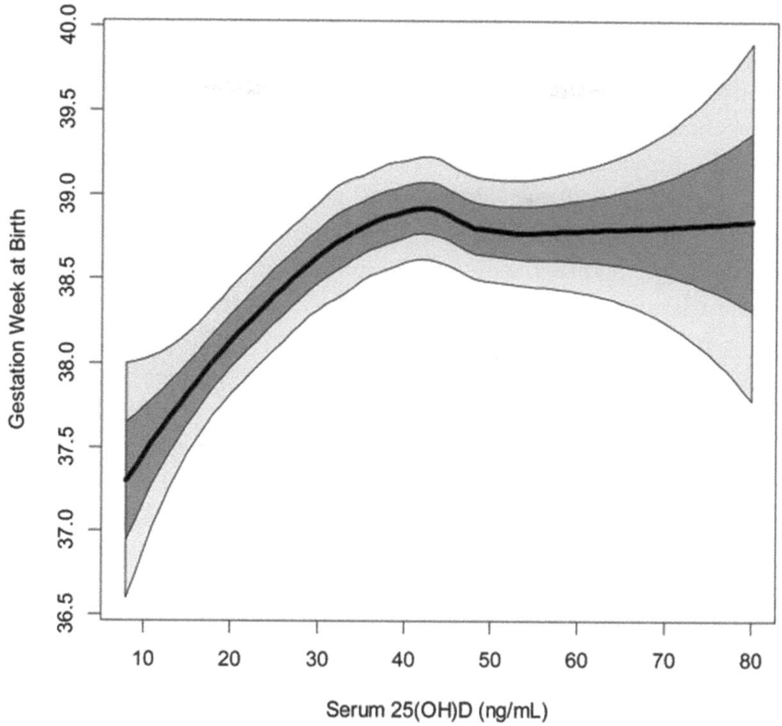

Figure 15.1 Relationship between Total Circulating 25(OH)D concentrations and gestational age at birth. Black *line* represents fitted LOESS curve; dark gray area represents 1 standard deviation; and light gray area represents 2 standard deviations. Multivariable log-binomial regression found that 25(OH)D concentrations ≥40 ng/mL reduce the risk of preterm birth by 59% compared to ≤20 ng/mL, adjusted for covariates. Zoom on the fitted LOESS curve of 25(OH)D concentration and gestational age (weeks) at birth to better show the change in average behavior with 1 and 2SD windows superimposed (NICHD and TRF, N = 509). *(From reproduced with permission CL. Wagner, C. Baggerly, S. McDonnell, KA. Baggerly, CB. French, L.Baggerly, SA. Hamilton, BW. Hollis. Post-hoc analysis of vitamin D status and reduced risk of preterm birth in two vitamin D pregnancy cohorts compared with South Carolina March of Dimes 2009-2011 rates. J Steroid Biochem Mol Biol 155 (2016);(Pt B):245-251. doi: 10.1016/j.jsbmb.2015.10.022. PubMed PMID: 26554936; PMCID: PMC5215876.)*

on preterm birth is exposed [76] (Fig. 15.1). The same associations from our VDAART trial also hold true for the prevention of preeclampsia [95]. How does this occur? Vitamin D supplementation during pregnancy appears to affect genetic information of several highly functional modules related to systemic inflammation and immune responses and implicates the emergence of a distinctive immune response in women destined to develop preeclampsia [26,64] and other comorbidities of pregnancy such as gestational diabetes [89,91,96] and infection [97,98].

A recent paper by Al-Garawi et al. [99], derived from the VDAART RCT study, provides direct proof of vitamin D's ability to induce genomic changes during pregnancy. Patterns of gene expression during human pregnancy are poorly understood. This study is an RCT of vitamin D supplementation in pregnancy for the reduction of pediatric asthma risk [85]. The trial enrolled 881 women at 10–18 weeks of gestation. Longitudinal gene expression measures were obtained on 30 pregnant women, using RNA isolated from peripheral blood samples obtained in the first and third trimesters. Differentially expressed genes were identified using significance of analysis of microarrays (SAM) and clustered using a weighted gene coexpression network analysis (WGCNA). Gene-set enrichment performed to identify major biological transcriptional profiles between first and third trimesters of pregnancy identified 5839 significantly differentially expressed genes. Weighted gene coexpression network analysis clustered these transcripts into 14 coexpression modules of which two showed significant correlation with maternal 25(OH)D concentrations (Table 15.1). Pathway analysis of these two modules revealed genes enriched in immune defense pathways and extracellular matrix reorganization as well as genes enriched in Notch signaling and transcription factor networks (Table 15.2, Figs. 15.2–15.5). These data suggest that maternal gene expression changes during pregnancy occur and that these changes are related to vitamin D supplementation that increase circulating 25(OH)D concentrations. What remains unclear is whether these changes in maternal 25(OH)D concentrations impact fetal development directly or through downstream effects, and whether there is any direct effect of maternal gene expression on the fetus. New data suggest that there are indeed direct genomic alterations induced by vitamin D administered during pregnancy that can alter birth outcomes [100].

Postnatal asthma prevention

Observational studies by Brehm et al. suggested that vitamin D supplementation during pregnancy could reduce childhood asthma rates [100]. A double-blind multicenter RCT conducted in the United States was performed involved giving supplemental vitamin D_3 (400 or 4400 IU/d) to pregnant women across the three major racial/ethnic groups in the United

Table 15.1 Top differentially expressed genes identified by SAM analysis (FDR <0.05).

Upregulated genes

Entrez ID	Gene	*P*-value	Adjusted *P*-value	Gene description
8451	CUL4A	<.0001	<.0001	Cullin 4A
83666	PARP9	<.0001	<.0001	Poly (ADP-ribose) polymerase family, member 9
4128	MAOA	<.0001	<.0001	Monoamine oxidase A
10935	PRDX3	<.0001	<.0001	Peroxiredoxin 3
948	CD36	<.0001	<.0001	CD36 molecule (thrombospondin receptor)
221895	JAZF1	<.0001	<.0001	JAZF zinc finger 1
6423	SFRP2	<.0001	<.0001	Secreted frizzled-related protein 2
56994	CHPT1	<.0001	<.0001	Choline phosphotransferase 1
10935	PRDX3	5.54E-08	7.80E-05	Peroxiredoxin 3
7027	TFDP1	5.54E-08	7.80E-05	Transcription factor Dp-1
4928	NUP98	1.11E-07	9.48E-05	Nucleoporin 98 kDa
440672	NUDT4P1	1.11E-07	9.48E-05	Nudix (nucleoside diphosphate linked moiety X)-type motif4
11171	STRAP	1.11E-07	9.48E-05	Serine/threonine kinase receptor associated protein
6772	STAT1	1.11E-07	9.48E-05	Signal transducer and activator of transcription 1
140739	UBE2F	1.11E-07	9.48E-05	Ubiquitin-conjugating enzyme E2F

Downregulated genes

Entrez ID	Gene	*P*-value	Adjusted *P*-value	Gene description
5333	PLCD1	<.0001	<.0001	Phospholipase C, delta 1
6844	VAMP2	<.0001	<.0001	Vesicle-associated membrane protein 2 (synaptobrevin 2)

(*Continued*)

Table 15.1 Top differentially expressed genes identified by SAM analysis (FDR <0.05).—cont'd

6689	SPIB	<.0001	<.0001	Spi-B transcription factor (spi-1/PU.1 related)
135	ADORA2A	<.0001	<.0001	Adenosine A2a receptor
2788	GNG7	5.54E-08	7.80E-05	Guanine nucleotide binding protein (G protein), gamma 7
3633	INPP5B	5.54E-08	7.80E-05	Inositol polyphosphate-5-phosphatase, 75 kDa
1359	CPA3	5.54E-08	7.80E-05	Carboxypeptidase A3 (mast cell)
84958	SYTL1	1.11E-07	9.48E-05	Synaptotagmin-like 1
26207	PITPNC1	1.11E-07	9.48E-05	Phosphatidylinositol transfer protein, cytoplasmic 1
326624	RAB37	1.11E-07	9.48E-05	RAB37, member RAS oncogene family
128637	TBC1D20	1.11E-07	9.48E-05	TBC1 domain family, member 20
9619	ABCG1	1.11E-07	9.48E-05	ATP-binding cassette, subfamily G
9813	EFCAB14	2.22E-07	0.000161771	KIAA0494
9619	ABCG1	2.77E-07	0.000161771	ATP-binding cassette, subfamily G
8498	RANBP3	2.77E-07	0.000161771	RAN binding protein 3

States from 16 weeks of gestation until delivery. The primary endpoint was prevention of asthma/wheeze in the infant/child at 1, 2, and 3 years post birth. Nearly 900 high-risk subjects were enrolled and completed the study, which recently was published [85]. The results of this study are quite clear: on the basis of maternal circulating 25(OH)D concentrations achieved, vitamin D supplementation during pregnancy will decrease asthma or recurrent wheezing rates in children. This positive finding, however, is dependent upon a circulating 25(OH)D concentration of at least 40 ng/mL at conception [71,72,85].

A nearly identical RCT study performed in Denmark also recently has been published [73]. The authors of these two RCTs performed a combined analysis [72]. The results from this combined RCT analysis is quite

Table 15.2 Enrichment analysis of key transcription factors that act on genes in green module (FDR <0.05).

Network	GO processes	Total nodes	Seed nodes	Adjusted *P*-value
CREB1	G1/S transition of mitotic cell cycle, metallo- and- iron-sulfur cluster assembly	73	73	3.980E-193
c-Myc	Modulation by virus of host morphology or physiology or of other organism involved in symbiotic interaction	49	48	8.490E-124
p53	Cell cycle process cellular response to glucose starvation, negative regulation of cell cycle	20	19	4.240E-48
ZNF143	Single-organism carbohydrate metabolic process, carbohydrate metabolic process, nucleotide metabolic process, nucleoside phosphate metabolic process, CMP-N-acetylneuraminate biosynthetic process	19	18	1.550E-45
GCR-alpha	Cellular component organization, cellular component organization or biogenesis, cellular amino acid biosynthetic process, rhythmic process, response to arsenic-containing substance	19	18	1.550E-45
Androgen receptor	Androgen receptor signaling pathway, intracellular steroid hormone receptor signaling pathway, positive regulation of transcription, DNA-dependent, positive regulation of RNA metabolic process, positive regulation of gene expression	16	15	7.080E-38
SP1	Response to arsenic-containing substance, cellular response to chemical stimulus, cellular nitrogen compound metabolic process, modulation by virus of host morphology or physiology, regulation of	15	14	2.490E-35

Continued

Table 15.2 Enrichment analysis of key transcription factors that act on genes in green module (FDR <0.05).—cont'd

Network	GO processes	Total nodes	Seed nodes	Adjusted *P*-value
	transcription from RNA polymerase II promoter in response to hypoxia			
ESR1 (nuclear)	Intracellular receptor signaling pathway, RNA metabolic process, intracellular steroid hormone receptor signaling pathway, gene expression, transcription from RNA polymerase II promoter	15	14	2.490E-35
E2F1	Cell cycle process, mitotic cell cycle, negative regulation of cellular process, cell cycle, negative regulation of biological process	14	13	8.650E-33

Top 10 significantly enriched transcription factor networks of the 202 annotated genes from the green module. For each network, the GO processes are shown along with the number of genes from the green network that are enriched within each network and the number of total nodes that define the network. Total nodes = total number of objects in the network (database); seed nodes = number of objects in green dataset. Hypergeometric test adjusted for multiple comparisons using Benjamini and Hochberg ($P < .05$).

clear: vitamin D_3 given to a pregnant woman will prevent asthma/wheeze in her child [71,72]. This revelation is displayed in Figs. 15.6 and 15.7.

Further analysis of the VDAART study published in JAMA revealed some highly relevant findings [71,72]. Figs. 15.6 and 15.7 detail these findings. What is explicitly demonstrated in the VDAART study is that a woman has to enter pregnancy with a circulating 25(OH)D levels of at least 30 ng/mL and then be given 4000 IU/d vitamin D_3 starting at approximately 16 weeks' post conception to provide maximum protection against asthma development in her infant following birth [71,72]. Further, these data suggest that vitamin D is strongly associated with very early in utero lung development in the fetus that cannot be reduced by starting vitamin D supplementation at the end of the first trimester. Vitamin D-related genes in early lung development and asthma pathogenesis have been described [33]. These developmental genes include LAMP1, PIP5-KIB, SCARB2, and TXNIP [99]. TXNIP, also known as vitamin D_3

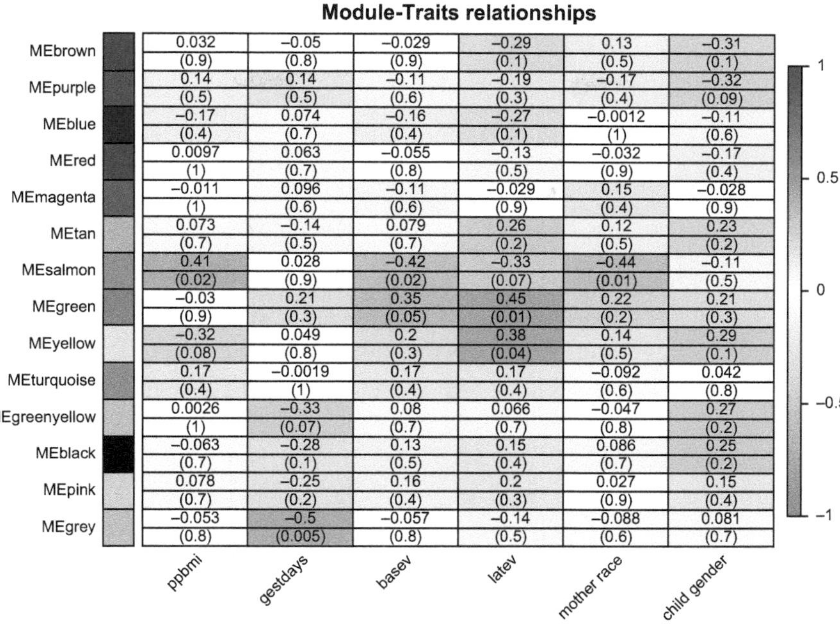

Figure 15.2 Weighted gene coexpression network analysis and associations with clinical traits. Weighted Co-Expression Network Analysis (WGCNAs) was carried out on 5839 differentially expressed probes identified by SigGenes. 14 coexpression modules were identified and, and correlated to various clinical traits. Gene network, represented by different colored-coded coexpression modules (y-axis) and their association with various clinical traits (x-axis). The intensity of the colors indicates the strength of the relationship, as indicated by the scale to the right. The range of the scale (+1 to −1) indicates either positive (+1) or negative (−1) correlation with a specific clinical trait. Top number in each box corresponds to the Pearson's correlation coefficient between a module and a specific trait, while the lower number represents its *P*-value. Traits: ppbmi = prepregnancy BMI; gestdays = gestational age; basev = Vitamin D levels in first trimester; latev = vitamin D levels in third trimester; mother.race = maternal race (White/African-American); Child.-gender = infant gender (boy/girl). Pearson's correlation ($P < .05$). *(From A. Al-Garawi, VJ. Carey, D. Chhabra, H. Mirzakhani, J. Morrow, J. Lasky-Su, W. Qiu, N. Laranjo, AA. Litonjua, ST. Weiss. The role of vitamin D in the transcriptional program of human pregnancy. PloS One 11(10) (2016):e0163832. doi: 10.1371/journal.pone.0163832. PubMed PMID: 27711190; PMCID: PMC5053446.reproduced with permission.)*

upregulated protein 1, is required for the development of natural killer cells. LAMP3 appears to be a marker of dendritic cell maturation. PIP5K1B regulates calcium signaling in mast cells. SCAR2B appears to modulate the normal maturation of phagosomes and autophagosomes [99].

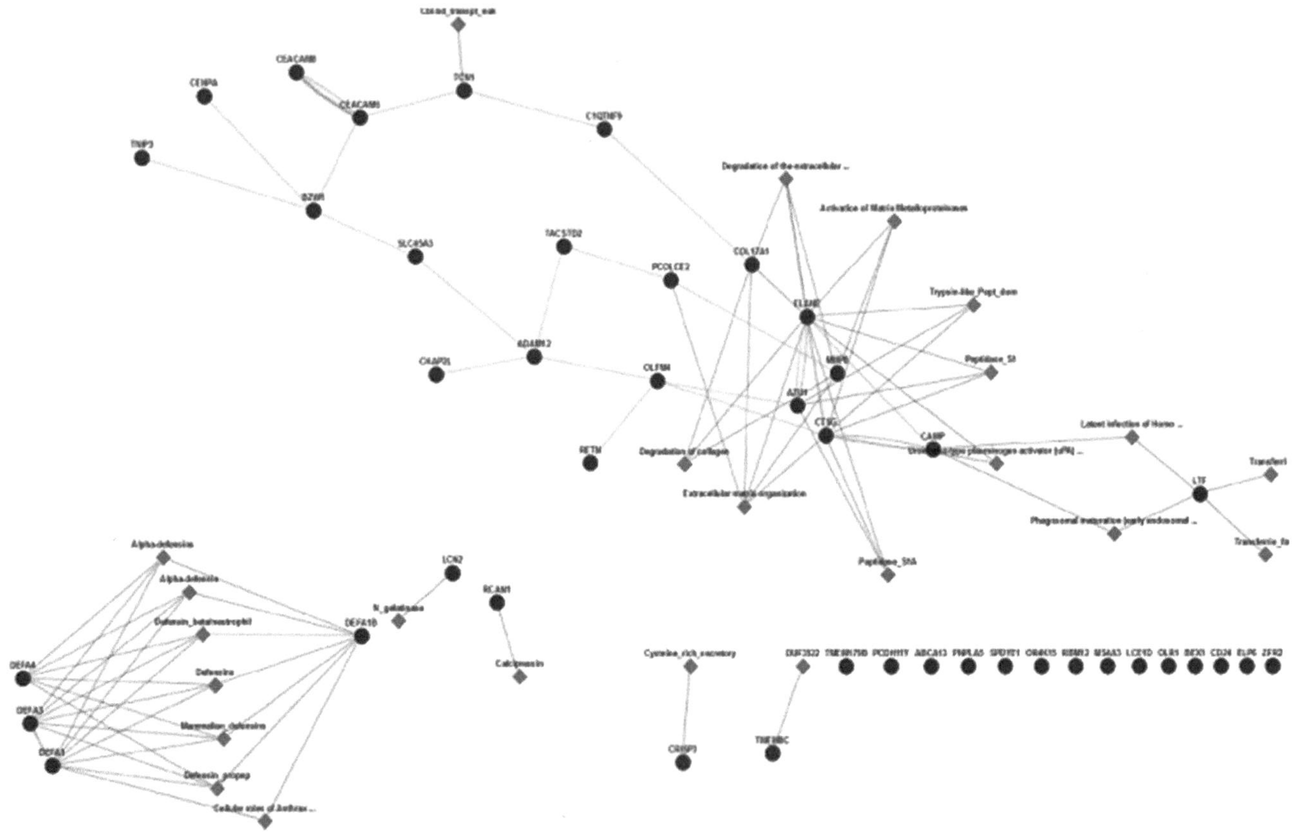

Figure 15.3 Functional pathway enrichment of genes in salmon module. Gene maps constructed based on evidence from genetic (green *line*: light gray line in printed version), physical (red *line*: dark gray line in printed version), and predicted (yellow *line*: gray line in printed version) interaction. The distance between groups of genes reflects the strength of their relationship and groups of genes that are more closely related are clustered together. Functional Pathway analysis revealing most enriched pathways based on InterPro, Pathway Commons, and Transcription Factor target databases. The resulting visual map represents known functional pathways involving salmon gene nodes. Black *circle* = nodes, gray diamonds = enriched functional pathways. Al-Garawi et al. 2016 [99]. *(reproduced with permission.)*

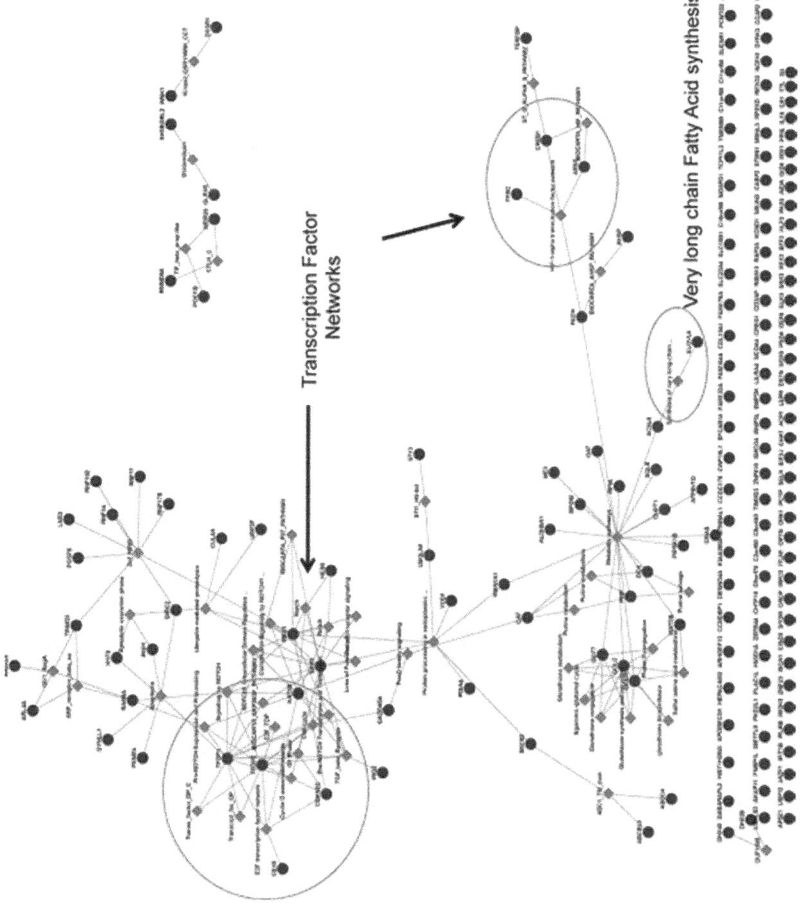

Figure 15.4 Functional pathway enrichment of genes in green module revealing most enriched pathways based on InterPro, Pathway Commons and Transcription Factor target databases. The distance between groups of genes reflects the strength of their relationship and groups of genes that are more closely related are clustered together. Black *circle* = nodes, gray diamonds = enriched functional pathways. Al-Garawi et al. 2016 [99]. *(reproduced with permission.)*

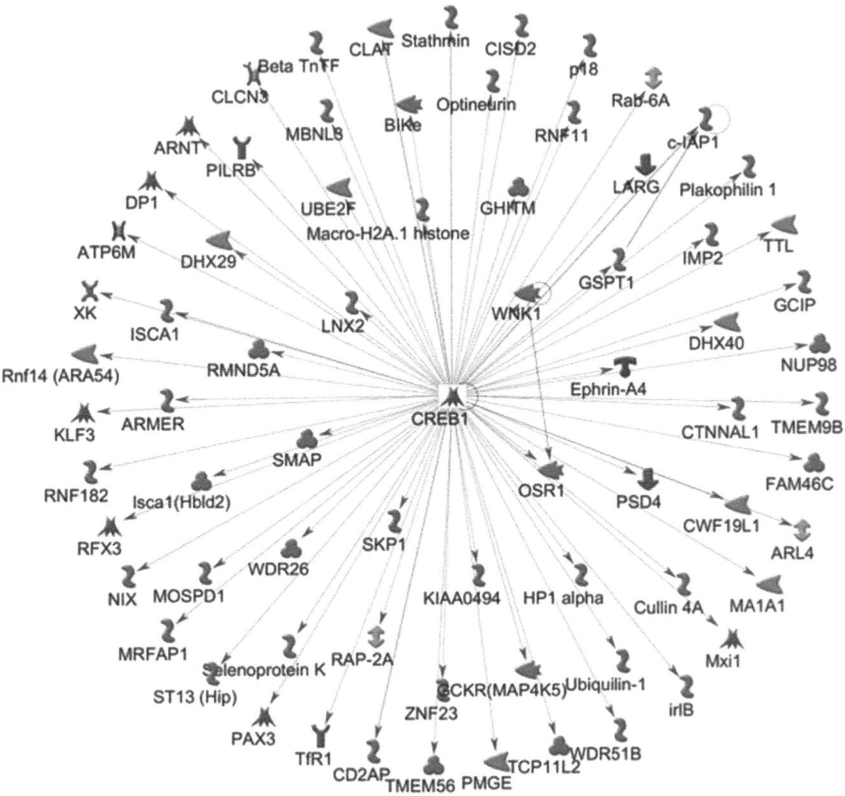

Figure 15.5 Transcription factor enrichment analysis of Green module genes. CREB1 transcription factor network depicting CREB1 in center and known interactions among 72 genes demonstrating various functionality within the green module. Hypergeometric test adjusted for multiple comparisons using Benjamini & Hochberg ($P < .05$). Al-Garawi et al. 2016 [99]. *(reproduced with permission.)*

Preeclampsia prevention

A recent study by Mirzakhani et al. [95] derived from the VDAART RCT presents interesting new data describing how maternal vitamin D when at adequate levels, through direct genomic alteration, basically eliminates preeclampsia. When the VDAART study was conceived, several assumptions were made. First, it was assumed that 4000 IU/d vitamin D_3 would normalize circulating 25(OH)D concentrations throughout pregnancy. Secondly, the assumption was made that supplementation beginning at approximately 14 weeks' gestation would impart the biological effects desired, that being decreased preeclampsia and childhood asthma rates. These assumptions assume that afflictions of vitamin D deficiency prior to

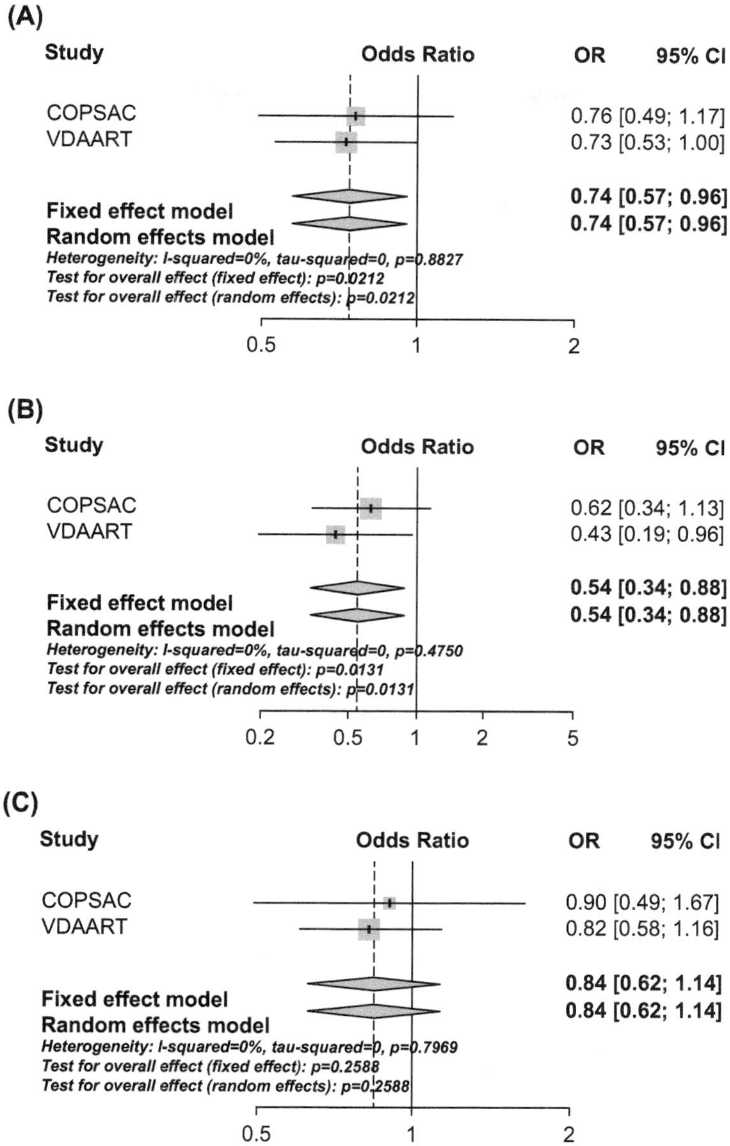

Figure 15.6 Combined analysis of two RCTs of vitamin D supplementation during pregnancy to prevent recurrent wheezing and asthma at 3 year of age. *(Data from the Vitamin D Antenatal Asthma Reduction Trial (VDAART) and Copenhagen Prospective Studies on Asthma in Childhood 2010 (COPSAC) studies were combined in this analysis. HM. Wolsk, BL. Chawes, AA. Litonjua, BW. Hollis, J. Waage, J. Stokholm, K. Bonnelykke, H. Bisgaard, ST. Weiss. Prenatal vitamin D supplementation reduces risk of asthma/ recurrent wheeze in early childhood: a combined analysis of two randomized controlled trials. PloS One 12(10) 2017:e0186657. doi: 10.1371/journal.pone.0186657. PubMed PMID: 2907771reproduced with permission.)*

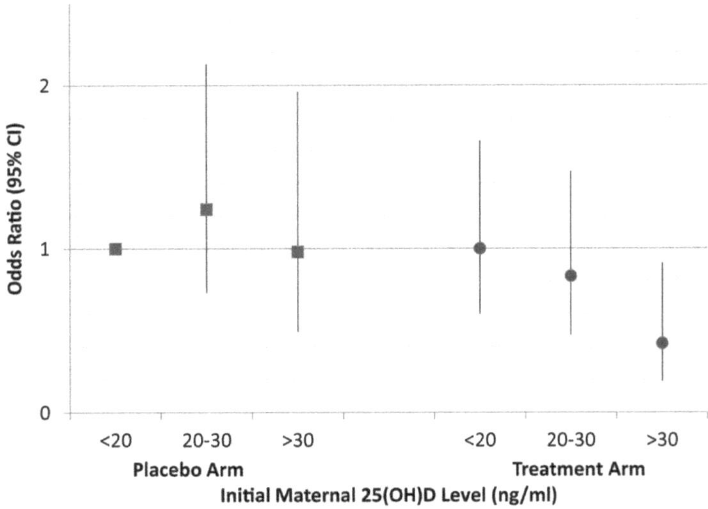

Figure 15.7 Odds Ratio (95% CI) of recurrent wheezing/asthma at three years as a function of maternal 25(OH)D concentration (ng/mL) at baseline by treatment group. *(Secondary Analysis of Data from the Vitamin D Antenatal Asthma Reduction Trial (VDAART). HM. Wolsk, BL. Chawes, AA. Litonjua, BW. Hollis, J. Waage, J. Stokholm, K. Bonnelykke, H. Bisgaard, ST. Weiss. Prenatal vitamin D supplementation reduces risk of asthma/recurrent wheeze in early childhood: a combined analysis of two randomized controlled trials. PloS One 12(10) (2007):e0186657. doi: 10.1371/journal.pone.0186657. PubMed PMID: 29077711. Reproduced with permission.)*

14 weeks of gestation could be corrected by the resulting supplementation for the duration of the pregnancy. This assumption turned out to be somewhat accurate with respect to childhood asthma formation [95] in the pregnancy period. Fig. 15.8 clearly demonstrates this fact, and tells us that the most import factor in preventing preeclampsia is to enter pregnancy with adequate vitamin D status. Entering pregnancy with a circulating 25(OH)D level of a least 40 ng/mL imparts perfect protection against development of preeclampsia (Fig. 15.8). In fact, this effect of vitamin D is predicted by experimental animal models, which collectively demonstrated vitamin D deficiency altered placental development and embryo implantation [25,101,102]. This effect is likely mediated by vitamin D through normalization of placental vascularization and angiogenesis during a very early point in pregnancy. Once this time point is passed, rescue by further vitamin D supplementation is futile as the results of Mirzakhani et al. imply [95]. What is equally remarkable is how this point is either missed or ignored by leading experts in the field [103]. Further, more supportive

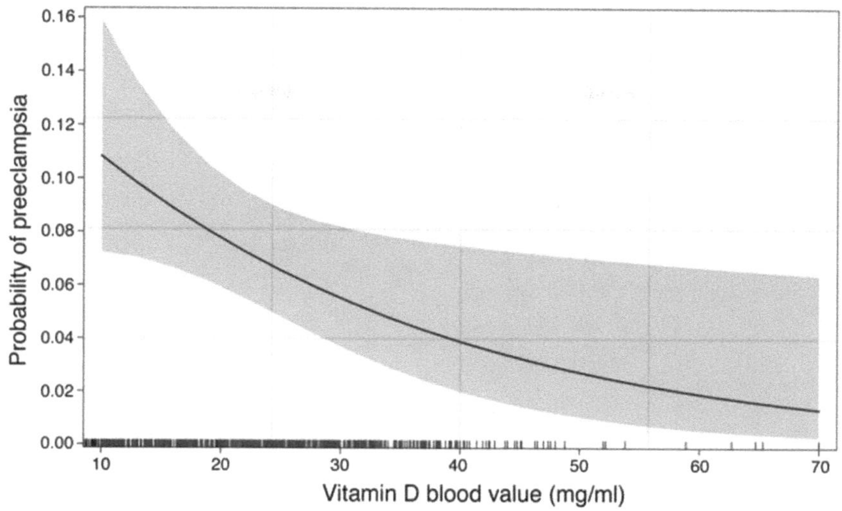

Figure 15.8 Dose–response association between maternal serum 25OHD concentrations at 10–18 weeks of gestation and the corresponding predicted probability of preeclampsia derived from a logistic regression model adjusted for the identified confounders. The gray zone indicates 0.95 confidence bands ($N_{preeclampsia} = 67$, $N_{healthy} = 749$). The minimum predicted risk for the population under study relative to the distribution of pregnant women (vertical tick marks on the x-axis) falls at the concentrations of 40–50 ng/mL total circulating 25(OH)D. Mirzakhani et al., 2016 [95]. *(reproduced with permission.)*

evidence concerning the role of vitamin D in the prevention of preeclampsia comes from a recent RCT study where the administration of vitamin D (50,000 IU/week that translates into ~7142 IU/day) during the prenatal period reduced the preeclamptic rate by half [94].

The basic question would be, what are the physiologic/genomic alterations responsible for this vitamin D-induced protection to preeclampsia? In the recent report by Mirzakhani et al. [95], a gene expression substudy identified a set of vitamin D-associated genes related to preeclampsia. The study demonstrated genomic connectivity to known vitamin D-signaling pathways indicating the functional cohesiveness of vitamin D to the preeclampsia disease model (Figs. 15.9 and 15.10). Most of the genes in this replication model were associated with maternal systemic changes in immune, both innate and humoral, and inflammatory responses (Figs. 15.9 and 15.10). A more detailed explanation of this interaction can be viewed within the publication [95]. This remarkable study is the first to explain how supplemental vitamin D can reduce the incidence of a serious condition at both the clinical and genomic level.

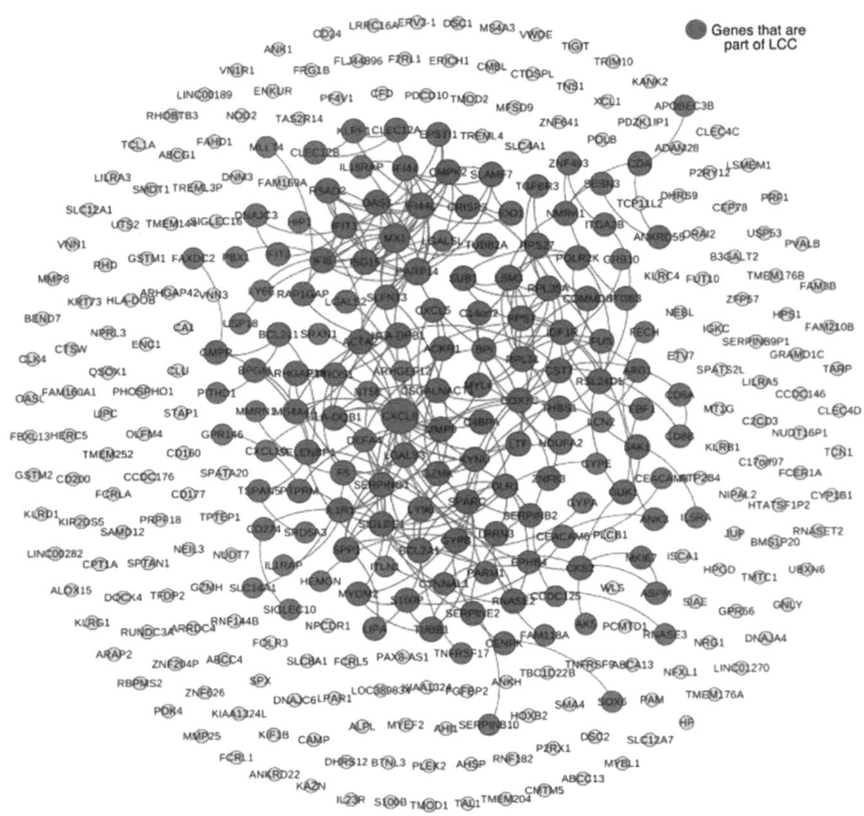

Term	No. of involved genes	Corrected *P* value
Immune system process	109	1.31×10^{-16}
Immune response	83	1.12×10^{-15}
Defense response	82	4.07×10^{-13}
Response to stress	125	1.28×10^{-9}
Response to biotic stimulus	50	5.27×10^{-9}
Regulation of immune system process	63	1.17×10^{-6}
Innate immune response	50	0.000001
Inflammatory response	35	0.0000042
Platelet degranulation	12	0.0000606
Immune effector process	36	0.000174
Cellular response to cytokine stimulus	34	0.000536
Leukocyte migration	22	0.000583
Negative regulation of immune system process	22	0.00102
Cytokine-mediated–signaling pathway	29	0.00139
Cell-surface receptor–signaling pathway	81	0.00143
IL-10 production	8	0.00157
Cellular response to type I IFN	10	0.00294
Type I IFN–signaling pathway	10	0.00294
Response to type I IFN	10	0.00411
Regulation of cell migration	29	0.00733
Cytokine production	28	0.0127
Lymphocyte-mediated immunity	15	0.0364
Adaptive immune response	19	0.043
Regulation of cytokine production	25	0.0498

Figure 15.9 From the vitamin D antenatal asthma reduction trial (VDAART), interactome mapping demonstrates immunomodulatory gene signatures in early pregnancy in women who developed preeclampsia. N = 323 of 348 (86.78%) replicated differentially expressed genes were mapped onto the interactome and demonstrated local clustering in the network (preeclampsia module vs. random expectation, $P < .0001$. LCC genes (143 genes, highlighted in red [dark gray in printed version]) corresponding to the "observable preeclampsia module" among the replicated differentially expressed genes (N = 348) and their biological processes. The connectivity of the replicated signatures was explored by mapping onto functional protein–protein interaction networks from HumanNet v.1. Mirzakhani et al., 2016[95]. *(reproduced with permission.)*

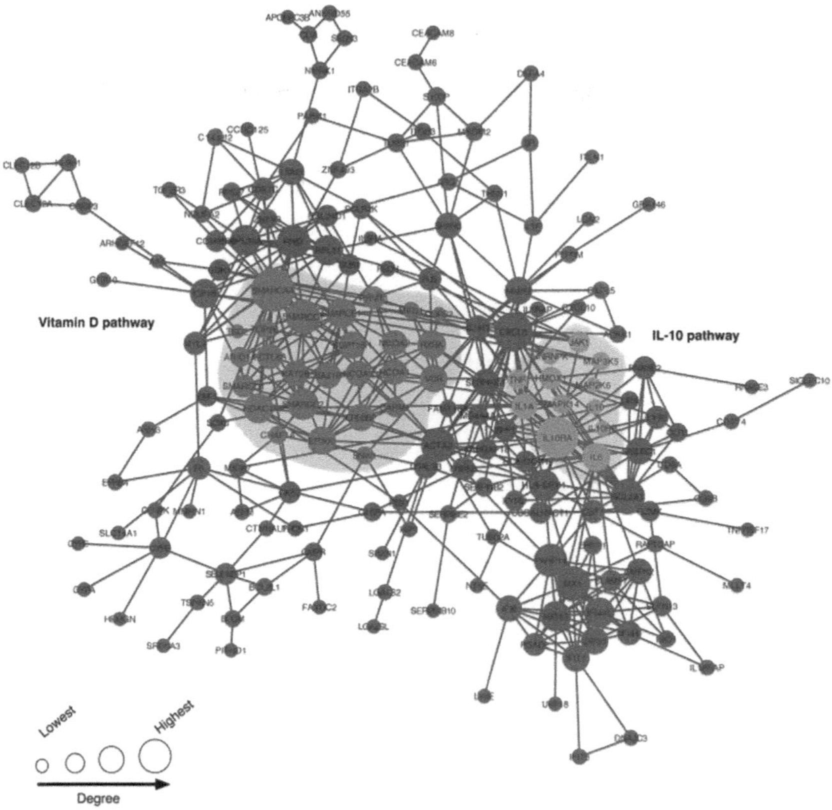

Figure 15.10 From the Vitamin D antenatal asthma reduction trial (VDAART), interactome mapping demonstrates immunomodulatory gene signatures in early pregnancy in women who developed preeclampsia. Connection among the vitamin D—and IL-10—signaling pathway genes (blue [gray in printed version] and yellow [light gray in printed version] modules, respectively) within the module. Mirzakhani et al., 2016[95]. *(reproduced with permission.)*

Maternal vitamin D supplementation is also involved in the epigenetic regulation, DNA methylation, in children. Pathways affected by this metabolic process include antigen processing and presentation, inflammation, regulation of cell death, cell proliferation, transmission of nerve impulse, neurogenesis, neuron differentiation, sensory organ development [104], and vitamin D metabolism [105]. The epigenetic effects of vitamin D have been demonstrated in experimental animal models [106,107], and preliminary findings have been reported in humans [104]. The total genomic effects of vitamin D are truly impressive by any standard.

What is clear from these recent RCTs is that a 4000 IU/d vitamin D_3 supplement is beneficial to both mother and child and these benefits have nothing to do with the classic role of vitamin D in calcium homeostasis. What is not resolved is the dose and time of administration to achieve optimum results. We believe that a target circulating 25(OH)D concentration of 40 ng/mL be achieved in pregnancy as early as possible. Because of biochemical heterogeneity in attaining a given concentration of 25(OH) D, we believe all women should consume at least 4000 IU/d vitamin D_3 prior to conception [10].

Neurodevelopment and autoimmune consequences

Can vitamin D deficiency and subsequent vitamin D supplementation during pregnancy impact autoimmune disease and neuropsychological development? To even raise this specter is a very scary consequence indeed.

It has long been thought that the development of MS is a result of a complex interaction between genes and environment with an important environmental factor being vitamin D deficiency [50]. It is not yet understood how and when vitamin D acts to modulate MS risk, although there is increasing evidence that this occurs through genetic alterations [49]. Data have emerged that demonstrate that vitamin D supplementation during pregnancy alters transcriptome and epigenetic alterations through DNA methylation in genes that regulate metabolic processes, antigen processing, inflammation, regulation of cell death, cell proliferation, transmission of nerve impulse, neurogenesis, neuron differentiation, and sensory organ development [104]. For now, what we have are observational studies strongly suggesting vitamin D deficiency during pregnancy and/or the early neonatal period as a strong causative agent in the development of MS in later life [46,48,108]. Agencies such as the IOM and Centers of Disease Control will say that these data must be confirmed by RCT. We state here that such an RCT will NEVER be performed because of the cost involved. How do we know that? A few years ago MS world experts were assembled by the National Multiple Sclerosis Society in Chicago to help design such a study. It was determined that the minimum dollar amount to conduct such an RCT would exceed 50 US million and would consume their entire budget for at least 5 years. While the study never went forth and never will, other randomized controlled trials of treatment to prevent progression of disease, for example, may be conducted. Further, an article by Mokry et al. on Mendelian randomization provides strong support of a causal association of vitamin D and lower MS risk in humans [109]. Health providers will have to make decisions on the data that are available that come from corollary studies such as these.

An even scarier prospect exists around vitamin D deficiency during pregnancy and neurologic disease and altered development [17,51,52]. Strong experimental animal evidence points to dire neurological consequences if vitamin D is restricted during pregnancy [110–113]. If one wants to read the biochemical basis for this, we suggest you read recent reviews by Patrick and Ames, who make an excellent case for intrauterine vitamin D deficiency as it relates to autism, attention deficit disorder, bipolar disorder, schizophrenia, and impulse behavior, through the control of serotonin synthesis in the neonatal brain [114]. There is also a fair amount of observational data available to support these claims. If that is not convincing, we suggest you read a recent prospective, interventional vitamin D trial during pregnancy for the prevention of autism in the newborn [51]. From these data, the authors suggest that even performing an RCT would be unethical based on the delay that would result to complete such a study, thus delaying supplementation implementation [51]. A recent study again strongly links vitamin D concentrations during pregnancy with the development of ASD [115].

Current recommendation for vitamin D supplementation

At this time, based on RCT data as well as substantial observational and interventional data, we suggest that all pregnant women maintain a circulating 25(OH)D concentration of a least 40 ng/mL during the earliest time points of pregnancy [76]. This will insure maximum protection from pregnancy complications, including preeclampsia in the mother and asthma formation in the infant. To achieve this, intakes of a least 4000 IU/d vitamin D_3 will be required because of variable individual abilities to convert vitamin D to 25(OH)D [6]. These supplements have proven to be safe in thousands of patients over the past 15 years, as not a single adverse event has been observed. Further, this level of supplementation lies within the safe intake level as defined by The Endocrine Society [8]. Also, our data agree with data derived from populations living in sun-rich environments where humans evolved over the past 200,000 years [116]. It is interesting that the blood concentrations of 25(OH)D achieved in our pregnancy RCTs are quite similar to those achieved in these indigenous populations during pregnancy simply from sun exposure [116,117].

Finally, does vitamin D qualify as a substance as described by the Barker Hypothesis? The clear answer is yes; it does because its absence during pregnancy imparts detrimental genetic alterations on both mother and fetus, and, at least in the case of asthma, phenotypic expression in the infant/child.

References

[1] Barker DJ, Osmond C. Diet and coronary heart disease in England and Wales during and after the second world war. J Epidemiol Community Health 1986;40(1):37–44. Epub 1986/03/01. PubMed PMID: 3711768; PMCID: 1052486.

[2] Daly S, Mills JL, Molloy AM, Conley M, Lee YJ, Kirke PN, Weir DG, Scott JM. Minimum effective dose of folic acid for food fortification to prevent neural-tube defects. Lancet 1997;350(9092):1666–9. Epub 1997/12/24. doi: 10.1016/S0140-6736(97)07247-4. PubMed PMID: 9400511.

[3] Hibbard ED, Smithells RW. Preliminary Communications. Folic acid metabolism and human embryopathy. Lancet 1965;285(6):1254.

[4] Smithells R, Sheppard S, Schorah C. Vitamin deficiencies and neural tube defects. Arch Dis Child 1976;51(1):944–50.

[5] Haddad JG, Chyu K. Competitive protein-binding radioassay for 25-hydroxycholecalciferol. J Clin Endocrinal Metab 1971;33:992–5.

[6] Heaney R, Davies K, Chen T, Holick M, Barger-Lux M. Human serum 25-hydroxycholecalciferol response to extended oral dosing with cholecalciferol. Am J Clin Nutr 2003;77:204–10.

[7] Food, Board N. Standing committee on the scientific evaluation of dietary reference intakes. Dietary reference intakes for vitamin D and calcium. Washington, D.C.: National Academy Press; 2010.

[8] Holick MF, Binkley NC, Bischoff-Ferrari HA, et al. Evaluation, treatment, and prevention of vitamin D deficiency: an Endocrine Society clinical practice guideline [published correction appears in J Clin Endocrinol Metab. 96 (12. J Clin Endocrinol Metab 2011;96(7):1911–30. https://doi.org/10.1210/jc.2011-0385. 2011, 3908].

[9] Wagner CL, Greer FR. Prevention of rickets and vitamin D deficiency in infants, children, and adolescents. Pediatrics 2008;122(5):1142–52. Epub 2008/11/04. doi: 122/5/1142 [pii] 10.1542/peds.2008-1862. PubMed PMID: 18977996.

[10] Hollis BW, Johnson D, Hulsey TC, Ebeling M, Wagner CL. Vitamin D supplementation during pregnancy: double-blind, randomized clinical trial of safety and effectiveness. J Bone Miner Res Offic J Am Soci Bone Miner Res 2011;26(10):2341–57. Epub 2011/06/28. doi: 10.1002/jbmr.463. PubMed PMID: 21706518; PMCID: 3183324.

[11] Wagner CL, Howard C, Hulsey TC, Lawrence RA, Taylor SN, Will H, Ebeling M, Hutson J, Hollis BW. Circulating 25-hydroxyvitamin D levels in fully breastfed infants on oral vitamin D supplementation. Int j endocrinol 2010;2010:235035. Epub 2010/01/06. doi: 10.1155/2010/235035. PubMed PMID: 20049156; PMCID: 2798111.

[12] Halloran BP, DeLuca HF. Skeletal changes during pregnancy and lactation: the role of vitamin D. Endocrinology 1980;107(6):1923–9. doi: 10.1210/endo-107-6-1923. PubMed PMID: 7428698.

[13] Eyles D, Smith S, Kinobeb R, Hewison M, McGrath J. Distribution of the vitamin D receptor and 1a-hydroxylase in human brain. J Chem Neuroanat 2005;29:21–30.

[14] Eyles D, Brown J, MacKay-Sim A, McGrath J, Feron F. Vitamin D3 and brain development. Neuroscience 2003;118(3):641–53.
[15] Ko P, Burkert R, McGrath J, Eyles D. Maternal vitamin D3 deprivation and the regulation of apoptosis and cell cyle during rat brain development. Dev Brain Res 2004;153:61–8.
[16] Hawes JE, Tesic D, Whitehouse AJ, Zosky GR, Smith JT, Wyrwoll CS. Maternal vitamin D deficiency alters fetal brain development in the BALB/c mouse. Behav Brain Res 2015;286:192–200. doi: 10.1016/j.bbr.2015.03.008. PubMed PMID: 25753408.
[17] Cannell JJ. Autism and vitamin D. Med Hypotheses 2008;70(4):750–9. doi: 10.1016/j.mehy.2007.08.016. PubMed PMID: 17920208.
[18] Grant WB, Soles CM. Epidemiologic evidence supporting the role of maternal vitamin D deficiency as a risk factor for the development of infantile autism. Derm Endocrinol 2009;1(4):223–8. PubMed PMID: 20592795; PMCID: PMC2835879.
[19] Vuillermot S, Luan W, Meyer U, Eyles D. Vitamin D treatment during pregnancy prevents autism-related phenotypes in a mouse model of maternal immune activation. Mol Autism 2017;8:9. doi: 10.1186/s13229-017-0125-0. PubMed PMID: 28316773; PMCID: PMC5351212.
[20] Al-Harbi AN, Khan KM, Rahman A. Developmental vitamin D deficiency affects spatial learning in wistar rats. J Nutr 2017;147(9):1795–805. doi: 10.3945/jn.117.249953. PubMed PMID: 28747485.
[21] Nicholas C, Davis J, Fisher T, Segal T, Petti M, Sun Y, Wolfe A, Neal-Perry G. Maternal vitamin D deficiency programs reproductive dysfunction in female mice offspring through adverse effects on the neuroendocrine Axis. Endocrinology 2016;157(4):1535–45. doi: 10.1210/en.2015-1638. PubMed PMID: 26741195; PMCID: PMC5393357.
[22] Behrman RE, Butler AS, Institute of Medicine (US). Institute of medicine (US), committee on understanding premature birth and assuring healthy outcomes. Preterm birth: causes, consequences, and prevention. Washington, DC: National Academics Press; 2007.
[23] Bodnar LM, Catov JM, Simhan HN, Holick MF, Powers RW, Roberts JM. Maternal vitamin D deficiency increases the risk of preeclampsia. J Clin Endocrinol Metabol 2007;92(9):3517–22. Epub 2007/05/31. doi: 10.1210/jc.2007-0718. PubMed PMID: 17535985.
[24] Steegers EA, von Dadelszen P, Duvekot JJ, Pijnenborg R. Pre-eclampsia. Lancet 2010;376(9741):631–44. doi: 10.1016/S0140-6736(10)60279-6. PubMed PMID: 20598363.
[25] Liu NQ, Ouyang Y, Bulut Y, Lagishetty V, Chan SY, Hollis BW, Wagner C, Equils O, Hewison M. Dietary vitamin D restriction in pregnant female mice is associated with maternal hypertension and altered placental and fetal development. Endocrinology 2013;154(7):2270–80. Epub 2013/05/17. doi: 10.1210/en.2012-2270. PubMed PMID: 23677931.
[26] Schulz EV, Cruze L, Wei W, Gehris J, Wagner CL. Maternal vitamin D sufficiency and reduced placental gene expression in angiogenic biomarkers related to comorbidities of pregnancy. J. Steroid Biochem. Mol. Biol 2017;173:273–9. https://doi.org/10.1016/j.jsbmb.2017.02.003.Ref.
[27] Roberts JM, Hubel CA. The two stage model of preeclampsia: variations on the theme. Placenta 2009;30(Suppl. A):S32–7. doi: 10.1016/j.placenta.2008.11.009. PubMed PMID: 19070896; PMCID: PMC2680383.

[28] Chan SY, Susarla R, Canovas D, Vasilopoulou E, Ohizua O, McCabe CJ, Hewison M, Kilby MD. Vitamin D promotes human extravillous trophoblast invasion in vitro. Placenta 2015;36(4):403–9. doi: 10.1016/j.placenta.2014.12.021. PubMed PMID: 25596923.
[29] Liu NQ, Larner DP, Yao Q, et al. Vitamin D-deficiency and sex-specific dysregulation of placental inflammation. J Steroid Biochem Mol Biol 2018;177:223–30. https://doi.org/10.1016/j.jsbmb.2017.06.012.
[30] Ma SL, Tian XY, Wang YQ, Zhang HF, Zhang L. Vitamin D supplementation prevents placental ischemia induced endothelial dysfunction by downregulating placental soluble FMS-like tyrosine kinase-1. DNA Cell Biol 2017;36(12):1134–41. https://doi.org/10.1089/dna.2017.3817.
[31] Chinellato I, Piazza M, Sandri M, Peroni D, Piacentini G, Boner AL. Vitamin D serum levels and markers of asthma control in Italian children. J Pediatr 2011;158(3):437–41. doi: 10.1016/j.jpeds.2010.08.043. PubMed PMID: 20870246.
[32] Janssens W, Bouillon R, Claes B, Carremans C, Lehouck A, Buysschaert I, Coolen J, Mathieu C, Decramer M, Lambrechts D. Vitamin D deficiency is highly prevalent in COPD and correlates with variants in the vitamin D-binding gene. Thorax 2010;65(3):215–20. doi: 10.1136/thx.2009.120659. PubMed PMID: 19996341.
[33] Foong RE, Bosco A, Jones AC, Gout A, Gorman S, Hart PH, Zosky GR. The effects of in utero vitamin D deficiency on airway smooth muscle mass and lung function. Am J Respir Cell Mol Biol 2015;53(5):664–75. doi: 10.1165/rcmb.2014-0356OC. PubMed PMID: 25867172.
[34] Zosky GR, Berry LJ, Elliot JG, James AL, Gorman S, Hart PH. Vitamin D deficiency causes deficits in lung function and alters lung structure. Am J Respir Crit Care Med 2011;183(10):1336–43. doi: 10.1164/rccm.201010-1596OC. PubMed PMID: 21297070.
[35] Yurt M, Liu J, Sakurai R, Gong M, Husain SM, Siddiqui MA, Husain M, Villarreal P, Akcay F, Torday JS, Rehan VK. Vitamin D supplementation blocks pulmonary structural and functional changes in a rat model of perinatal vitamin D deficiency. Am J Physiol Lung Cell Mol Physiol 2014;307(11):L859–67. doi: 10.1152/ajplung.00032.2014. PubMed PMID: 25305247; PMCID: PMC4254963.
[36] Dankers W, Colin EM, van Hamburg JP, Lubberts E. Vitamin D in autoimmunity: molecular mechanisms and therapeutic potential. Front Immunol 2016;7:697. doi: 10.3389/fimmu.2016.00697. PubMed PMID: 28163705; PMCID: PMC5247472.
[37] Simpson Jr S, der Mei IV, Taylor B. The role of vitamin D in multiple sclerosis: biology and biochemistry, epidemiology and potential roles in treatment. Med Chem 2018;14(2):129–43. https://doi.org/10.2174/1573406413666170921143600.
[38] Lassmann H, Bradl M. Multiple sclerosis: experimental models and reality. Acta Neuropathol 2017;133(2):223–44. doi: 10.1007/s00401-016-1631-4. PubMed PMID: 27766432; PMCID: PMC5250666.
[39] Fernandes de Abreu DA, Ibrahim EC, Boucraut J, Khrestchatisky M, Feron F. Severity of experimental autoimmune encephalomyelitis is unexpectedly reduced in mice born to vitamin D-deficient mothers. J Steroid Biochem Mol Biol 2010;121(1–2):250–3. doi: 10.1016/j.jsbmb.2010.03.006. PubMed PMID: 20214984.
[40] Fernandes de Abreu DA, Landel V, Barnett AG, McGrath J, Eyles D, Feron F. Prenatal vitamin D deficiency induces an early and more severe experimental autoimmune encephalomyelitis in the second generation. Int J Mol Sci 2012;13(9):10911–9. doi: 10.3390/ijms130910911. PubMed PMID: 23109828; PMCID: PMC3472720.

[41] Li B, Wang X, Choi IY, Wang YC, Liu S, Pham AT, Moon H, Smith DJ, Rao DS, Boldin MP, Yang L. miR-146a modulates autoreactive Th17 cell differentiation and regulates organ-specific autoimmunity. J Clin Invest 2017;127(10):3702–16. doi: 10.1172/JCI94012. PubMed PMID: 28872459; PMCID: PMC5617680.

[42] Cooper C, Harvey NC, Bishop NJ, Kennedy S, Papageorghiou AT, Schoenmakers I, Fraser R, Gandhi SV, Carr A, D'Angelo S, Crozier SR, Moon RJ, Arden NK, Dennison EM, Godfrey KM, Inskip HM, Prentice A, Mughal MZ, Eastell R, Reid DM, Javaid MK, Group MS. Maternal gestational vitamin D supplementation and offspring bone health (MAVIDOS): a multicentre, double-blind, randomised placebo-controlled trial. Lancet Diabetes endocrinol 2016;4(5):393–402. doi: 10.1016/S2213-8587(16)00044-9. PubMed PMID: 26944421; PMCID: PMC4843969.

[43] Olsen SF, Secher NJ. A possible preventive effect of low-dose fish oil on early delivery and pre-eclampsia: indications from a 50-year-old controlled trial. Br J Nutr 1990;64(3):599–609. PubMed PMID: 2265175.

[44] Camargo Jr CA, Ingham T, Wickens K, Thadhani R, Silvers KM, Epton MJ, Town GI, Pattemore PK, Espinola JA, Crane J. Cord-blood 25-hydroxyvitamin D levels and risk of respiratory infection, wheezing, and asthma. Pediatrics 2011;127(1):e180–7. Epub 2010/12/29. doi: peds.2010-0442 [pii] 10.1542/peds.2010-0442. PubMed PMID: 21187313.

[45] Litonjua AA. Childhood asthma may be a consequence of vitamin D deficiency. Curr Opin Allergy Clin Immunol 2009;9(3):202–7. doi: 10.1097/ACI.0b013e32832b36cd. PubMed PMID: 19365260; PMCID: PMC2897155.

[46] Munger KL, Aivo J, Hongell K, Soilu-Hanninen M, Surcel HM, Ascherio A. Vitamin D status during pregnancy and risk of multiple sclerosis in offspring of women in the Finnish maternity cohort. JAMA Neurol 2016;73(5):515–9. doi: 10.1001/jamaneurol.2015.4800. PubMed PMID: 26953778; PMCID: PMC4861670.

[47] Greenberg BM. Vitamin D during pregnancy and multiple sclerosis: an evolving association. JAMA Neurol 2016;73(5):498–9. doi: 10.1001/jamaneurol.2016.0018. PubMed PMID: 26953523.

[48] Dobson R, Giovannoni G, Ramagopalan S. The month of birth effect in multiple sclerosis: systematic review, meta-analysis and effect of latitude. J Neurol Neurosurg Psychiatr 2013;84(4):427–32. doi: 10.1136/jnnp-2012-303934. PubMed PMID: 23152637.

[49] Berlanga-Taylor AJ, Disanto G, Ebers GC, Ramagopalan SV. Vitamin D-gene interactions in multiple sclerosis. J Neurol Sci 2011;311(1–2):32–6. doi: 10.1016/j.jns.2011.08.041. PubMed PMID: 22000399.

[50] Ebers G. Interactions of environment and genes in multiple sclerosis. J Neurol Sci 2013;334(1–2):161–3. doi: 10.1016/j.jns.2013.08.018. PubMed PMID: 24007873.

[51] Stubbs G, Henley K, Green J. Autism: will vitamin D supplementation during pregnancy and early childhood reduce the recurrence rate of autism in newborn siblings? Med Hypotheses 2016;88:74–8. doi: 10.1016/j.mehy.2016.01.015. PubMed PMID: 26880644.

[52] McGrath JJ, Feron FP, Burne TH, Mackay-Sim A, Eyles DW. Vitamin D3-implications for brain development. J Steroid Biochem Mol Biol 2004;89–90(1–5):557–60. doi: 10.1016/j.jsbmb.2004.03.070. PubMed PMID: 15225838.

[53] Robinson CJ, Alanis MC, Wagner CL, Hollis BW, Johnson DD. Plasma 25-hydroxyvitamin D levels in early-onset severe preeclampsia. Am J Obstet Gynecol 2010;203(4):366 e1–6. Epub 2010/08/10. doi: S0002-9378(10)00811-2 [pii] 10.1016/j.ajog.2010.06.036. PubMed PMID: 20692641.

[54] Baker AM, Haeri S, Camargo Jr CA, Espinola JA, Stuebe AM. A nested case-control study of midgestation vitamin D deficiency and risk of severe preeclampsia. J Clin Endocrinol Metabol 2010;95(11):5105−9. Epub 2010/08/20. doi: jc.2010-0996 [pii] 10.1210/jc.2010-0996. PubMed PMID: 20719829; PMCID: 2968727.
[55] Bodnar LM, Simhan HN, Catov JM, Roberts JM, Platt RW, Diesel JC, Klebanoff MA. Maternal vitamin D status and the risk of mild and severe preeclampsia. Epidemiology 2014;25(2):207−14. doi: 10.1097/EDE.0000000000000039. PubMed PMID: 24457526; PMCID: 4053531.
[56] Gernand AD, Bodnar LM, Klebanoff MA, Parks WT, Simhan HN. Maternal serum 25-hydroxyvitamin D and placental vascular pathology in a multicenter US cohort. Am J Clin Nutr 2013;98(2):383−8. doi: 10.3945/ajcn.112.055426. PubMed PMID: 23803889; PMCID: PMC3712548.
[57] Merewood A, Mehta SD, Chen TC, Bauchner H, Holick MF. Association between vitamin D deficiency and primary cesarean section. J Clin Endocrinol Metabol 2009;94(3):940−5. Epub 2008/12/25. doi: jc.2008-1217 [pii] 10.1210/jc.2008-1217. PubMed PMID: 19106272; PMCID: 2681281.
[58] Zhang Q, Cheng Y, He M, Li T, Ma Z, Cheng H. Effect of various doses of vitamin D supplementation on pregnant women with gestational diabetes mellitus: a randomized controlled trial. Exp Ther Med 2016;12(3):1889−95. doi: 10.3892/etm.2016.3515. PubMed PMID: 27588106; PMCID: PMC4998009.
[59] Bodnar LM, Simhan HN. Vitamin D may be a link to black-white disparities in adverse birth outcomes. Obstet Gynecol Surv 2010;65(4):273−84. Epub 2010/04/21. doi: 0006254-201004000-00023 [pii] 10.1097/OGX.0b013e3181dbc55b. PubMed PMID: 20403218.
[60] Pal L, Zhang H, Williams J, Santoro NF, Diamond MP, Schlaff WD, Coutifaris C, Carson SA, Steinkampf MP, Carr BR, McGovern PG, Cataldo NA, Gosman GG, Nestler JE, Myers E, Legro RS, Reproductive Medicine N. Vitamin D status relates to reproductive outcome in women with polycystic ovary syndrome: secondary analysis of a multicenter randomized controlled trial. J Clin Endocrinol Metabol 2016;101(8):3027−35. doi: 10.1210/jc.2015-4352. PubMed PMID: 27186859; PMCID: PMC4971341.
[61] Miliku K, Vinkhuyzen A, Blanken LM, McGrath JJ, Eyles DW, Burne TH, Hofman A, Tiemeier H, Steegers EA, Gaillard R, Jaddoe VW. Maternal vitamin D concentrations during pregnancy, fetal growth patterns, and risks of adverse birth outcomes. Am J Clin Nutr 2016;103(6):1514−22. doi: 10.3945/ajcn.115.123752. PubMed PMID: 27099250; PMCID: PMC5410992.
[62] Hou W, Yan XT, Bai CM, Zhang XW, Hui LY, Yu XW. Decreased serum vitamin D levels in early spontaneous pregnancy loss. Eur J Clin Nutr 2016;70(9):1004−8. doi: 10.1038/ejcn.2016.83. PubMed PMID: 27222154; PMCID: PMC5023787.
[63] Lindqvist PG, Silva AT, Gustafsson SA, Gidlof S. Maternal vitamin D deficiency and fetal distress/birth asphyxia: a population-based nested case-control study. BMJ open 2016;6(9):e009733. doi: 10.1136/bmjopen-2015-009733. PubMed PMID: 27660312; PMCID: PMC5051327.
[64] Kiely ME, Zhang JY, Kinsella M, Khashan AS, Kenny LC. Vitamin D status is associated with uteroplacental dysfunction indicated by pre-eclampsia and small-for-gestational-age birth in a large prospective pregnancy cohort in Ireland with low vitamin D status. Am J Clin Nutr 2016;104(2):354−61. doi: 10.3945/ajcn.116.130419. PubMed PMID: 27357092.
[65] Gernand AD, Simhan HN, Baca KM, Caritis S, Bodnar LM. Vitamin D, pre-eclampsia, and preterm birth among pregnancies at high risk for pre-eclampsia: an analysis of data from a low-dose aspirin trial. BJOG An Int J Obstet Gynaecol 2017;124(12):1874−82. doi: 10.1111/1471-0528.14372. PubMed PMID: 27704679.

[66] Baca KM, Simhan HN, Platt RW, Bodnar LM. Low maternal 25-hydroxyvitamin D concentration increases the risk of severe and mild preeclampsia. Ann Epidemiol 2016;26(12):853–857 e1. doi: 10.1016/j.annepidem.2016.09.015. PubMed PMID: 27818017.
[67] Qin LL, Lu FG, Yang SH, Xu HL, Luo BA. Does maternal vitamin D deficiency increase the risk of preterm birth: ameta-analysis of observational studies. Nutrients 2016;8(5). doi: 10.3390/nu8050301. PubMed PMID: 27213444; PMCID: PMC4882713.
[68] Heaney RP. Guidelines for optimizing design and analysis of clinical studies of nutrient effects. Nutr Rev 2014;72(1):48–54. doi: 10.1111/nure.12090. PubMed PMID: 24330136.
[69] Hollis B, Wagner C. The role of the parent compound vitamin D with respect to metabolism and function: why clinical dose intervals can affect clinical outcomes. J Clin Endocrinol Metabol 2013;98(12):4619–28. doi: doi:10.1210/jc.2013-2653. PubMed PMID: 24106283.
[70] Hollis B, Wagner C. Assessment of dietary vitamin D requirements during pregnancy and Lactation. Am J Clin Nutr 2004;79:717–26.
[71] Wolsk HM, Harshfield BJ, Laranjo N, Carey VJ, O'Connor G, Sandel M, Strunk RC, Bacharier LB, Zeiger RS, Schatz M, Hollis BW, Weiss ST, Litonjua AA. Vitamin D supplementation in pregnancy, prenatal 25(OH)D levels, race, and subsequent asthma or recurrent wheeze in offspring: secondary analyses from the Vitamin D Antenatal Asthma Reduction Trial. J Allergy Clin Immunol 2017;140(5):1423–9. e5. doi: 10.1016/j.jaci.2017.01.013. PubMed PMID: 28285844.
[72] Wolsk HM, Chawes BL, Litonjua AA, Hollis BW, Waage J, Stokholm J, Bonnelykke K, Bisgaard H, Weiss ST. Prenatal vitamin D supplementation reduces risk of asthma/recurrent wheeze in early childhood: a combined analysis of two randomized controlled trials. PloS One 2017;12(10):e0186657. doi: 10.1371/journal.pone.0186657. PubMed PMID: 29077711.
[73] Chawes BL, Bonnelykke K, Stokholm J, Vissing NH, Bjarnadottir E, Schoos AM, Wolsk HM, Pedersen TM, Vinding RK, Thorsteinsdottir S, Arianto L, Hallas HW, Heickendorff L, Brix S, Rasmussen MA, Bisgaard H. Effect of vitamin D3 supplementation during pregnancy on risk of persistent wheeze in the offspring: arandomized clinical trial. J Am Med Assoc J Am Med Associ 2016;315(4):353–61. 10.1001/jama.2015.18318. PubMed PMID: 26813208.
[74] Vahdaninia M, Mackenzie H, Helps S, Dean T. Prenatal intake of vitamins and allergic outcomes in the offspring: asystematic review and meta-analysis. J Allergy Clin Immunol Pract 2017;5(3):771–778 e5. doi: 10.1016/j.jaip.2016.09.024. PubMed PMID: 27888033.
[75] Wagner CL, McNeil R, Hamilton SA, Winkler J, Rodriguez Cook C, Warner G, Bivens B, Davis DJ, Smith PG, Murphy M, Shary JR, Hollis BW. A randomized trial of vitamin D supplementation in 2 community health center networks in South Carolina. Am J Obstet Gynecol 2013;208(2):137 e1–e13. Epub 2012/11/08. doi: 10.1016/j.ajog.2012.10.888. PubMed PMID: 23131462.
[76] Wagner CL, Baggerly C, McDonnell S, Baggerly KA, French CB, Baggerly L, Hamilton SA, Hollis BW. Post-hoc analysis of vitamin D status and reduced risk of preterm birth in two vitamin D pregnancy cohorts compared with South Carolina March of Dimes 2009-2011 rates. J Steroid Biochem Mol Biol 2016;155(Pt B):245–51. doi: 10.1016/j.jsbmb.2015.10.022. PubMed PMID: 26554936; PMCID: PMC5215876.

[77] McDonnell SL, Baggerly KA, Baggerly CA, Aliano JL, French CB, Baggerly LL, Ebeling MD, Rittenberg CS, Goodier CG, Mateus Nino JF, Wineland RJ, Newman RB, Hollis BW, Wagner CL. Maternal 25(OH)D concentrations >/=40 ng/mL associated with 60% lower preterm birth risk among general obstetrical patients at an urban medical center. PloS One 2017;12(7):e0180483. doi: 10.1371/journal.pone.0180483. PubMed PMID: 28738090; PMCID: PMC5524288.

[78] Liu PT, Stenger S, Li H, Wenzel L, Tan BH, Krutzik SR, Ochoa MT, Schauber J, Wu K, Meinken C, Kamen DL, Wagner M, Bals R, Steinmeyer A, Zugel U, Gallo RL, Eisenberg D, Hewison M, Hollis BW, Adams JS, Bloom BR, Modlin RL. Toll-like receptor triggering of a vitamin D-mediated human antimicrobial response. Science 2006;311(5768):1770–3. PubMed PMID: 16497887.

[79] Fabri M, Stenger S, Shin DM, Yuk JM, Liu PT, Realegeno S, Lee HM, Krutzik SR, Schenk M, Sieling PA, Teles R, Montoya D, Iyer SS, Bruns H, Lewinsohn DM, Hollis BW, Hewison M, Adams JS, Steinmeyer A, Zugel U, Cheng G, Jo EK, Bloom BR, Modlin RL. Vitamin D is required for IFN-{gamma}-Mediated antimicrobial activity of human macrophages. Sci Transl Med 2011;3(104):104ra2. Epub 2011/10/15. doi: 10.1126/scitranslmed.3003045. PubMed PMID: 21998409.

[80] Liu NQ, Hewison M. Vitamin D, the placenta and pregnancy. Arch Biochem Biophys 2012;523(1):37–47. Epub 2011/12/14. doi: 10.1016/j.abb.2011.11.018. PubMed PMID: 22155151.

[81] Lagishetty V, Liu NQ, Hewison M. Vitamin D metabolism and innate immunity. Mol Cell Endocrinol 2011;347(1–2):97–105. Epub 2011/06/15. doi: 10.1016/j.mce.2011.04.015. PubMed PMID: 21664425; PMCID: 3200473.

[82] Liu NQ, Kaplan AT, Lagishetty V, Ouyang YB, Ouyang Y, Simmons CF, Equils O, Hewison M. Vitamin D and the regulation of placental inflammation. J Immunol 2011;186(10):5968–74. Epub 2011/04/13. doi: 10.4049/jimmunol.1003332. PubMed PMID: 21482732.

[83] Vieth R, Chan PC, MacFarlane GD. Efficacy and safety of vitamin D3 intake exceeding the lowest observed adverse effect level. Am J Clin Nutr 2001;73(2):288–94. Epub 2001/02/07. PubMed PMID: 11157326.

[84] Souberbielle JC, Cormier C, Kindermans C, Gao P, Cantor T, Forette F, Baulieu EE. Vitamin D status and redefining serum parathyroid hormone reference range in the elderly. J Clin Endocrinol Metabol 2001;86(7):3086–90. doi: 10.1210/jcem.86.7.7689. PubMed PMID: 11443171.

[85] Litonjua AA, Carey VJ, Laranjo N, Harshfield BJ, McElrath TF, O'Connor GT, Sandel M, Iverson Jr RE, Lee-Paritz A, Strunk RC, Bacharier LB, Macones GA, Zeiger RS, Schatz M, Hollis BW, Hornsby E, Hawrylowicz C, Wu AC, Weiss ST. Effect of prenatal supplementation with vitamin D on asthma or recurrent wheezing in offspring by age 3 Years: the VDAART randomized clinical trial. J Am Med Assoc J Am Med Associ 2016;315(4):362–70. doi: 10.1001/jama.2015.18589. PubMed PMID: 26813209.

[86] Hollis BW, Wagner CL. Vitamin d and pregnancy: skeletal effects, nonskeletal effects, and birth outcomes. Calcif Tissue Int 2013;92(2):128–39. Epub 2012/05/25. doi: 10.1007/s00223-012-9607-4. PubMed PMID: 22623177.

[87] Goldring ST, Griffiths CJ, Martineau AR, Robinson S, Yu C, Poulton S, Kirkby JC, Stocks J, Hooper R, Shaheen SO, Warner JO, Boyle RJ. Prenatal vitamin d supplementation and child respiratory health: a randomised controlled trial. PloS One 2013;8(6):e66627. doi: 10.1371/journal.pone.0066627. PubMed PMID: 23826104; PMCID: PMC3691177.

[88] Sablok A, Batra A, Thariani K, Batra A, Bharti R, Aggarwal AR, Kabi BC, Chellani H. Supplementation of vitamin D in pregnancy and its correlation with feto-maternal outcome. Clin Endocrinol 2015;83(4):536–41. doi: 10.1111/cen.12751. PubMed PMID: 25683660.
[89] Mojibian M, Soheilykhah S, Fallah Zadeh MA, Jannati Moghadam M. The effects of vitamin D supplementation on maternal and neonatal outcome: a randomized clinical trial. Iran J Reproductive Med 2015;13(11):687–96. PubMed PMID: 26730243; PMCID: PMC4695683.
[90] Grant CC, Crane J, Mitchell EA, Sinclair J, Stewart A, Milne T, Knight J, Gilchrist C, Camargo Jr CA. Vitamin D supplementation during pregnancy and infancy reduces aeroallergen sensitization: a randomized controlled trial. Allergy 2016;71(9):1325–34. doi: 10.1111/all.12909. PubMed PMID: 27060679.
[91] Zhang C, Qiu C, Hu FB, David RM, van Dam RM, Bralley A, Williams MA. Maternal plasma 25-hydroxyvitamin D concentrations and the risk for gestational diabetes mellitus. PloS One 2008;3(11):e3753. doi: 10.1371/journal.pone.0003753. PubMed PMID: 19015731; PMCID: PMC2582131.
[92] Zerofsky M, Ryder M, Bhatia S, Stephensen CB, King J, Fung EB. Effects of early vitamin D deficiency rickets on bone and dental health, growth and immunity. Matern Child Nutr 2016;12(4):898–907. doi: 10.1111/mcn.12187. PubMed PMID: 25850574; PMCID: PMC4610869.
[93] Hornsby PE, Pfeffer N, Laranjo W, Cruikshank M, Tuzova AA, Litonjua ST, Weiss VJ, Carey G, O'Connor, Hawrylowicz C. Vitamin D supplementation during pregnancy: effect on the neonatal immune system in a randomized controlled trial. J Allergy Clin Immunol 2017. https://doi.org/10.1016/j.jaci.2017.02.039. PubMed PMID: 28552588.
[94] Behjat Sasan S, Zandvakili F, Soufizadeh N, Baybordi E. The effects of vitamin D supplement on prevention of recurrence of preeclampsia in pregnant women with a history of preeclampsia. Obstet Gynecol Int 2017;2017:8249264. doi: 10.1155/2017/8249264. PubMed PMID: 28912817; PMCID: PMC5585545.
[95] Mirzakhani H, Litonjua AA, McElrath TF, O'Connor G, Lee-Parritz A, Iverson R, Macones G, Strunk RC, Bacharier LB, Zeiger R, Hollis BW, Handy DE, Sharma A, Laranjo N, Carey V, Qiu W, Santolini M, Liu S, Chhabra D, Enquobahrie DA, Williams MA, Loscalzo J, Weiss ST. Early pregnancy vitamin D status and risk of preeclampsia. J Clin Invest 2016;126(12):4702–15. 10.1172/JCI89031. PubMed PMID: 27841759; PMCID: PMC5127689.
[96] Parlea L, Bromberg IL, Feig DS, Vieth R, Merman E, Lipscombe LL. Association between serum 25-hydroxyvitamin D in early pregnancy and risk of gestational diabetes mellitus. Diabetic medicine : a journal of the British Diabetic Association. 2011. Epub 2011/12/14. doi: 10.1111/j.1464-5491.2011.03550.x. PubMed PMID: 22150870.
[97] Bodnar LM, Krohn MA, Simhan HN. Maternal vitamin D deficiency is associated with bacterial vaginosis in the first trimester of pregnancy. J Nutr 2009;139(6):1157–61. Epub 2009/04/10. doi: 10.3945/jn.108.103168. PubMed PMID: 19357214; PMCID: 2682987.
[98] Hensel KJ, Randis TM, Gelber SE, Ratner AJ. Pregnancy-specific association of vitamin D deficiency and bacterial vaginosis. Am J Obstet Gynecol 2011;204(1):41 e1–9. Epub 2010/10/05. doi: 10.1016/j.ajog.2010.08.013. PubMed PMID: 20887971.
[99] Al-Garawi A, Carey VJ, Chhabra D, Mirzakhani H, Morrow J, Lasky-Su J, Qiu W, Laranjo N, Litonjua AA, Weiss ST. The role of vitamin D in the transcriptional program of human pregnancy. PloS One 2016;11(10):e0163832. doi: 10.1371/journal.pone.0163832. PubMed PMID: 27711190; PMCID: PMC5053446.

[100] Brehm JM, Celedon JC, Soto-Quiros ME, Avila L, Hunninghake GM, Forno E, Laskey D, Sylvia JS, Hollis BW, Weiss ST, Litonjua AA. Serum vitamin D levels and markers of severity of childhood asthma in Costa Rica. Am J Respir Crit Care Med 2009;179(9):765–71. Epub 2009/01/31. doi: 10.1164/rccm.200808-1361OC. PubMed PMID: 19179486; PMCID: 2675563.
[101] Faulkner JL, Cornelius DC, Amaral LM, Harmon AC, Cunningham Jr MW, Darby MM, Ibrahim T, Thomas DS, Herse F, Wallukat G, Dechend R, LaMarca B. Vitamin D supplementation improves pathophysiology in a rat model of preeclampsia. Am J Physiol Regul Integr Comp Physiol 2016;310(4):R346–54. doi: 10.1152/ajpregu.00388.2015. PubMed PMID: 26676250; PMCID: PMC4796742.
[102] Song J, Li Y, An R. Vitamin D restores angiogenic balance and decreases tumor necrosis factor-alpha in a rat model of pre-eclampsia. J Obstet Gynaecol Res 2017;43(1):42–9. doi: 10.1111/jog.13186. PubMed PMID: 27862673.
[103] Grotegut CA. Prevention of preeclampsia. J Clin Invest 2016;126(12):4396–8. doi: 10.1172/JCI91300. PubMed PMID: 27841760; PMCID: PMC5127661.
[104] Zhu H, Wagner C, Pan Y, Wang X, Shary J, Hollis B, Dong Y, editors. Maternal vitamin D supplementation and cord blood genome-wide DNA methylation analysis. (abstract). Vitamin D workshop; 2016. March 29-31, 2016; Boston, MA, www.vitaminDworkshop.org.
[105] Anderson CM, Ralph JL, Johnson L, Scheett A, Wright ML, Taylor JY, Ohm JE, Uthus E. First trimester vitamin D status and placental epigenomics in preeclampsia among Northern Plains primiparas. Life Sci 2015;129:10–5. doi: 10.1016/j.lfs.2014.07.012. PubMed PMID: 25050465.
[106] Meems LM, Mahmud H, Buikema H, Tost J, Michel S, Takens J, Verkaik-Schakel RN, Vreeswijk-Baudoin I, Mateo-Leach IV, van der Harst P, Plosch T, de Boer RA. Parental vitamin D deficiency during pregnancy is associated with increased blood pressure in offspring via Panx1 hypermethylation. Am J Physiol Heart Circ Physiol 2016;311(6):H1459–69. doi: 10.1152/ajpheart.00141.2016. PubMed PMID: 27769995.
[107] Xue J, Schoenrock SA, Valdar W, Tarantino LM, Ideraabdullah FY. Maternal vitamin D depletion alters DNA methylation at imprinted loci in multiple generations. Clin Epigenet 2016;8:107. doi: 10.1186/s13148-016-0276-4. PubMed PMID: 27777636; PMCID: PMC5062906.
[108] Nielsen NM, Munger KL, Koch-Henriksen N, Hougaard DM, Magyari M, Jorgensen KT, Lundqvist M, Simonsen J, Jess T, Cohen A, Stenager E, Ascherio A. Neonatal vitamin D status and risk of multiple sclerosis: a population-based case-control study. Neurology 2017;88(1):44–51. doi: 10.1212/WNL.0000000000003454. PubMed PMID: 27903815; PMCID: PMC5200855.
[109] Mokry LE, Ross S, Ahmad OS, Forgetta V, Smith GD, Goltzman D, Leong A, Greenwood CM, Thanassoulis G, Richards JB. Vitamin D and risk of multiple sclerosis: amendelian randomization study. PLoS Med 2015;12(8):e1001866. doi: 10.1371/journal.pmed.1001866. PubMed PMID: 26305103; PMCID: PMC4549308.
[110] Whitehouse AJ, Holt BJ, Serralha M, Holt PG, Kusel MM, Hart PH. Maternal serum vitamin d levels during pregnancy and offspring neurocognitive development. Pediatrics 2012;129(3):485–93. Epub 2012/02/15. doi: 10.1542/peds.2011-2644. PubMed PMID: 22331333.
[111] Chen J, Xin K, Wei J, Zhang K, Xiao H. Lower maternal serum 25(OH) D in first trimester associated with higher autism risk in Chinese offspring. J Psychosom Res 2016;89:98–101. doi: 10.1016/j.jpsychores.2016.08.013. PubMed PMID: 27663117.

[112] Gould JF, Anderson AJ, Yelland LN, Smithers LG, Skeaff CM, Zhou SJ, Gibson RA, Makrides M. Association of cord blood vitamin D with early childhood growth and neurodevelopment. J Paediatr Child Health 2017;53(1):75–83. doi: 10.1111/jpc.13308. PubMed PMID: 27566125.
[113] Murthi P, Davies-Tuck M, Lappas M, Singh H, Mockler J, Rahman R, Lim R, Leaw B, Doery J, Wallace EM, Ebeling PR. Maternal 25-hydroxyvitamin D is inversely correlated with foetal serotonin. Clin Endocrinol 2017;86(3):401–9. doi: 10.1111/cen.13281. PubMed PMID: 27862146.
[114] Patrick RP, Ames BN. Vitamin D hormone regulates serotonin synthesis. Part 1: relevance for autism. Faseb J 2014;28(6):2398–413. doi: 10.1096/fj.13-246546. PubMed PMID: 24558199.
[115] Wu D-M, Wen X, Xan X-R, Wang S, Wang Y-J, Shen M, Fan S-H, Zhuang J, Li M-Q, Hu B, Sun C-H, Bao Y-X, Yan J, Lu J. Relationship between neonatal vitamin D at birth and risk of autism spectrum disorders: the NBSIB Study. J Bus Manag Res 2017. https://doi.org/10.1002/jbmr.3326.
[116] Luxwolda MF, Kuipers RS, Kema IP, van der Veer E, Dijck-Brouwer DA, Muskiet FA. Vitamin D status indicators in indigenous populations in East Africa. Eur J Nutr 2013;52(3):1115–25. Epub 2012/08/11. doi: 10.1007/s00394-012-0421-6. PubMed PMID: 22878781.
[117] Luxwolda MF, Kuipers RS, Kema IP, Janneke Dijck-Brouwer DA, Muskiet FA. Traditionally living populations in East Africa have a mean serum 25-hydroxyvitamin D concentration of 115 nmol/l. Br J Nutr 2012:1–5. Epub 2012/01/24. doi: 10.1017/S0007114511007161. PubMed PMID: 22264449.

CHAPTER 16

Nutritional influence on miRNA epigenetic regulation

Effect of maternal diet and miRNAs on the fetal metabolic programming

Sunitha Meruvu, Luis F. Schutz, Mahua Choudhury
Department of Pharmaceutical Sciences, Irma Lerma Rangel College of Pharmacy, Texas A&M Health Science Center, College Station, TX, United States

Contents

Introduction

Noncommunicable diseases such as obesity, type 2 diabetes, cardiovascular diseases, and several types of cancer represent a growing public health burden [1–3]. An unhealthy diet is well established as an important contributor to noncommunicable diseases, with adverse effect to human health [2,4–6]. Nevertheless, lifestyle alone does not account for the prevention of chronic diseases [7]. Epidemic associations between birth weight and diseases susceptibility have drawn the attention of researchers for several decades [7,8]. Following these observations, a series of studies led to the hypothesis that maternal undernutrition during the intrauterine and infancy periods permanently alter the physiology of the body, influencing the risks of diseases such as coronary heart disease in adult life [6,7,9,10]. This hypothesis emerged more than two decades ago, and it is known as the

Molecular Nutrition
ISBN 978-0-12-813862-5
https://doi.org/10.1016/B978-0-12-813862-5.00016-5

"fetal origin hypothesis," also called as the "Barker's hypothesis," named after the influential epidemiologist David Barker, who provided valuable contributions to the field [10].

The ideas behind the "fetal origin hypothesis" had an important impact in the field and were expanded with studies discovering that the developmental plasticity could occur before or after the fetal period [8,11,12]. Such studies led to the foundation of an international society for the study of developmental origins of health and disease (DOHaD) in the recent years [10]. Studies of DOHaD served to strengthen the theory that stimuli during several developmental periods, from the oocyte to the infancy and even later, could have crucial effects to future disease susceptibility [10].

Advances in molecular biology have brought enormous contributions to the understanding of how diet influences the health of individuals [13] and of factors influencing developmental origins of chronic diseases [8,14,15]. Indeed, in the recent years, molecular studies have unveiled the role of epigenetics in the pathogenesis of chronic diseases and in the interaction between maternal nutrition and chronic metabolic diseases of the offspring [16–19]. Epigenetics refers to the heritable changes in the phenotype without alteration in the DNA sequence [20]. Epigenetic mechanisms include processes that alter the chromatin structure, such as DNA methylation and histone modifications, and processes that act to modulate protein activity, such as microRNAs (miRNAs) [20,21]. These epigenetic mechanisms are influenced by several environmental factors, including exercise, alcohol consumption, and nutrition [13,22]. In early life, the fetal epigenome is highly susceptible to the outside environment and is consistently altered by the maternal diet [23]. This chapter will focus on how the maternal nutrition influences the miRNA epigenetic regulation with an impact on development and health of the offspring.

MiRNAs characterization

MiRNAs are a large family of small noncoding RNAs that are 18–25 nucleotides long [24,25]. These molecules act mainly at the post-transcriptional level by binding to 3′ untranslated regions of target mRNA, therefore regulating translation [24,26,27]. Nevertheless, some miRNAs can prevent translation through the degradation of target mRNA [1,24]. The synthesis of mature miRNAs in mammalian cells follows a sequence of processes involving both the nucleus and the cytoplasm [19]. Initially, miRNAs are transcribed by RNA polymerase II as primary transcripts (pri-miRNAs) that possess stem-loop structures [25,28]. The pri-miRNAs, which are several nucleotides long, are then recognized and cleaved by the type III RNase Drosha and its associated protein DiGeorge syndrome critical region 8 (DGCR8) to give rise to the pre-miR, the precursor miRNA [19,28]. After formed, the pre-miR is transported from the nucleus to the cytoplasm by the nuclear export protein exportin 5 [25,29]. In the cytoplasm, the pre-miR is cleaved by the enzyme Dicer (another type III RNase) to form a duplex of miRNAs [28]. This duplex is then unraveled by the protein Argonaute 2 into two strands: one strand, called passenger strand, is usually degraded, whereas the other strand is the mature miRNA [19,29,30]. The mature miRNA is incorporated into an RNA-induced silencing complex composed of Dicer and other associated proteins and is then ready to target mRNAs [25,29].

A single mRNA may be regulated by more than one miRNA, and each miRNA can target several mRNAs, demonstrating a complex and important role for miRNAs to modulate genes expression [27,31]. Indeed, it is currently believed that miRNAs regulate the majority of the human genes and have critical importance in the regulation of many biological processes [25,32,33]. Interestingly, miRNAs can either have functions inside the cells or be exported from the cells within exosomes to exert both short- and long-ranged communication between cells [24,34]. Therefore, for their participation in the regulation of gene expression, with consequences to several biological functions, and their ability to exert both intra- and extracellular communication, miRNAs are now recognized as important regulators of human health [25].

Among several biological functions, miRNAs have been reported to regulate development, differentiation, cell cycle, cell proliferation, and apoptosis [25,31,35]. Some miRNAs have also been described as regulators of important metabolic processes, including insulin signaling and glucose homeostasis [36,37]. Hence, the fact that dysregulation of miRNAs has been associated with the development of chronic diseases such as cancer [31,38], cardiovascular disease [25,35], and type 2 diabetes [25,36,39] is not surprising. Furthermore, various studies have shown alterations of miRNAs in the offspring in response to maternal diet with potential consequences for the development of chronic diseases in the adult life [40]. Furthermore, extracellular circulating miRNAs resist adverse physiological conditions and can be found abundantly in biological fluids such as blood, saliva, cerebrospinal fluid, urine, and breast milk [25,41]; they are now considered important biomarkers for chronic diseases [24,29].

Effect of maternal overnutrition or undernutrition on miRNA regulation in the offspring

Various dietary factors, including carbohydrates, amino acids, vitamins, fatty acids, and polyphenols, have been associated with miRNAs levels in mammals [1,36]. Several dietary compounds play a role in prevention of noncommunicable diseases through epigenetics [13,14,36] and studies are now reporting an association between maternal diet, miRNAs, and chronic diseases in the offspring [40]. It is now accepted that miRNAs expression is associated with lifestyle factors, including diet and weight loss [24]. Maternal overnutrition (Table 16.1) or undernutrition (Table 16.2) can greatly influence the fetal miRNAs that can target the key developmental proteins, leading to diseases like obesity and diabetes later in life [19]. In many animal models of maternal overnutrition or maternal low protein diet, miRNAs have been shown to be differentially regulated in the offspring in multiple tissues like liver, heart, and skeletal muscle [19,42].

Maternal overnutrition and offspring miRNA regulation of insulin signaling pathway and fat metabolism

Maternal obesity during pregnancy can often result in adverse pregnancy outcomes, affecting mother (maternal insulin resistance and hyperglycemia) as well as the offspring (large-for-gestation age infants and metabolic syndrome later in life). A recent study on obese ewes demonstrated that high calorie diet during the periconceptual period increased the fetal hepatic miR-29b, miR-103, and miR-107 expression levels which decreased IR, Akt2 (in female offspring only), Ser473 phospho-Akt, and Thr24 phospho-FoxO1 expression as well as a decrease in 11 betaHSD1, PEPCK-C, and PEPCK-M expression in the 4-month-old offsprings [43]. An increase in miR-29b expression levels was previously reported in different tissues including liver [44,45], beta cells [46,47], kidney [48], skeletal muscle [49], and adipose tissue [49] of diabetic rodent models and humans. An increase in miR-29a levels is also observed in the serum of children diagnosed with T1DM [50] and adult patients with T2DM [51]. An increase in the miR-29b in 3T3-L1 cells repressed insulin-stimulated glucose uptake by inhibiting Akt activation [49] indicating insulin resistance. Based on these observations, this study on obese ewes indicates that high calorie diet during periconceptual period may negatively influence glucose uptake in the livers of the offspring. Maternal obesity also decreased the constitutively expressed PEPCK-M in liver suggesting that these lambs have a decreased basal gluconeogenic capacity.

Table 16.1 Maternal overnutrition and related miRNAs in offspring.

Maternal diet	miRNAs	Gene targets and sites of action/pathways in offspring
High fat diet	miR-29b, miR-103, miR-107↑	Signaling molecules in the insulin signaling pathway and gluconeogenic factors such as IR, phospho-Akt, phospho-FoxO1, 11b HSD1, PEPCK-C, and PEPCK-M are decreased in offspring liver in the lamb [43].
High fat diet	miR-709, miR-122, miR-192, miR-194, miR-26a, let-7a, let7b, let-7c, miR-494, and miR-483* ↓	Insulin-growth factor 2 (Igf2) and fat metabolic genes such as PPARs and CPT1a increased in the fetal liver in mice [53].
High fat diet	let-7g ↓	FST and TNFRSF4 were upregulated in fetal muscle in sheep leading to stem cell proliferation and adipogenic differentiation [63].
High fat diet	miR-615-5p, miR-3079-5p, miR-124*, and miR-101b* ↓ miR-143*↑	Proinflammatory factors, tumor necrosis factor-α (TNF-α) and mitogen-activated protein kinase 1 (MAPK1) in livers of offspring leading to higher body weight, hepatic inflammation, and impaired glucose metabolism in mice [66].
High fat diet	miR-122 ↓ miR-370 ↑	Hepatic fatty acid synthesis (de novo) and β-oxidation pathway—related genes like SCD1 and AGPAT1 increased, while expression levels of the β-oxidation-related genes ACADVL and CPT1 were decreased in the offspring in mice [60].

↑,↓ Increase and decrease respectively.

Interestingly, miR-103/107, which is usually upregulated in obese mice, is also increased in the livers of these lambs. Mir-103/107 plays key role in regulating insulin sensitivity [52] indicating that the lambs born from obese ewes may have impaired insulin signaling pathway.

In another study, in mice where the dams were fed high fat diet (HFD) before conception, during pregnancy, and lactation induced changes in the IGF2, fat metabolic genes, and miRNAs in the liver of adult offspring [53].

Table 16.2 Maternal undernutrition and related miRNAs in offspring.

Maternal diet	miRNAs	Gene targets and sites of action/pathways in offspring
Low protein diet	miR-483-3p ↑	Repression of growth/differentiation factor-3, a target of miR-483-3p limits storage of lipids in adipose tissue, causing lipotoxicity and insulin resistance and increasing susceptibility to metabolic disease in rats [70].
Low protein diet	miR-615, miR-124, miR-376b, and let-7e↓ miR-708 and miR-879 ↑	Serum tumor necrosis factor-α (TNF-α), interleukin 6 (IL-6) levels were higher in the offspring in mice [76].
Low protein diet	miR-130b, miR-374b ↑	PPAR-γ and CCAAT/enhancer-binding protein-β (C/EBP-β) protein expression in subcutaneous fat leading to altered offspring lipid metabolism in pigs [73].
Low protein diet	miR-27a and 27b ↑ miR-330 ↓	Fetal brains showed increased expression of angiotensinogen and angiotensin-converting enzyme-1 (ACE-1), with a decrease in expression of angiotensin II type-2 (AT2) receptors which lead to significant alterations in the systemic renin—angiotensin system (RAS) in the mice fetus [85].
Undernutrition	miR-29c ↓	ECM genes are the targets of miR-29c and expression levels of elastin (ELN), MMP2, Col3A1, and Col4A5 increased in fetal carotids in rats [81]

↑,↓ Increase and decrease respectively.

Maternal HFD fed offspring have altered expression of a small percentage (around 5.7%) miRNAs involved in developmental timing and fat oxidation. These mice also have altered gene expression levels of IGF2 (which regulates fetal growth), PPARalpha, and CPT1a (which regulates fat metabolism) in the liver. Among the altered miRNAs, miR-709, miR-122, miR-192, miR-194, miR-26a, let-7a, let-7b, and let-7c, miR-494, and miR-483* were reduced nearly fivefold in the livers of offspring. Let-7c belongs to the let-7 miRNA gene family and regulates developmental timing, playing an important role in growth regulation [54]. Reduced expression of let-7c in the livers of maternal HFD fed offspring favored hepatic growth. In contrast, overexpression of let-7c suppresses the growth of hepatocytes by decreasing c-myc and miR-17 [55]. IGF2 which is also involved in fetal growth is increased in livers of the offspring. These mice have a significant increase in liver weights (nearly 16% increase) compared to control mice. This result was also observed in a similar study in rats, where maternal HFD during gestation increased offspring liver weight with associated increase in body weight and percentage body fat [56]. Interestingly, in IGF2 knockout mice, expression of let-7c levels is significantly increased (around 31% increase) suggesting an inverse correlation between IGF2 and let-7c expression [53]. Further studies are required to determine if there is a direct regulation between let-7c and IGF2.

Among significantly altered miRNAs in the above study, miR-122 is highly expressed in the liver (around 70% of total miRNA population). It is involved in various metabolic processes including cholesterol synthesis and fat metabolism [57]. Repression of miR-122 resulted in hepatic insulin resistance through protein-tyrosine phosphatase 1B induction. However, in the maternal HFD offspring, hepatic expression of miR-122 decreased along with an increased expression of hepatic fatty acid oxidation genes such as PPARalpha and CPT1alpha. Few studies also showed that increased PPARalpha levels could inhibit let-7c expression in the liver [55,58]. These results suggest that maternal HFD induces coordinated changes in expression levels of IGF2, PPARalpha, and let-7c expression to promote hepatic growth. In addition to miRNA regulation, maternal HFD can also regulate DNA methylation in the offspring through miRNAs. As several miRNAs can act together, and a small set of miRNAs can account for most of the differences, this study found that five miRNAs in the subset of regulated miRNAs target MECP2. MECP2 is essential to maintain CpG status of genomic DNA [59]. Target Scan also showed that some of the predicated targets of let-7c are proteins involved in methylation such as hypermethylated in cancer 2 (HIC2), chromodomain helicase 4, and DOT1-like histone H3 methyltransferase. Thus, maternal HFD before conception, during pregnancy, and lactation may induce coordinated changes in the epigenome which may have long-lasting effects on the health of offspring.

In a similar study, maternal consumption of an HFD during pregnancy and lactation resulted in insulin resistance, hepatic lipid accumulation, and increased serum cytokine levels in offspring and also into their adulthood [60]. De novo hepatic fatty acid synthesis, beta-oxidation pathways, and expression levels of miR-122 and miRNA-370 expression levels were altered in weaned offspring (28 days). These mice weighed more, had a larger adipose tissue mass, and were more intolerant to glucose and insulin. The expression of miR-122 was reduced, and miR-370 was increased in the livers of the offspring. Liver-specific deletion of miR-122 results in the upregulation of genes involved in lipid synthesis such as acylglycerolphosphate acyltransferase (AGPAT), phosphatidic acid phosphatase type 2A (PPAP2a), and monoacylglycerol transferase (MOGAT) as well as accumulation of triacylglycerides in the hepatocytes [60]. Additionally, miR-122-deficient mice showed an increase in the number of infiltrating inflammatory cells in the liver, suggesting a proinflammatory effect of reduced expression of miR-122 [61]. Interestingly, the maternal HFD fed offspring exhibited reduced miR-122, increased TAG deposition in liver, and increased liver inflammation. Alternatively, miR-370 is expressed more in the livers of the maternal HFD fed offspring compared to control mice [62]. MiR-370 controls the expression of miR-122 and affects lipid metabolism by activating lipogenic genes indirectly through miR-122 and downregulates beta-oxidation by decreasing CPT1alpha. Hence, maternal HFD caused hepatic lipid accumulation, changes in oxidative pathways, and increased liver inflammation in the offspring. These studies indicate that maternal obesity can lead to the changes in miRNAs known to regulate hepatic insulin signaling pathways and fat metabolism in the livers of offspring.

Maternal overnutrition and offspring miRNA regulation: Effect on stem cell proliferation, adipogenic differentiation, and inflammatory pathways

Maternal obesity predisposes offspring to obesity as studies have shown that myogenesis is impaired in fetal muscle while adipogenesis is increased along with chronic inflammation in the ewes fed obesogenic diet [63]. MiRNA microarray analysis of midgestational fetal longissimus dorsi muscle indicated differential expression of 155 miRNAs between obese fetuses compared to control. Of these miRNAs, let-7g, an abundantly expressed miRNA, is significantly decreased in the fetal muscle of obese ewes which correlated with the increased expression of its target genes, tumor necrosis factor receptor superfamily, member 4 (TNFRSF4), and follistatin (FST). Let-7g plays an important role in stem cell proliferation and differentiation, especially in adipogenesis [63]. FST is a myostatin-binding protein which inhibits the activity of myostatin, induces satellite proliferation, which then leads to muscle hypertrophy [64]. Less let-7g expression in fetal muscle promoted FST expression leading to higher muscle weights in the fetal muscle in obese ewes compared to control ewes. Let-7g also affects adipogenesis and in vitro overexpression of let-7g in mesenchymal stem cells decreased the expression of adipogenic markers. The results of this study also implicated let-7g in inflammation. TNF-alpha and IL-6 mRNA were upregulated in the fetal muscle of obese ewes indicating the role of let-7g in the inflammatory response. Therefore, let-7g can be a key mediator linking obesity, inflammation, and adipose tissue development [63].

Inflammatory signaling has been recently identified as an epigenetic mediator [65]. A recent study in mice showed that maternal high calorie diet impaired metabolic health by modulating hepatic miRNA expression and increasing the markers of hepatic inflammation in offspring as early as weaning age [66]. Microarray analysis in livers from offspring from high calorie fed dams indicated that miR-615-5p, miR-3079-5p, miR-124*, and miR-101b* were downregulated, whereas miR-143* was upregulated. Functional enrichment analysis mapped these differentially expressed miRNAs to inflammatory pathways including TNF-alpha and mitogen-activated protein kinase 1 (MAPK1). Both the mRNA and protein levels of these proinflammatory factors increased in the liver of offspring from high calorie fed dams. Additionally, miR-101b* also targets TNF-alpha and MAPK1 and may play an intermediary role in the development of hepatic inflammation [66]. In conclusion, these results demonstrate that maternal high calorie diet induces an inflammatory state in offspring at weaning age. Since low-grade inflammation is associated with T2DM; maternal high calorie diet impairs offspring metabolic health.

Maternal undernutrition and miRNA expression in offspring: Effect on adipogenesis, lipid metabolism, and inflammation

Several human and rodent studies reveal that maternal dietary insufficiency can lead to the poor intrauterine environment and that can cause metabolic diseases such as insulin resistance, impaired glucose tolerance, and T2DM, in the offspring during adulthood [67−69]. Maternal protein restriction models are the most commonly used models to study maternal undernutrition, where 5%−9% protein is used in the maternal diet instead of the normal 20% protein in the diet. In a recent study on a rat model of maternal protein restriction, the offspring exhibited similar phenotypic characteristics of low birth weight humans, including insulin resistance in muscle and adipose tissue and age-dependent glucose intolerance in late adulthood [70] indicating that both adipose and skeletal muscle can be nutritionally programmed. At 3 months, the offspring of low protein fed mothers had reduced body weight, body fat with a decrease in white adiposity due to the smaller size of adipocytes compared to controls. This study also demonstrated changes in miR-483-3p in adipose tissue which linked early life nutrition to long-term health. Increase in the miR-483-3p expression limited the lipid storage in the adipose tissue causing lipotoxicity and insulin resistance in offspring leading to increased susceptibility to metabolic disease later in life. The expression of miR-483-3p demonstrated a sustained programmed event as it was expressed in the epididymal adipose tissue at 22 days as well as at 3 months of age of offspring from low protein fed mothers. Interestingly, an increase in miR-483-3p expression was also observed in adipose biopsies from low birth weight men compared to controls indicating a modulation of miR-483-3p by poor nutrition is a conserved phenomenon. Both the rat and the human genomes show that miR-483-3p sequence lies within an intron of the IGF2 gene, essential for growth and development. Growth Differentiation Factor 3 (GDF3) which is expressed at high levels in adipose tissue is found to be one of the targets of miR-483-3p. It is implicated in the regulation of adiposity and energy expenditure, and a 40% decrease in the GDF3 protein was observed in the adipose tissue of maternal low protein offspring. A similar decrease in the expression levels of GDF3 protein was also observed in the adipose tissues of low birth weight humans compared to controls. These observations reveal that GDF3 modulates the adipose tissue expandability and in turn lipid storage which would then promote ectopic triglyceride storage and lipotoxicity. It is observed that in the low protein rat models, older mice exhibit increased hepatic lipid accumulation instead of increased adiposity and obesity [71]. This similarity was also observed in the low birth weight men who show an increased risk of nonalcoholic liver disease with age [72]. This study demonstrates that the nutrition during early mammalian development can program miRNA changes. These changes can permanently influence the health of the adult increasing the risk of T2DM and coronary heart diseases.

In a study in Meishan pigs, the effect of maternal low dietary protein on offspring lipid metabolism is mediated by the miRNAs, miR-130b and miR-374b, which target PPARgamma and C/EBPbeta, respectively [73]. PPARgamma and C/EBPbeta are important transcriptional factors involved in adipocyte differentiation and lipid metabolism. While PPARgamma-deficient mice exhibit small adipocytes and reduced fat mass, C/EBPbeta-deficient mice fail to accumulate lipid in the adipocytes [74,75] leading to ectopic fat deposition. The results from this study demonstrate that maternal low protein diet can increase the expression levels of key miRNAs which in turn can downregulate important transcriptional factors involved in adipogenesis and lipid metabolism.

A recent study in mice provided novel evidence that maternal low protein diet during pregnancy and lactation can regulate miRNAs that are associated with chronic inflammation leading to impaired metabolic health as early as at weaning age [76]. Microarray analysis of the offspring's liver indicated that miR-165, miR-124, miR-376b, and let-7e were significantly downregulated, while miR-708 and miR-879 were upregulated with a low protein diet. Bioinformatics analysis of the target genes were all mapped to inflammation responses that include MAPK, TGF-beta, Jak-STAT, chemokine, an adipocytokine, and Toll-like receptor signaling pathways as well as cytokine—cytokine receptor interactions. IL-6 and TNF-alpha, proinflammatory factors, were significantly elevated in the serum of the low protein diet male offspring [76]. Recent advances supported that the epigenetics could regulate inflammatory gene expression and more specifically, miRNAs play an important role in the progression and management of inflammatory response, ultimately resulting in adverse physiological changes [77]. This is the first study that showed evidence that maternal low protein feeding regulates miRNAs associated with inflammation showing similarities with studies on maternal high calorie diet [66]. The results of this study indicate that maternal undernutrition is associated with inflammation and may be associated with aberrant metabolic health in offspring.

Maternal undernutrition and miRNA expression in offspring: Effect on cardiovascular remodeling

Maternal undernutrition has been implicated in the fetal programming of adult-onset hypertension in several animal studies [78—80]. Studies now show that maternal undernutrition can alter offspring's vascular miRNAs which in turn regulate genes involved in angiogenesis and carotid artery remodeling [81,82]. In a recent study, maternal undernutrition altered several miRNAs in aortas, including miR-29c whose expression was inhibited in rats. MiR-29c targets elastin (ELN), collagens (Col4A5a, Col3A1), and matrix metalloproteinases (MMP2), proteins associated with the extracellular matrix (ECM) indicating that maternal undernutrition can alter offspring vascular contractility through miR-29c. ELN along with other proteins maintain the elastic function of blood vessels, while aging, hypertension, and atherosclerosis decrease ELN content and compliance. Interestingly, maternal undernutrition offspring showed hypertension and decreased vascular compliance. However, these animals showed increased ELN indicating that ELN organization or cross-linking with other myofibrillar proteins maybe disrupted. Another important component of vascular ECM is collagen. Col3A1 and Col4A5 are also targeted by miR-29c. These structural proteins provide tensile strength and rigidity to blood vessels. Maternal undernutrition increases collagen by inhibiting miR-29c in offspring carotid arteries which may lead to blood vessel stiffening. An increase in collagen and ELN was also observed in ischemic stroke which may promote the formation of carotid plaques leading to cerebral ischemia [83,84]. Along with ELN and collagens, MMPs are important for vascular stiffness [84]. MMPs selectively degrade the structural proteins like ELN and collagen to maintain vascular stiffness and compliance. Though the expression of MMP2 is increased with maternal undernutrition, the significance of this increase in vascular stiffness is still unknown. In conclusion, this study provides evidence that maternal undernutrition can alter miR-29c which has a significant inverse correlation with ECM proteins.

Maternal undernutrition and miRNA expression in offspring: Effect on brain renin—angiotensin system

Epidemiological and animal studies show that maternal protein deprivation results in the development of hypertension, stroke, depression, schizophrenia, obesity, diabetes, and other diseases in offspring. Renin—angiotensin system (RAS) which regulates blood pressure and fluid balance exists in various organs including the brain. Alterations in RAS in the brain lead to stroke, hypertension, depression, and Alzheimer disease. The effect of maternal low protein diet on fetal programming can lead to changes in RAS in the brain through epigenetics. A study in mice demonstrated that antenatal maternal protein deprivation led to changes in fetal brain miRNAs, namely miR-27a, miR-27b, and miR-330 [85]. Maternal low protein diet decreased the protein expression levels of angiotensin-converting enzyme (ACE-1) and angiotensin II type-2 (AT2) receptors. Mir-27a and miR-27b which regulate ACE-1 mRNA translation are significantly upregulated, while miR-330 which regulates AT2 receptor is downregulated. This study supports the hypothesis that fetal programming which occurs during gestation is capable of epigenetic modifications which can persist lifelong and can lead to the delayed manifestation of hypertension and other diseases in adults.

Effect of maternal consumption of dietary factors on epigenetics in the offspring

In addition to maternal over- or undernutrition, several nutrients are critically important to the health of the offspring. The importance of dietary supplementation with dietary factors during gestation is well established and the relationship between maternal consumption of dietary factors and its effects on the epigenome of the offspring is now being unveiled [30].

Effects of maternal consumption of vitamins in fetal miRNAs expression

Vitamins are micronutrients critically important for several biochemical reactions in the body [19]. These nutrients are known for numerous physiological functions, including metabolism regulation and diseases prevention [86]. Water-soluble vitamins include vitamin C and members of the B complex, whereas lipid-soluble vitamins include vitamin A, D, E, and K [19]. There is now increasing evidence that maternal vitamin status is associated with developmental origins of chronic diseases [87—89].

The influence of vitamins on miRNAs expression and health has been reported in several species, including humans [90,91]. Recently, studies have started to unveil the effects maternal concentrations of the vitamin on long-term effects in the health of the offspring. In a clinical study, the expression of miRNAs involved in the regulation of several cellular functions, including inflammation and metabolic processes, was shown to be altered in the peripheral blood of pregnant women with low vitamin D concentrations with potential detrimental effects on the development of chronic diseases of the offspring [92]. In another study, the expression of miRNAs associated with regulation of adipogenesis and insulin metabolism was altered in plasma of pregnant women with low levels of vitamin B12, which may lead to obesity and metabolic disease of the offspring [93].

Effects of maternal consumption of polyphenols in fetal miRNAs expression

Polyphenols are abundant micronutrients that have attracted the attention of the scientific community for their antioxidants effects and their potential to prevent chronic conditions associated with oxidative stress, including cardiovascular disease and cancer [94]. These phytochemicals are found in fruits and beverages derived from plants, including tea, coffee, fruit juices, and red wine, besides being present in vegetables, dry legumes, cereals, and chocolates [95]. The types of polyphenols present in our diet include phenolic acids, flavonoids, stilbenes, and lignans [94].

Various polyphenols have been reported to modulate the expression of miRNAs associated with insulin signaling, glucose homeostasis, oxidative stress, and inflammation, which may affect diabetes and cardiovascular disease [36,96]. For example, flavonoids and the stilbene resveratrol have been shown to modulate miRNAs expression with potential beneficial effects on the etiopathogenesis of chronic diseases [97–100].

The metabolic programming of the offspring in response to maternal diet has been shown to be affected by polyphenols by several studies [101]. Many of these studies present beneficial effects of maternal consumption of polyphenols such as flavonoids in the health of the offspring [102,103]. Nevertheless, observations of detrimental effects on the offspring in response to maternal consumption of flavonoids have also been reported [104]. Recently, a study using rats as a model has reported that maternal consumption of grape seed procyanidin extract, a flavonoid, reduces the expression of miR-33a, a key regulator of cholesterol metabolism, in the liver of offsprings, with potentially detrimental effects on the etiopathogenesis of cardiovascular disease [101]. Therefore, the effects of maternal consumption of polyphenols on the study of the development of chronic diseases via miRNAs modulation are still in need of experimental and clinical investigation.

Conclusion

The theory behind the developmental origins of disease is well established. Advances in the field of epigenetics are bringing important contributions to how the maternal diet influences the health of the offspring. To date, several studies have reported the effects of maternal dietary factors and nutritional status on miRNAs expression of the offspring with subsequent effects on inflammation, metabolism, and cardiovascular remodeling. Because epigenetic modifications are reversible, future research shows a promise for the use of miRNAs in the diagnosis, prevention, and treatment of health conditions of the offspring.

Acknowledgments

Mahua Choudhury is supported by the Morris L. Lichtenstein Jr. Medical Research Foundation for diabetes and obesity research and Texas A&M Health Science Center Faculty Development Fund.

References

[1] McKay JA, Mathers JC. Diet induced epigenetic changes and their implications for health. Acta Physiol 2011;202:103–18.
[2] Ronto R, Wu JH, Singh GM. The global nutrition transition: trends, disease burdens and policy interventions. Publ Health Nutr 2018:1–4.
[3] WHO. Diet, nutrition and the prevention of chronic diseases. World Health Organ Tech Rep Ser 2003;916(i-viii):1–149 [backcover].
[4] Sofi F, Macchi C, Abbate R, Gensini GF, Casini A. Mediterranean diet and health. Biofactors 2013;39:335–42.
[5] Szostak-Wegierek D, Klosiewicz-Latoszek L, Szostak WB, Cybulska B. The role of dietary fats for preventing cardiovascular disease. A review. Rocz Panstw Zakl Hig 2013;64:263–9.
[6] Zimmet P, Alberti KG, Shaw J. Global and societal implications of the diabetes epidemic. Nature 2001;414:782–7.
[7] Barker DJ. The origins of the developmental origins theory. J Intern Med 2007;261:412–7.
[8] Waterland RA, Michels KB. Epigenetic epidemiology of the developmental origins hypothesis. Annu Rev Nutr 2007;27:363–88.
[9] Beauchamp B, Harper ME. In utero undernutrition programs skeletal and cardiac muscle metabolism. Front Physiol 2015;6:401.
[10] Wadhwa PD, Buss C, Entringer S, Swanson JM. Developmental origins of health and disease: brief history of the approach and current focus on epigenetic mechanisms. Semin Reprod Med 2009;27:358–68.
[11] Costa-Silva JH, Simoes-Alves AC, Fernandes MP. Developmental origins of cardiometabolic diseases: role of the maternal diet. Front Physiol 2016;7:504.
[12] Gluckman PD, Hanson MA. Developmental origins of disease paradigm: a mechanistic and evolutionary perspective. Pediatr Res 2004;56:311–7.
[13] Tokunaga M, Takahashi T, Singh RB, De Meester F, Wilson DW. Nutrition and epigenetics. Medical Epigenetics 2013;1:70–7.
[14] Chen PY, Ganguly A, Rubbi L, Orozco LD, Morselli M, Ashraf D, Jaroszewicz A, Feng S, Jacobsen SE, Nakano A, Devaskar SU, Pellegrini M. Intrauterine calorie restriction affects placental DNA methylation and gene expression. Physiol Genom 2013;45:565–76.
[15] Junien C. Impact of diets and nutrients/drugs on early epigenetic programming. J Inherit Metab Dis 2006;29:359–65.
[16] Dhobale M, Joshi S. Altered maternal micronutrients (folic acid, vitamin B(12)) and omega 3 fatty acids through oxidative stress may reduce neurotrophic factors in preterm pregnancy. J Matern Fetal Neonatal Med 2012;25:317–23.
[17] Handy DE, Castro R, Loscalzo J. Epigenetic modifications: basic mechanisms and role in cardiovascular disease. Circulation 2011;123:2145–56.
[18] Smith CJ, Ryckman KK. Epigenetic and developmental influences on the risk of obesity, diabetes, and metabolic syndrome. Diabetes Metab Syndr Obes 2015;8:295–302.
[19] Wang J, Wu Z, Li D, Li N, Dindot SV, Satterfield MC, Bazer FW, Wu G. Nutrition, epigenetics, and metabolic syndrome. Antioxid Redox Signal 2012;17:282–301.
[20] Ho DH, Burggren WW. Epigenetics and transgenerational transfer: a physiological perspective. J Exp Biol 2010;213:3–16.
[21] Tammen SA, Friso S, Choi SW. Epigenetics: the link between nature and nurture. Mol Aspect Med 2013;34:753–64.
[22] Bishop KS, Ferguson LR. The interaction between epigenetics, nutrition and the development of cancer. Nutrients 2015;7:922–47.

[23] Lee HS. Impact of maternal diet on the epigenome during in utero life and the developmental programming of diseases in childhood and adulthood. Nutrients 2015;7:9492–507.
[24] Flowers E, Won GY, Fukuoka Y. MicroRNAs associated with exercise and diet: a systematic review. Physiol Genom 2015;47:1–11.
[25] Ross SA, Davis CD. The emerging role of microRNAs and nutrition in modulating health and disease. Annu Rev Nutr 2014;34:305–36.
[26] He L, Hannon GJ. MicroRNAs: small RNAs with a big role in gene regulation. Nat Rev Genet 2004;5:522–31.
[27] Stefani G, Slack F. MicroRNAs in search of a target. Cold Spring Harbor Symp Quant Biol 2006;71:129–34.
[28] Kim VN, Han J, Siomi MC. Biogenesis of small RNAs in animals. Nat Rev Mol Cell Biol 2009;10:126–39.
[29] Wagner AE, Piegholdt S, Ferraro M, Pallauf K, Rimbach G. Food derived microRNAs. Food Funct 2015;6:714–8.
[30] Chango A, Pogribny IP. Considering maternal dietary modulators for epigenetic regulation and programming of the fetal epigenome. Nutrients 2015;7:2748–70.
[31] Li C, Hashimi SM, Good DA, Cao S, Duan W, Plummer PN, Mellick AS, Wei MQ. Apoptosis and microRNA aberrations in cancer. Clin Exp Pharmacol Physiol 2012;39:739–46.
[32] Cui J, Zhou B, Ross SA, Zempleni J. Nutrition, microRNAs, and human health. Adv Nutr 2017;8:105–12.
[33] Friedman RC, Farh KK, Burge CB, Bartel DP. Most mammalian mRNAs are conserved targets of microRNAs. Genome Res 2009;19:92–105.
[34] Makarova JA, Shkurnikov MU, Wicklein D, Lange T, Samatov TR, Turchinovich AA, Tonevitsky AG. Intracellular and extracellular microRNA: an update on localization and biological role. Prog Histochem Cytochem 2016;51:33–49.
[35] Qin DN, Qian L, Hu DL, Yu ZB, Han SP, Zhu C, Wang X, Hu X. Effects of miR-19b overexpression on proliferation, differentiation, apoptosis and Wnt/beta-catenin signaling pathway in P19 cell model of cardiac differentiation in vitro. Cell Biochem Biophys 2013;66:709–22.
[36] Berna G, Oliveras-Lopez MJ, Jurado-Ruiz E, Tejedo J, Bedoya F, Soria B, Martin F. Nutrigenetics and nutrigenomics insights into diabetes etiopathogenesis. Nutrients 2014;6:5338–69.
[37] Zhu H, Shyh-Chang N, Segre AV, Shinoda G, Shah SP, Einhorn WS, Takeuchi A, Engreitz JM, Hagan JP, Kharas MG, Urbach A, Thornton JE, Triboulet R, Gregory RI, Consortium D, Investigators M, Altshuler D, Daley GQ. The Lin28/let-7 axis regulates glucose metabolism. Cell 2011;147:81–94.
[38] Mitchell PS, Parkin RK, Kroh EM, Fritz BR, Wyman SK, Pogosova-Agadjanyan EL, Peterson A, Noteboom J, O'Briant KC, Allen A, Lin DW, Urban N, Drescher CW, Knudsen BS, Stirewalt DL, Gentleman R, Vessella RL, Nelson PS, Martin DB, Tewari M. Circulating microRNAs as stable blood-based markers for cancer detection. Proc Natl Acad Sci U S A 2008;105:10513–8.
[39] Zampetaki A, Kiechl S, Drozdov I, Willeit P, Mayr U, Prokopi M, Mayr A, Weger S, Oberhollenzer F, Bonora E, Shah A, Willeit J, Mayr M. Plasma microRNA profiling reveals loss of endothelial miR-126 and other microRNAs in type 2 diabetes. Circ Res 2010;107:810–7.
[40] Casas-Agustench P, Iglesias-Gutierrez E, Davalos A. Mother's nutritional miRNA legacy: nutrition during pregnancy and its possible implications to develop cardiometabolic disease in later life. Pharmacol Res 2015;100:322–34.

[41] Turchinovich A, Samatov TR, Tonevitsky AG, Burwinkel B. Circulating miRNAs: cell-cell communication function? Front Genet 2013;4:119.
[42] Neri C, Edlow AG. Effects of maternal obesity on fetal programming: molecular approaches. Cold Spring Harb Perspect Med 2015;6:a026591.
[43] Nicholas LM, Rattanatray L, MacLaughlin SM, Ozanne SE, Kleemann DO, Walker SK, Morrison JL, Zhang S, Muhlhausler BS, Martin-Gronert MS, McMillen IC. Differential effects of maternal obesity and weight loss in the periconceptional period on the epigenetic regulation of hepatic insulin-signaling pathways in the offspring. FASEB J 2013;27:3786−96.
[44] Liang J, Liu C, Qiao A, Cui Y, Zhang H, Cui A, Zhang S, Yang Y, Xiao X, Chen Y, Fang F, Chang Y. MicroRNA-29a-c decrease fasting blood glucose levels by negatively regulating hepatic gluconeogenesis. J Hepatol 2013;58:535−42.
[45] Pandey AK, Verma G, Vig S, Srivastava S, Srivastava AK, Datta M. miR-29a levels are elevated in the db/db mice liver and its overexpression leads to attenuation of insulin action on PEPCK gene expression in HepG2 cells. Mol Cell Endocrinol 2011;332:125−33.
[46] Bagge A, Clausen TR, Larsen S, Ladefoged M, Rosenstierne MW, Larsen L, Vang O, Nielsen JH, Dalgaard LT. MicroRNA-29a is up-regulated in beta-cells by glucose and decreases glucose-stimulated insulin secretion. Biochem Biophys Res Commun 2012;426:266−72.
[47] Roggli E, Gattesco S, Caille D, Briet C, Boitard C, Meda P, Regazzi R. Changes in microRNA expression contribute to pancreatic beta-cell dysfunction in prediabetic NOD mice. Diabetes 2012;61:1742−51.
[48] Long J, Wang Y, Wang W, Chang BH, Danesh FR. MicroRNA-29c is a signature microRNA under high glucose conditions that targets sprouty homolog 1, and its in vivo knockdown prevents progression of diabetic nephropathy. J Biol Chem 2011;286:11837−48.
[49] He A, Zhu L, Gupta N, Chang Y, Fang F. Overexpression of micro ribonucleic acid 29, highly up-regulated in diabetic rats, leads to insulin resistance in 3T3-L1 adipocytes. Mol Endocrinol 2007;21:2785−94.
[50] Nielsen LB, Wang C, Sorensen K, Bang-Berthelsen CH, Hansen L, Andersen ML, Hougaard P, Juul A, Zhang CY, Pociot F, Mortensen HB. Circulating levels of microRNA from children with newly diagnosed type 1 diabetes and healthy controls: evidence that miR-25 associates to residual beta-cell function and glycaemic control during disease progression. Exp Diabetes Res 2012;2012:896362.
[51] Kong L, Zhu J, Han W, Jiang X, Xu M, Zhao Y, Dong Q, Pang Z, Guan Q, Gao L, Zhao J, Zhao L. Significance of serum microRNAs in pre-diabetes and newly diagnosed type 2 diabetes: a clinical study. Acta Diabetol 2011;48:61−9.
[52] Trajkovski M, Hausser J, Soutschek J, Bhat B, Akin A, Zavolan M, Heim MH, Stoffel M. MicroRNAs 103 and 107 regulate insulin sensitivity. Nature 2011;474:649−53.
[53] Zhang J, Zhang F, Didelot X, Bruce KD, Cagampang FR, Vatish M, Hanson M, Lehnert H, Ceriello A, Byrne CD. Maternal high fat diet during pregnancy and lactation alters hepatic expression of insulin like growth factor-2 and key microRNAs in the adult offspring. BMC Genom 2009;10:478.
[54] Lee H, Han S, Kwon CS, Lee D. Biogenesis and regulation of the let-7 miRNAs and their functional implications. Protein Cell 2016;7:100−13.
[55] Shah YM, Morimura K, Yang Q, Tanabe T, Takagi M, Gonzalez FJ. Peroxisome proliferator-activated receptor alpha regulates a microRNA-mediated signaling cascade responsible for hepatocellular proliferation. Mol Cell Biol 2007;27:4238−47.
[56] Guo F, Jen KL. High-fat feeding during pregnancy and lactation affects offspring metabolism in rats. Physiol Behav 1995;57:681−6.

[57] Wen J, Friedman JR. miR-122 regulates hepatic lipid metabolism and tumor suppression. J Clin Invest 2012;122:2773–6.
[58] Gonzalez FJ, Shah YM. PPARalpha: mechanism of species differences and hepatocarcinogenesis of peroxisome proliferators. Toxicology 2008;246:2–8.
[59] Bogdanovic O, Veenstra GJ. DNA methylation and methyl-CpG binding proteins: developmental requirements and function. Chromosoma 2009;118:549–65.
[60] Benatti RO, Melo AM, Borges FO, Ignacio-Souza LM, Simino LA, Milanski M, Velloso LA, Torsoni MA, Torsoni AS. Maternal high-fat diet consumption modulates hepatic lipid metabolism and microRNA-122 (miR-122) and microRNA-370 (miR-370) expression in offspring. Br J Nutr 2014;111:2112–22.
[61] Li C, Deng M, Hu J, Li X, Chen L, Ju Y, Hao J, Meng S. Chronic inflammation contributes to the development of hepatocellular carcinoma by decreasing miR-122 levels. Oncotarget 2016;7:17021–34.
[62] de Paula Simino LA, de Fante T, Figueiredo Fontana M, Oliveira Borges F, Torsoni MA, Milanski M, Velloso LA, Souza Torsoni A. Lipid overload during gestation and lactation can independently alter lipid homeostasis in offspring and promote metabolic impairment after new challenge to high-fat diet. Nutr Metab 2017;14:16.
[63] Yan X, Huang Y, Zhao JX, Rogers CJ, Zhu MJ, Ford SP, Nathanielsz PW, Du M. Maternal obesity downregulates microRNA let-7g expression, a possible mechanism for enhanced adipogenesis during ovine fetal skeletal muscle development. Int J Obes 2013;37:568–75.
[64] Lee SJ, McPherron AC. Regulation of myostatin activity and muscle growth. Proc Natl Acad Sci U S A 2001;98:9306–11.
[65] Backdahl L, Bushell A, Beck S. Inflammatory signalling as mediator of epigenetic modulation in tissue-specific chronic inflammation. Int J Biochem Cell Biol 2009;41:176–84.
[66] Zheng J, Zhang Q, Mul JD, Yu M, Xu J, Qi C, Wang T, Xiao X. Maternal high-calorie diet is associated with altered hepatic microRNA expression and impaired metabolic health in offspring at weaning age. Endocrine 2016;54:70–80.
[67] de Rooij SR, Painter RC, Phillips DI, Osmond C, Michels RP, Godsland IF, Bossuyt PM, Bleker OP, Roseboom TJ. Impaired insulin secretion after prenatal exposure to the dutch famine. Diabetes Care 2006;29:1897–901.
[68] Kahn HS. Glucose tolerance in adults after prenatal exposure to famine. Lancet 2001;357:1798–9.
[69] Zohdi V, Lim K, Pearson JT, Black MJ. Developmental programming of cardiovascular disease following intrauterine growth restriction: findings utilising a rat model of maternal protein restriction. Nutrients 2014;7:119–52.
[70] Ferland-McCollough D, Fernandez-Twinn DS, Cannell IG, David H, Warner M, Vaag AA, Bork-Jensen J, Brons C, Gant TW, Willis AE, Siddle K, Bushell M, Ozanne SE. Programming of adipose tissue miR-483-3p and GDF-3 expression by maternal diet in type 2 diabetes. Cell Death Differ 2012;19:1003–12.
[71] Erhuma A, Salter AM, Sculley DV, Langley-Evans SC, Bennett AJ. Prenatal exposure to a low-protein diet programs disordered regulation of lipid metabolism in the aging rat. Am J Physiol Endocrinol Metab 2007;292:E1702–14.
[72] Fraser A, Ebrahim S, Smith GD, Lawlor DA. The associations between birthweight and adult markers of liver damage and function. Paediatr Perinat Epidemiol 2008;22:12–21.
[73] Pan S, Zheng Y, Zhao R, Yang X. MicroRNA-130b and microRNA-374b mediate the effect of maternal dietary protein on offspring lipid metabolism in Meishan pigs. Br J Nutr 2013;109:1731–8.

[74] Gray SL, Dalla Nora E, Vidal-Puig AJ. Mouse models of PPAR-gamma deficiency: dissecting PPAR-gamma's role in metabolic homoeostasis. Biochem Soc Trans 2005;33:1053–8.
[75] Tanaka T, Yoshida N, Kishimoto T, Akira S. Defective adipocyte differentiation in mice lacking the C/EBPbeta and/or C/EBPdelta gene. EMBO J 1997;16:7432–43.
[76] Zheng J, Xiao X, Zhang Q, Wang T, Yu M, Xu J. Maternal low-protein diet modulates glucose metabolism and hepatic MicroRNAs expression in the early life of offspring dagger. Nutrients 2017;9.
[77] Zhou D, Pan YX. Pathophysiological basis for compromised health beyond generations: role of maternal high-fat diet and low-grade chronic inflammation. J Nutr Biochem 2015;26:1–8.
[78] Gardner DS, Jackson AA, Langley-Evans SC. Maintenance of maternal diet-induced hypertension in the rat is dependent on glucocorticoids. Hypertension 1997;30:1525–30.
[79] Langley-Evans SC. Hypertension induced by foetal exposure to a maternal low-protein diet, in the rat, is prevented by pharmacological blockade of maternal glucocorticoid synthesis. J Hypertens 1997;15:537–44.
[80] McMillen IC, Robinson JS. Developmental origins of the metabolic syndrome: prediction, plasticity, and programming. Physiol Rev 2005;85:571–633.
[81] Khorram O, Chuang TD, Pearce WJ. Long-term effects of maternal undernutrition on offspring carotid artery remodeling: role of miR-29c. J Dev Orig Health Dis 2015;6:342–9.
[82] Khorram O, Han G, Bagherpour R, Magee TR, Desai M, Ross MG, Chaudhri AA, Toloubeydokhti T, Pearce WJ. Effect of maternal undernutrition on vascular expression of micro and messenger RNA in newborn and aging offspring. Am J Physiol Regul Integr Comp Physiol 2010;298:R1366–74.
[83] Goncalves I, Moses J, Dias N, Pedro LM, Fernandes e Fernandes J, Nilsson J, Ares MP. Changes related to age and cerebrovascular symptoms in the extracellular matrix of human carotid plaques. Stroke 2003;34:616–22.
[84] Pelisek J, Eckstein HH, Zernecke A. Pathophysiological mechanisms of carotid plaque vulnerability: impact on ischemic stroke. Arch Immunol Ther Exp 2012;60:431–42.
[85] Goyal R, Goyal D, Leitzke A, Gheorghe CP, Longo LD. Brain renin-angiotensin system: fetal epigenetic programming by maternal protein restriction during pregnancy. Reprod Sci 2010;17:227–38.
[86] Balogun OO, da Silva Lopes K, Ota E, Takemoto Y, Rumbold A, Takegata M, Mori R. Vitamin supplementation for preventing miscarriage. Cochrane Database Syst Rev 2016;5:CD004073.
[87] Aleliunas RE, Aljaadi AM, Laher I, Glier MB, Green TJ, Murphy M, Miller JW, Devlin AM. Folic acid supplementation of female mice, with or without vitamin B-12, before and during pregnancy and lactation programs adiposity and vascular health in adult male offspring. J Nutr 2016;146(4):688–96.
[88] Reichetzeder C, Chen H, Foller M, Slowinski T, Li J, Chen YP, Lang F, Hocher B. Maternal vitamin D deficiency and fetal programming–lessons learned from humans and mice. Kidney Blood Press Res 2014;39:315–29.
[89] Rush EC, Katre P, Yajnik CS. Vitamin B12: one carbon metabolism, fetal growth and programming for chronic disease. Eur J Clin Nutr 2014;68:2–7.
[90] Garcia-Segura L, Perez-Andrade M, Miranda-Rios J. The emerging role of MicroRNAs in the regulation of gene expression by nutrients. J Nutrigenet Nutrigenomics 2013;6:16–31.

[91] Wang WL, Welsh J, Tenniswood M. 1,25-Dihydroxyvitamin D3 modulates lipid metabolism in prostate cancer cells through miRNA mediated regulation of PPARA. J Steroid Biochem Mol Biol 2013;136:247–51.
[92] Enquobahrie DA, Williams MA, Qiu C, Siscovick DS, Sorensen TK. Global maternal early pregnancy peripheral blood mRNA and miRNA expression profiles according to plasma 25-hydroxyvitamin D concentrations. J Matern Fetal Neonatal Med 2011;24:1002–12.
[93] Adaikalakoteswari A, Vatish M, Alam MT, Ott S, Kumar S, Saravanan P. Low vitamin B12 in pregnancy is associated with adipose-derived circulating miRs targeting PPARgamma and insulin resistance. J Clin Endocrinol Metab 2017;102:4200–9.
[94] Manach C, Scalbert A, Morand C, Remesy C, Jimenez L. Polyphenols: food sources and bioavailability. Am J Clin Nutr 2004;79:727–47.
[95] Scalbert A, Johnson IT, Saltmarsh M. Polyphenols: antioxidants and beyond. Am J Clin Nutr 2005;81:215S–7S.
[96] Blade C, Baselga-Escudero L, Salvado MJ, Arola-Arnal A. miRNAs, polyphenols, and chronic disease. Mol Nutr Food Res 2013;57:58–70.
[97] Arola-Arnal A, Blade C. Proanthocyanidins modulate microRNA expression in human HepG2 cells. PLoS One 2011;6:e25982.
[98] Boesch-Saadatmandi C, Wagner AE, Wolffram S, Rimbach G. Effect of quercetin on inflammatory gene expression in mice liver in vivo - role of redox factor 1, miRNA-122 and miRNA-125b. Pharmacol Res 2012;65:523–30.
[99] Milenkovic D, Deval C, Gouranton E, Landrier JF, Scalbert A, Morand C, Mazur A. Modulation of miRNA expression by dietary polyphenols in apoE deficient mice: a new mechanism of the action of polyphenols. PLoS One 2012;7:e29837.
[100] Tome-Carneiro J, Larrosa M, Yanez-Gascon MJ, Davalos A, Gil-Zamorano J, Gonzalvez M, Garcia-Almagro FJ, Ruiz Ros JA, Tomas-Barberan FA, Espin JC, Garcia-Conesa MT. One-year supplementation with a grape extract containing resveratrol modulates inflammatory-related microRNAs and cytokines expression in peripheral blood mononuclear cells of type 2 diabetes and hypertensive patients with coronary artery disease. Pharmacol Res 2013;72:69–82.
[101] Del Bas JM, Crescenti A, Arola-Arnal A, Oms-Oliu G, Arola L, Caimari A. Intake of grape procyanidins during gestation and lactation impairs reverse cholesterol transport and increases atherogenic risk indexes in adult offspring. J Nutr Biochem 2015;26:1670–7.
[102] Resende AC, Emiliano AF, Cordeiro VS, de Bem GF, de Cavalho LC, de Oliveira PR, Neto ML, Costa CA, Boaventura GT, de Moura RS. Grape skin extract protects against programmed changes in the adult rat offspring caused by maternal high-fat diet during lactation. J Nutr Biochem 2013;24:2119–26.
[103] Wu Z, Zhao J, Xu H, Lyv Y, Feng X, Fang Y, Xu Y. Maternal quercetin administration during gestation and lactation decrease endoplasmic reticulum stress and related inflammation in the adult offspring of obese female rats. Eur J Nutr 2014;53:1669–83.
[104] Zielinsky P, Piccoli Jr AL, Manica JL, Nicoloso LH. New insights on fetal ductal constriction: role of maternal ingestion of polyphenol-rich foods. Expert Rev Cardiovasc Ther 2010;8:291–8.

Index

Note: 'Page numbers followed by "f" indicate figures and "t" indicates tables'.

G

H

I

L

M

R

FSC
www.fsc.org
MIX
Papier | Fördert
gute Waldnutzung
FSC® C083411

Kolibri 360 GmbH
Ferdinand-Jühlke-Straße 7
99095 Erfurt, Deutschland
produktsicherheit@kolibri360.de